Diagnosis and Treatment in Pediatrics

Diagnosis and Treatment in Pediatrics

Edited by Vanessa Stevens

AMERICAN
MEDICAL PUBLISHERS
www.americanmedicalpublishers.com

American Medical Publishers,
41 Flatbush Avenue,
1st Floor, New York,
NY 11217, USA

Visit us on the World Wide Web at:
www.americanmedicalpublishers.com

ISBN: 978-1-63927-420-8

Cataloging-in-Publication Data

Diagnosis and treatment in pediatrics / edited by Vanessa Stevens.
p. cm.
Includes bibliographical references and index.
ISBN 978-1-63927-420-8
1. Pediatrics. 2. Children--Diseases--Diagnosis. 3. Children--Diseases--Treatment. I. Stevens, Vanessa.
RJ47 .D53 2022
618.92--dc23

Table of Contents

Preface

Pediatrics is a branch of medicine which is concerned with the medical care of infants, children and adolescents. A child has unique medical requirements as compared to an adult, owing to their immature physiology and maturation changes. Pediatricians address the assessment and management of injuries, infections, organ dysfunctions and cancer. Complex issues like genetic variance, developmental delays and disorders, behavioral and functional disabilities and congenital defects in children are also under the scope of pediatrics. Specialties within pediatrics include neonatology, pediatric critical care, pediatric endocrinology, pediatric hematology, pediatric cardiology, pediatric oncology, etc. This book presents the complex subject of pediatrics in the most comprehensible and easy to understand language. Different approaches, evaluations, methodologies and advanced studies on pediatrics have been included herein. This book is appropriate for students seeking detailed information in this area as well as for experts.

In the end, I would like to extend my heartiest thanks to the authors who worked with great determination on their chapters. I also appreciate the publisher's support in the course of the book. I would also like to deeply acknowledge my family who stood by me as a source of inspiration during the project.

Editor

1

A pediatric death audit in a large referral hospital in Malawi

Elizabeth Fitzgerald[1*], Rachel Mlotha-Mitole[2], Emily J. Ciccone[3], Alyssa E. Tilly[3], Jennie M. Montijo[4], Hans-Joerg Lang[5] and Michelle Eckerle[6]

Abstract

Background: Death audits have been used to describe pediatric mortality in under-resourced settings, where record keeping is often a challenge. This information provides the cornerstone for the foundation of quality improvement initiatives. Malawi, located in sub-Saharan Africa, currently has an Under-5 mortality rate of 64/1000. Kamuzu Central Hospital, in the capital city Lilongwe, is a busy government referral hospital, which admits up to 3000 children per month. A study published in 2013 reported mortality rates as high as 9%. This is the first known audit of pediatric death files conducted at this hospital.

Methods: A retrospective chart review on all pediatric deaths that occurred at Kamuzu Central Hospital (excluding deaths in the neonatal nursery) during a 13-month period was done using a standardized death audit form. A descriptive analysis was completed, including patient demographics, HIV and nutritional status, and cause of death. Modifiable factors were identified that may have contributed to mortality, including a lack of vital sign collection, poor documentation, and delays in the procurement or results of tests, studies, and specialist review.

Results: Seven hundred forty three total pediatric deaths were recorded and 700 deceased patient files were reviewed. The mortality rate by month ranged from a low of 2.2% to a high of 4.4%. Forty-four percent of deaths occurred within the first 24 h of admission, and 59% occurred within the first 48 h. The most common causes of death were malaria, malnutrition, HIV-related illnesses, and sepsis.

Conclusions: The mortality rate for this pediatric referral center has dramatically decreased in the 6 years since the last published mortality data, but remains high. Areas identified for continued development include improved record keeping, improved patient assessment and monitoring, and more timely and reliable provision of testing and treatment. This study demonstrates that in low-resource settings, where reliable record keeping is often difficult, death audits are useful tools to describe the sickest patient population and determine factors possibly contributing to mortality that may be amenable to quality improvement interventions.

Keywords: Pediatric emergency medicine, Global Health, Death audits

Background

The path to pediatric mortality in the developing world is complex, with myriad modifiable factors that can serve as public health intervention points. Programs directed at reducing child mortality have traditionally focused on the areas of prevention and improving access to care. More recently, the impact that acute and inpatient hospital care has on child mortality has been recognized, and opportunities for improvement have been described [1–5]. To successfully implement care improvement plans, existing systems must be objectively assessed and components amenable to intervention identified. However, accurate record keeping is often a challenge in low-resource settings. The paucity of reliable information about in-hospital care leads to further challenges in evaluating barriers to treatment, and in creating and assessing quality improvement interventions. The lack of valid vital statistics in the developing world often leaves many deaths unaccounted for, and the lack of accurate information regarding patient's cause

* Correspondence: efitzgerald@med.unc.edu
[1]Assistant Professor of Pediatrics, University of North Carolina at Chapel Hill, Chapel Hill, USA

of death complicates the ability to plan for, fund, and assess interventions [6, 7]. Audits of deceased pediatric patient files have been shown to be a useful tool in creating sustainable hospital Quality Improvement initiatives in low-resource settings [8–10].

Malawi is a resource-poor, malaria-endemic country in sub-Saharan Africa, consistently ranked among the least developed in the world. Approximately 62% of its 16.7 million inhabitants live below the international poverty line of $1.25 USD (US Dollar) per day. Despite its challenges, great strides have been made in improving the health of children in Malawi in the last few decades. Malawi has reached its fourth Millennium Development Goal, a two-thirds reduction in childhood mortality, before the target date of 2015 [11]. The World Health Organization (WHO) reports that Under-five mortality was 71/1000 in 2013, compared to 245/1000 in 1990. However, although Malawian pediatric patients are accessing clinical care at an increasing rate, the clinical standards set forth by the WHO for some common illnesses are being inconsistently adhered to in hospitals nationwide [11].

Kamuzu Central Hospital (KCH) is a tertiary referral hospital in Lilongwe, Malawi, which serves the central region of the country and a population of approximately 5 million people. The pediatric ward of the hospital admits between 40 and 120 patients per day, with significant seasonal variation related to malaria burden and food insecurity. Medical record keeping has traditionally been inconsistent; charts are hand-written when paper is available and held by the pediatric patient's caregiver. There is no electronic medical record. Deaths are recorded in a ledger by an administrative layperson, with a presumed cause of death as diagnosed by the evaluating clinician. To date, no comprehensive effort has been made at investigating modifiable factors that may contribute to pediatric mortality at KCH. We report the results of the first known audit of pediatric death files conducted at this hospital. In the absence of reliable record-keeping, the objective of this study was to describe the patients who died in the hospital, evaluate the emergency and inpatient care provided to them, and identify gaps in their care that may have contributed to their mortality.

Methods

A retrospective chart review was conducted by a team of two pediatricians and two University of North Carolina (UNC) Medicine-Pediatric residents on behalf of the Pediatric Department at KCH. Each member of the team was responsible for the review of a portion of the death files, and the entry of the collected data into an Excel spreadsheet. Hospital charts for all pediatric deaths that occurred at Kamuzu Central Hospital during a 13-month period were reviewed using a standardized death audit form, created and approved by the KCH medical staff for data collection. The data was de-identified and recorded in an electronic database. Variables extracted are listed in Table 1. Data collected included patient date of birth or approximate age (if the patient's date of birth was unknown), gender, address, date and time of admission and death, HIV and immunization status, nutritional state, and presumed cause of death. Patient weights were

Table 1 Patient Characteristics ($N = 700$)

	Number (%)
Age	
Median	24 months
Range	1 day to 16.5 years
Gender	
Male	353 (50.4)
Female	353 (50.4)
Unknown	14 (2)
Nutritional status	
Unknown (not documented)	535 (76.4)
Newborn	24 (3.4)
Malnourished	141 (20)
Marasmus	65 (9.3)
Kwashiorkor	36 (5.1)
Marasmic Kwashiorkor	31 (4.4)
Unknown type	9 (1.3)
HIV status	
Non-reactive	222 (31.6)
Reactive	40 (5.7)
Unknown	413
Deceased on arrival	86 (12.2)
Died before testing could be completed	204 (29)
Untested	126 (18)
Presumed Severe HIV disease	24 (3.4)
Immunization status	
Unknown (undocumented)	495 (70.9)
Vaccines up to date	82 (11.7)
Vaccines deficient	4 (0.6)
Not applicable (neonate)	33 (4.7)
Deceased on arrival	86 (12.2)
Referral History	
Referred from outside health facility	464 (66.3)
Referral note in chart	100 (21.4)
No referral note	333 (71.3)
Unknown	31 (6.8)
Self-referred	157 (22.4)
Unknown	79 (11.3)

frequently estimated by clinicians, and it was uncommon for a formal nutritional assessment to have been completed. Therefore, in order to avoid over-estimating the impact of malnutrition, nutritional state was assumed to be normal unless a formal nutritional assessment indicating malnutrition had been completed, or a provider had clinically assessed the patient to be malnourished. Cause of death was extrapolated based on recorded information, but was often difficult to definitively diagnose given the limited diagnostic tools. A combination of recorded history, including the diagnosis recorded by the clinician who declared the patient dead, physical exam findings, and test results were used to infer the cause of death. If a patient had an underlying disease process such as HIV or malnutrition and a secondary illness such as malaria, the cause of death was considered to be the primary disease process. Additionally, we reviewed the initial patient assessment and noted whether any vital signs were recorded at first encounter. The pediatric ward admission sheet contains an assessment tool meant to approximate an Emergency Triage and Assessment Tool (ETAT) evaluation and determine patient acuity. Percent completion of this form was reviewed. Further data was collected about whether any vital signs were recorded during the first twenty-four hours of hospitalization, and whether a complete set of vital signs (temperature, heart rate, respiratory rate, oxygen saturation) was obtained at least once each day during the hospitalization. A complete review of each chart was then conducted, with a focus on identifying delays in the assessment or management of patients. We specifically noted delays in the procurement of radiology studies, specialist consultation, nutritional assessment and treatment, initiation of TB treatment, and HIV testing. A delay was defined as greater than 24 h between the ordering and completion of a diagnostic test, evaluation, or treatment. Ethical approval was not required, as this was considered a KCH Pediatric department audit.

Results

A total of 743 total pediatric deaths were recorded in the hospital death registry during the audit period, and 700 deceased patient files were reviewed. Forty-three charts (5.8%) were missing and unable to be reviewed. Total inpatient admissions to the pediatric ward ranged from 956 to 2866 per month (Fig. 1). The monthly mortality rate ranged from a low of 2.2% in October 2015 to a high of 4.4% in August 2015. The mean was 3.3%. Patient ages at admission ranged from 1 day to 16.5 years, with a median age of 24 months. Eighty-six patients were brought to the hospital already deceased. Thirty-seven percent of deaths occurred within the first 24 h of admission, and 53% occurred within the first 48 h. The nutritional status of the majority of the patients was not noted in the chart, but 19% were either reported by the clinician or assessed by the Nutritional Rehabilitation Unit to have some form of malnutrition. Kwashiorkor was the most prevalent form. HIV status was determined in 38% of patients, with 5.7% positive and a further 4% with presumed severe HIV disease based on their mother's HIV status and the clinical criteria determined by the WHO Staging guidelines. No vital signs were done at initial presentation in 44% of patients, and 49% did not have any recorded vital signs within the first twenty-four hours of hospitalization

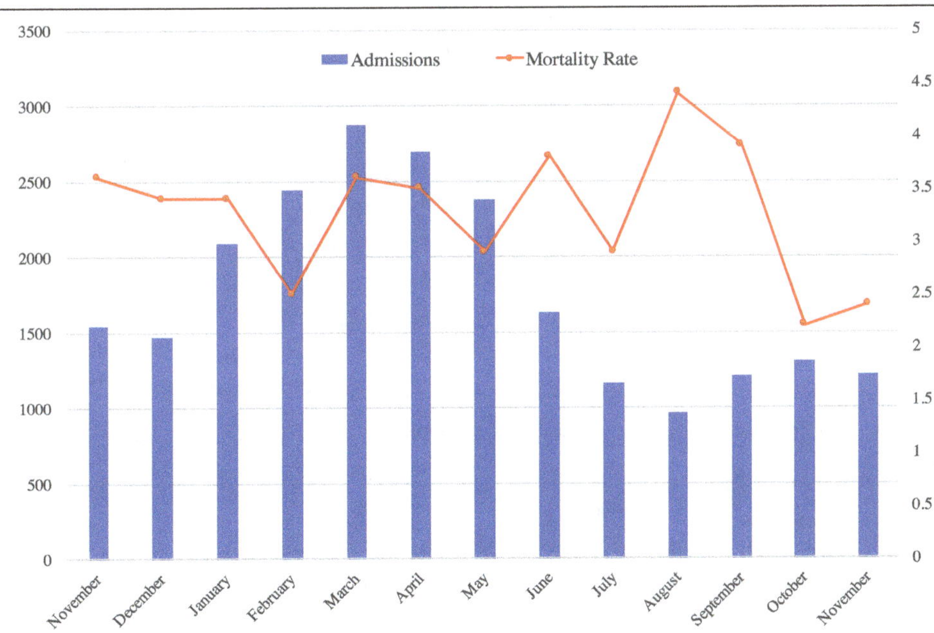

Fig. 1 Admissions and deaths in the Pediatric department at KCH November 2014 to November 2015

(Table 2). Documentation deficiencies were noted in 58% of the charts reviewed, with missing admission sheets being the most common deficiency (16%). Thirteen percent of patients were missing a note, and presumably a review, from a clinician on at least one day of hospitalization. There were one hundred and two cases where at least one radiology study was ordered and not completed within 24 h, most frequently chest X-rays and ultrasounds of the heart or abdomen. Of the 392 patients alive at 24 h after admission, 56 (14.3%) had an HIV test ordered but not done within 24 h. There was a delay of greater than 24 h in obtaining a Nutritional Rehabilitation Unit (NRU) evaluation or consultant review in 13% and 11% of cases, respectively. The most frequent consultant delay was in surgical review. The most common cause of death was malaria, with malnutrition, HIV, and sepsis being the next most common causes of death (Table 3).

Table 2 Characteristics of care provided

	Number (%)
Vital signs obtained at admission	
At least one vital sign obtained	303/614 (49.3)
Temperature	212 (34.5)
Heart rate	203 (33.0)
Respiratory rate	101 (16.4)
Oxygen saturation	219 (35.6)
Blood pressure	25 (4.1)
No vital signs obtained	311 (50.1)
Use of the initial assessment tool	
Some use	439/614 (71.2)
Not used	175 (28.5)
Vital signs obtained within the first 24 h of admission	
At least one vital sign obtained	343/614 (55.9)
Temperature	249 (40.1)
Heart rate	262 (42.7)
Respiratory rate	98 (16)
Oxygen saturation	304 (49.5)
Blood pressure	23 (3.7)
No vital signs obtained	271 (44.1)
Complete set of vital signs obtained at least once each 24 h	
At least one complete set per day	154/614 (25)
At least one day without a complete set of vital signs	462 (75.2)
Delays in assessment/care	
HIV testing	56/392 (14.3)
NRU assessment	51/392 (13)
TB treatment	26/392 (6.6)
Specialist consultation	43/392 (11)
Radiology studies	102/700 (14.6)

Discussion

Worldwide, there are large numbers of pediatric patients presenting to hospitals for emergency care, most of whom are previously healthy [12, 13]. Improvement in the mortality of these patients contributes to life-years saved and productivity. Yet it is well-recognized that there is a lack of basic data in emergency settings in low- and middle-income countries (LMCI's), and that this has made the assessment of systems and identification of priorities challenging [12–14]. As was noted by the World Health Organization in 2005, "epidemiology, demography and biostatistics are the key disciplines of public health," and lack of data, especially in the inpatient setting, has hampered progress [7]. In 2010, eight agencies in Global Health put out a call to action on health data, specifically including health-facility reporting, to inform decision-making and assess interventions [6]. Use of death audits is one approach that has been used to evaluate hospital care when poor record-keeping, high volume, and inadequate staffing make assessment difficult [9, 10, 15]. Kamuzu Central Hospital is no exception to the challenges of monitoring and evaluation of its pediatric systems. This retrospective review of the files of deceased pediatric patients at KCH was undertaken in an effort to describe the care provided to a cohort of patients who presented to the pediatric department emergently, and identify gaps in their care.

The results of this retrospective 13-month review of pediatric death audits reveal that mortality at KCH has dramatically improved since the last published review in

Table 3 Presumed Cause of Death

	Number (%)
Malaria	183 (26.1)
Malnutrition	95 (13.6)
HIV-related illness	69 (9.9)
Sepsis	62 (8.9)
Unknown	39 (5.6)
Respiratory disease	35 (5.0)
Meningitis/encephalitis	34 (4.9)
Perinatal death	31 (4.4)
Gastroenteritis	27 (3.9)
Heart disease	25 (3.6)
Surgical complication/missed surgery	22 (3.1)
Cancer	19 (2.7)
Anemia/blood disorder	18 (2.6)
Renal failure	13 (1.9)
Seizures	10 (1.4)
Trauma/burns	9 (1.3)
Tetanus/poisoning	7 (1.0)
Liver failure	2 (0.3)

2012, when it was as high as 9.3% [16], however it still remains significant, with an average monthly mortality of 3.3%. Without more information about the number of admissions and the care provided during the 2012 study, it is difficult to directly compare these statistics. A number of interventions have occurred in the pediatric department since that publication, including improved consultant-level coverage and a restructuring of the triage and emergency areas, which may have contributed to this substantial decrease in inpatient mortality. Further efforts should be made to investigate and describe the changes made, and to determine the impact that these efforts may have had on mortality.

The mortality rate in our study was somewhat variable, with a monthly range from 2.2% to 4.4%, and surprisingly the month with the highest rate of deaths was not the one with the highest number of admissions. This mortality rate is similar to one seen in a 2015 systematic review of emergency care in LMCI's that showed the median pediatric mortality rate among fourteen sub-Saharan African hospitals was 5.1% [12]. The majority of deaths in our review occurred in patients younger than 24 months, and most occurred within the first 48 h of admission. Multiple studies of inpatient mortality in pediatric public hospitals in Africa have demonstrated similarly that the majority of deaths occur within the first hours of admission [17–19]. It is unusual that there were not more neonatal deaths reported, however this is likely due to the infrastructure of the pediatric department at KCH. Most neonatal deaths occur in the newborn ward or the infant nursery, and so information about their care is not accurately reflected in this review. Inclusion of this data would certainly both increase the overall mortality rate and change the age distribution of deceased patients.

This investigation reveals multiple modifiable factors that, if addressed, may reduce pediatric inpatient mortality at Kamuzu Central Hospital. Vital sign collection was often inadequate, a finding demonstrated in previous descriptions of pediatric acute care facilities in LMIC's. A 2001 review of 21 such hospitals demonstrated that 30% of inpatients were not monitored or reassessed [13]. It is difficult to prove definitively that inadequate monitoring was associated with mortality without reviewing the charts of age- and disease-matched controls, an effort that was beyond the scope of our review. However, earlier and more frequent patient assessment has been demonstrated to improve outcomes [20].

Multiple studies have shown the benefit of early recognition and treatment of critically ill children through use of Emergency Triage Assessment and Treatment [16, 19, 21, 22]. Our review showed that, despite inclusion of an initial assessment tool on the admission form (meant to approximate an ETAT assessment), documentation of a complete initial evaluation was inconsistent. Previous research has shown that interventions as simple as providing a pre-printed standardized admission form improves data collection [14], and it was rare that any of the 115 charts with missing admission forms contained any initial vital signs or ETAT assessment. It is possible that assessments of our patients were completed but not documented.

Nutritional review of our patients, including an accurate weight and Mean Upper Arm Circumference (MUAC), was rarely completed, despite the fact that nutritional status is a key factor associated with morbidity and mortality in the developing world [23, 24]. When malnutrition was identified by a clinician, there were often delays in initiating nutritional therapy. Our decision to exclude patients who did not have a formal nutritional assessment completed or who were not noted by the clinician to be malnourished likely underestimated the degree to which poor baseline nutritional status contributed to mortality. Similarly, HIV status was not determined in a significant number of children, although the evidence supporting the routine testing of inpatients is clear [25, 26]. It is possible that patients who were not tested were HIV reactive, and that our assessment of the contribution of HIV to the mortality rates of our patient population was underestimated.

Referral notes from providers outside the hospital were often missing from the chart, and documentation deficiencies were frequent. There were multiple instances of delays in the procurement of radiology studies, initiation of TB treatment, initiation of NRU assessment and treatment, and consultant review. Comparing the outcomes of a matched cohort of patients for whom timely care was provided would strengthen the implication that these delays contributed to mortality, but that effort was beyond the scope of our study due to the high number of patient charts that would need to be reviewed.

Determining the actual cause of death in a setting where clinicians are unable to perform diagnostic tests is inherently difficult. With such limited access to radiologic or laboratory investigations, cause of death is often based on clinical judgement, and may be inaccurate [27]. The diagnosis of sepsis is often made in patients with undifferentiated shock when more accurate diagnoses cannot be made, and is likely over-estimated in our review. For similar reasons, the contribution of malaria to the mortality rates is likely overestimated. The diagnosis of malaria at KCH is typically made based on positive Malaria Rapid Diagnostic Testing (MRDT), as peripheral smears are more difficult to obtain. These positive MRDTs could simply reflect a recent infection, and do not confirm that malaria was the cause of death [28, 29]. Future studies that more specifically diagnose malaria based on plasma PfHRP2 concentration, or that include confirmatory evaluation of parasite density on peripheral blood smears, would certainly enhance understanding of the extent to which malaria contributes to mortality at this hospital.

Finally, our decision to base the cause of death on known primary disease processes such as HIV or malnutrition, when there were often other etiologies that contributed to their deaths, may overestimate their contribution to patient mortality rates.

Although this audit clearly demonstrates several opportunities for improvement, it is also likely that the data underestimates the need, while simultaneously serving as a reminder of the "real-world" conditions in under-resourced settings. The poor quality of patient charts makes evaluation difficult, as data are often missing or illegible [6]. Furthermore, this data reflects delays in completion of requested interventions, but we did not measure delays in ordering studies, treatments, or specialist care. Our review does not include delays or deficiencies in medication administration or laboratory testing, which are essential components of treatment whose measurement was beyond the scope of this study, but which have been demonstrated to be deficient in similar setting [13, 30, 31]. Further chart reviews, including a comprehensive review of the care provided to and mortality rates in the newborn nursery, need to be done in order to render a more complete assessment of the quality of pediatric care and possible areas for intervention. This study should serve as the first step in what must be an ongoing process of hospital evaluation, so that modifiable barriers to standards of care can be continually identified, efforts at improvement can be rendered, and the impact of interventions can be demonstrated. As stated in the 2005 WHO Bulletin, "It is not because countries are poor that they cannot afford good health information; it is because they are poor that they cannot afford to be without it." [7].

Conclusion

The use of death audits to evaluate inpatient care in low and middle-income countries, where record keeping is often variable or inadequate, has proven to be beneficial. This study demonstrates improved mortality at a busy pediatric referral center in central Malawi, but also reveals gaps in care that may be contributing to the high percentage of deaths that occur in the first 48 h of admission. Identified gaps include poor documentation, inadequate patient assessment and monitoring, and delays in standard care.

Abbreviations

ETAT: Emergency Triage and Assessment Tool; HIV: Human Immunodeficiency Virus; KCH: Kamuzu Central Hospital; MUAC: Mean Upper Arm Circumference; NRU: Nutritional Rehabilitation Unit; TB: Tuberculosis; UNC: University of North Carolina at Chapel Hill; USD: US Dollar; WHO: World Health Organization

Acknowledgements

The authors would like to acknowledge the support and contribution of Dr. Peter Kazembe, Dr. Charles Schubert, and Mr. Irving Hoffman, who provided mentorship and advice throughout the process.

Funding

Grants were provided from the Benjamin Josephson fund and the Office of International Activities at the University of North Carolina at Chapel Hill. The funders did not contribute to the design of the study. The funders contributed to the collection of the data by facilitating travel for the authors. They did not contribute to data analysis or to the writing of the manuscript.

Authors' contributions

EF helped collect data, then compiled and analyzed it. EF wrote the manuscript, which was edited by each author. EC, AT, HJL, and JM provided substantial contribution to the acquisition and interpretation of data. HJL, RM and ME were instrumental in the concept and design of the study and the procurement of data. ME was also critically involved in the interpretation of the data and the writing and editing of the manuscript. All authors read and approved the final manuscript.

Competing interests

The authors declare that they have no competing interests.

Author details

[1]Assistant Professor of Pediatrics, University of North Carolina at Chapel Hill, Chapel Hill, USA. [2]University of Malawi College of Medicine, Blantyre, Malawi. [3]University of North Carolina at Chapel Hill, Chapel Hill, USA. [4]Hawaii Permanente Medical Group, Maui, Hawaii, USA. [5]Médecins sans Frontières – Belgium, Paediatric Referent, Brussels, Belgium. [6]Assistant Professor of Pediatrics, Cincinnati Children's Hospital Medical Center, Cincinnati, Ohio, USA.

References

1. Maitland K, Kiguli S, Opoka RO, Engoru C, Olupot-Olupot P, Akech SO, et al. Mortality after fluid bolus in African children with severe infection. N Engl J Med. 2011;364:2483–95.
2. Campbell H, Duke T, Weber M, English M, Carai S, Tamburlini G, et al. Global initiatives for improving hospital care for children: state of the art and future prospects. Pediatrics. 2008;121:e984–92.
3. Molyneux EM. Paediatric emergency care in resource-constrained health services is usually neglected: time for change. Ann Trop Paediatr. 2010;30:165–76.
4. Razzak JA, Kellermann AL. Emergency medical care in developing countries: is it worthwhile? Bull World Health Organ. 2002;80:900–5.
5. Maclennan C, von Xylander S, Weber MW. Improving the quality of emergency care for children in developing countries. Bull World Health Organ. 2006;84:258.
6. Chan M, Kazatchkine M, Lob-Levyt J, Obaid T, Schweizer J, Sidibe M, et al. Meeting the demand for results and accountability: a call for action on health data from eight global health agencies. PLoS Med. 2010;7:e1000223.
7. AbouZahr C, Boerma T. Health information systems: the foundations of public health. Bull World Health Organ. 2005;83:578–83.
8. Setel PW, Macfarlane SB, Szreter S, Mikkelsen L, Jha P, Stout S, et al. A scandal of invisibility: making everyone count by counting everyone. Lancet Lond Engl. 2007;370:1569–77.
9. South Africa Every Death Counts Writing Group, Bradshaw D, Chopra M, Kerber K, Lawn JE, Bamford L, et al. Every death counts: use of mortality audit data for decision making to save the lives of mothers, babies, and children in South Africa. Lancet Lond Engl. 2008;371:1294–304.
10. Krug A, Patrick M, Pattinson RC, Stephen C. Childhood death auditing to improve paediatric care. Acta Paediatr Oslo Nor. 2006;95:1467–73.

11. Kanyuka M, Ndawala J, Mleme T, Chisesa L, Makwemba M, Amouzou A, et al. Malawi and millennium development goal 4: a countdown to 2015 country case study. Lancet Glob Health. 2016;4:e201–14.
12. Obermeyer Z, Abujaber S, Makar M, Stoll S, Kayden SR, Wallis LA, et al. Emergency care in 59 low- and middle-income countries: a systematic review. Bull World Health Organ. 2015;93:577–86G.
13. Nolan T, Angos P, Cunha AJ, Muhe L, Qazi S, Simoes EA, et al. Quality of hospital care for seriously ill children in less-developed countries. Lancet Lond Engl. 2001;357:106–10.
14. Gathara D, Nyamai R, Were F, Mogoa W, Karumbi J, Kihuba E, et al. Moving towards routine evaluation of quality of inpatient pediatric care in Kenya. PLoS One. 2015;10:e0117048.
15. Hodkinson P, Argent A, Wallis L, Reid S, Perera R, Harrison S, et al. Pathways to Care for Critically ill or injured children: a cohort study from first presentation to healthcare services through to admission to intensive care or death. PLoS One. 2016;11:e0145473.
16. Robison JA, Ahmad ZP, Nosek CA, Durand C, Namathanga A, Milazi R, et al. Decreased pediatric hospital mortality after an intervention to improve emergency Care in Lilongwe. Malawi PEDIATRICS. 2012;130:e676–82.
17. Robison J, Ahmed Z, Durand C, Nosek C, Namathanga A, Milazi R, et al. Implementation of ETAT (emergency triage assessment and treatment) in a central hospital in malawi. Arch Dis Child. 2011;96(Supplement 1):A74–5.
18. Berkley JA, Ross A, Mwangi I, Osier FHA, Mohammed M, Shebbe M, et al. Prognostic indicators of early and late death in children admitted to district hospital in Kenya: cohort study. BMJ. 2003;326:361.
19. Ralston ME, Day LT, Slusher TM, Musa NL, Doss HS. Global paediatric advanced life support: improving child survival in limited-resource settings. Lancet Lond Engl. 2013;381:256–65.
20. Olson D, Preidis GA, Milazi R, Spinler JK, Lufesi N, Mwansambo C, et al. Task shifting an inpatient triage, assessment and treatment programme improves the quality of care for hospitalised Malawian children. Trop Med Int Health TM IH. 2013;18:879–86.
21. Molyneux E, Ahmad S, Robertson A. Improved triage and emergency care for children reduces inpatient mortality in a resource-constrained setting. Bull World Health Organ. 2006;84:314–9.
22. Tamburlini G, Di Mario S, Maggi RS, Vilarim JN, Gove S. Evaluation of guidelines for emergency triage assessment and treatment in developing countries. Arch Dis Child. 1999;81:478–82.
23. Ahmed T, Ali M, Ullah MM, Choudhury IA, Haque ME, Salam MA, et al. Mortality in severely malnourished children with diarrhoea and use of a standardised management protocol. Lancet Lond Engl. 1999;353:1919–22.
24. Preidis GA, McCollum ED, Mwansambo C, Kazembe PN, Schutze GE, Kline MW. Pneumonia and malnutrition are highly predictive of mortality among African children hospitalized with human immunodeficiency virus infection or exposure in the era of antiretroviral therapy. J Pediatr. 2011;159:484–9.
25. Ahmad S, Ellis JC, Kamwendo H, Molyneux EM. Impact of HIV infection and exposure on survival in critically ill children who attend a paediatric emergency department in a resource-constrained setting. Emerg Med J EMJ. 2010;27:746–9.
26. Preidis GA, McCollum ED, Kamiyango W, Garbino A, Hosseinipour MC, Kazembe PN, et al. Routine inpatient provider-initiated HIV testing in Malawi, compared with client-initiated community-based testing, identifies younger children at higher risk of early mortality. J Acquir Immune Defic Syndr. 2013;63:e16–22.
27. English M, Esamai F, Wasunna A, Were F, Ogutu B, Wamae A, et al. Assessment of inpatient paediatric care in first referral level hospitals in 13 districts in Kenya. Lancet Lond Engl. 2004;363:1948–53.
28. Hendriksen ICE, Mtove G, Pedro AJ, Gomes E, Silamut K, Lee SJ, et al. Evaluation of a PfHRP2 and a pLDH-based rapid diagnostic test for the diagnosis of severe malaria in 2 populations of African children. Clin Infect Dis Off Publ Infect Dis Soc Am. 2011;52:1100–7.
29. Hendriksen ICE, White LJ, Veenemans J, Mtove G, Woodrow C, Amos B, et al. Defining falciparum-malaria-attributable severe febrile illness in moderate-to-high transmission settings on the basis of plasma PfHRP2 concentration. J Infect Dis. 2013;207:351–61.
30. English M, Esamai F, Wasunna A, Were F, Ogutu B, Wamae A, et al. Delivery of paediatric care at the first-referral level in Kenya. Lancet Lond Engl. 2004; 364:1622–9.
31. Hategeka C, Shoveller J, Tuyisenge L, Kenyon C, Cechetto DF, Lynd LD. Pediatric emergency care capacity in a low-resource setting: an assessment of district hospitals in Rwanda. PLoS One. 2017;12:e0173233.

2

Vitamin D in children with growth hormone deficiency due to pituitary stalk interruption syndrome

Cécile Delecroix[1], Raja Brauner[1*] and Jean-Claude Souberbielle[2]

Abstract

Background: Recent studies have shown a relationship between vitamin D status and growth hormone (GH) and insulin-like growth factor 1 (IGF1). The objective of this study was to assess vitamin D status in children with GH deficiency due to pituitary stalk interruption syndrome (PSIS) and to investigate the relationship between 25-hydroxyvitamin D (25OHD) and 1,25-dihydroxyvitamin D (1,25 (OH) $_2$D) serum levels and patient characteristics.

Methods: A retrospective single-center study of 25OHD and 1,25(OH)$_2$D serum concentrations in 50 children with PSIS at the initial evaluation before treatment.

Results: Mean concentrations of 33.2 ± 18.0 ng/mL for 25OHD and 74.5 ± 40.7 ng/L for 1,25(OH)$_2$D were measured. Additionally, 25OHD concentrations were significantly higher in boys than in girls ($p = 0.04$) and lower in the cold season than in the sunny season ($p = 0.03$). Significant positive correlations were observed between the GH peak and serum 1,25 (OH) $_2$D concentrations (Rho = 0.35; $p = 0.015$) and the 1,25(OH)$_2$D/25OHD ratio (Rho = 0.29; $p < 0.05$). No correlation was found for other characteristics, including IGF1.

Conclusions: Vitamin D status in children with hypothalamic-pituitary deficiency due to PSIS was similar to that reported in national and European studies in healthy children. The positive significant correlations between the GH peak and the 1,25 (OH)$_2$D concentration as well as with the 1,25 (OH)$_2$D/25OHD ratio suggest that even in these patients who had severely impaired GH secretion and low IGF1 levels, an interplay between the GH/IGF1 axis and the vitamin D system still exists.

Keywords: 1,25(OH)$_2$D, 1,25-dihydroxyvitamin D, 25OHD, 25-hydroxyvitamin D, Growth hormone, Growth hormone deficiency, Insulin-like growth factor 1, Pituitary stalk interruption syndrome, Vitamin D

Background

Growth hormone (GH) deficiency (GHD) can be congenital or acquired. Pituitary stalk interruption syndrome (PSIS), a sign of congenital and permanent GHD, is an anomaly of the pituitary gland characterized by a combination of specific findings on magnetic resonance imaging, including an interrupted pituitary stalk, an absent or ectopic posterior pituitary and anterior pituitary hypoplasia [1]. Because of the heterogeneity in clinical, biological and imaging presentations, recent efforts have focused on discriminating patients with multiple hypothalamic-pituitary (HP) deficiencies from those with isolated GHD [2]. Previous studies have shown an association between PSIS and other syndromes and/or malformations, and occurrence of familial forms have led to identification of gene mutations [3–7].

Humans mainly acquire vitamin D from exposure to sunlight, but it can also be obtained from food (oily fish). Vitamin D is first metabolized to 25-hydroxyvitamin D (25OHD) in the liver and then to its active form, 1,25-dihydroxyvitamin D (1,25(OH)$_2$D), in the kidneys. Overall, the concentration of serum 25OHD reflects the vitamin D status of an individual. Although debate remains regarding the 25OHD level that defines the optimal level, vitamin D deficiency is considered to be common worldwide in both adults and children [8–11]. Vitamin D has a well-known

* Correspondence: raja.brauner@wanadoo.fr
[1]Fondation Ophtalmologique Adolphe de Rothschild and Université Paris Descartes, Paris, France

role in bone development in utero and in childhood, and it maintains bone health in adults through effective calcium regulation and bone mineralization [12]. Because vitamin D receptors are present in many tissues, vitamin D may also have "non-classical" effects. Indeed, vitamin D deficiency has been associated with obesity in children [13], cardiovascular disease, type 2 diabetes, cancers (colon, prostate or breast) and auto-immune disorders [14–16].

Recent studies have shown a relationship between vitamin D status and GH and insulin-like growth factor 1 (IGF1). For example, initiation of cholecalciferol treatment increases serum IGF1 levels in children and adults with vitamin D deficiency [17, 18], and Wei et al. and Saggese et al. showed that six and 12 months of GH treatment, respectively, raised $1,25(OH)_2D$ concentrations in children with GHD [19, 20].

The first objective of the present study was to assess vitamin D status at the initial evaluation before GH treatment in a large series of children with GHD due to PSIS attended by a single endocrinologist. The second objective was to investigate the relationship between 25OHD and $1,25\ (OH)\ _2D$ serum levels and patient characteristics, mainly the GH peak and serum IGF1 level.

Methods

Patients

This retrospective single-center study included 50 children (28 boys and 22 girls) of a total of 86 (58%) PSIS patients monitored for HP deficiency by a senior pediatric endocrinologist (R. Brauner) between 1982 and 2016 and for whom a serum sample preserved at the initial evaluation at − 22 °C was still available. Patients with a syndrome that can interfere with their growth rate, i.e., Fanconi or Diamond-Blackfan anemia, were excluded (Fig. 1). At the initial evaluation, the characteristics of the 50 patients were similar to those of the 36 without available samples (Table 1). The criterion for GHD was a GH peak response of less than 20 mU/L or 6.7 ng/mL after two pharmacological stimulation tests.

Methods

The following data were collected at the initial clinical evaluation: age, height, growth rate during the previous year and body mass index (BMI), all expressed in standard deviation scores (SDS) according to chronological age [21, 22]. Bone age was assessed by R. Brauner according to the Greulich and Pyle method [23]. The initial biological evaluation included the IGF1 plasma concentration (expressed in ng/mL and SDS according to age and pubertal stage) and the GH peak level after a stimulation test (ornithine, arginine-insulin and/or glucagon test) or during spontaneous hypoglycemia in a few neonates. As we used various GH assays over the study period, we expressed the GH peak concentration in mU/L using conversion factors (ng/mL ⇔ mU/L) that were specific of the international standard used to calibrate the GH assay (i.e., 1 ng/mL = 2 mU/L for the assay calibrated with the old 66/217 international standard composed of poorly purified pituitary GH; 1 ng/mL = 2.6 mU/L for the assay calibrated against the 80/505 international standard composed of highly purified pituitary GH; 1 ng/mL = 3 mU/L for the assay calibrated against the 98/574 international standard composed of recombinant human (h)GH).

Multiple HP deficiency was diagnosed by GH deficiency in association with one or multiple deficiencies in the following: thyroid-stimulating hormone,

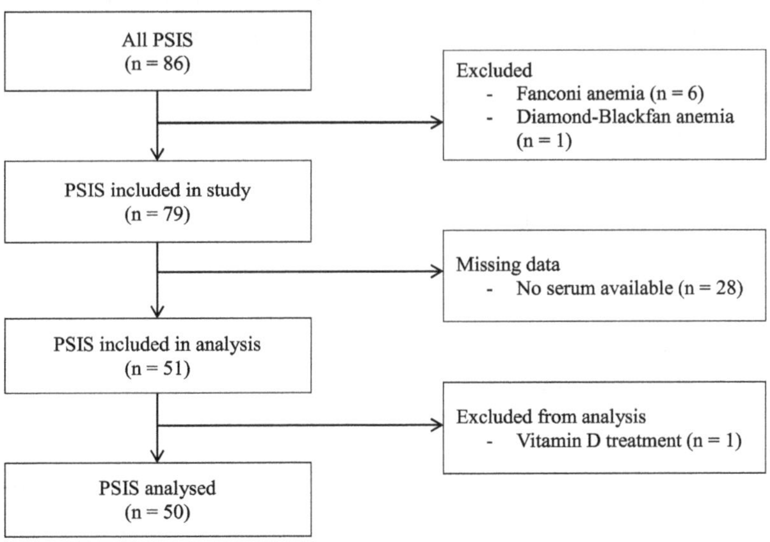

Fig. 1 Flowchart of the inclusion in the study

Table 1 Characteristics of the included and excluded patients with PSIS

	All PSIS ($n = 86$)		PSIS included ($n = 50$)		PSIS excluded ($n = 36$)		p
Boys	54	63%	28	56%	26	72%	0.9
Girls	32	37%	22	44%	10	28%	
Isolated GH deficiency	39	47%	22	44%	17	47%	0.8
Multiple HP deficiency	47	43%	28	56%	19	53%	
	Mean ± SD		Mean ± SD		Mean ± SD		
Age at diagnosis, years	4.9 ± 4.8		5.4 ± 4.9		4.2 ± 4.2		0.1
Bone age, years	3.7 ± 3.9		3.3 ± 4.1		3.8 ± 3.5		0.8
Height, SDS	−3.1 ± 1.5		−2.8 ± 1.1		−3.2 ± 1.8		0.7
BMI, SDS	0.2 ± 2.8		0.2 ± 2.2		0.2 ± 3.4		0.2
Growth rate, SDS	− 2.7 ± 1.4		−2.8 ± 1.4		−3 ± 1.4		0.6
GH peak, mU/L	5.9 ± 6.7		6.3 ± 6.0		4.1 ± 4.6		0.3
IGF1, SDS	− 3.6 ± 1.5		−3.6 ± 1.6		−3.6 ± 1.1		0.8
Free thyroxin, pmol/L	12.3 ± 7.8		12.1 ± 7.8		12.6 ± 10.8		0.5

adrenocorticotropic hormone, and/or luteinizing hormone and follicle-stimulating hormone [2]. Pituitary functions other than GH were evaluated by basal blood cortisol at 08.00 h, free thyroxin, prolactin, and the thyroid stimulating hormone response to thyrotropin releasing hormone; the plasma and urinary osmolalities after water deprivation for 12-h were normal in the first 29 patients evaluated, showing a normal concentration capacity. The normal limits were 12 to 28 pmol/L for plasma free thyroxin, and 0.6 to 4 mU/L for basal plasma thyroid stimulating hormone, 14 ± 7 mU/L for its peak, and < 10 mU/L for its value at 120 min after the thyrotropin releasing hormone test; and 5–25 μg/L for basal prolactin, except for neonates, who had higher concentrations. Adrenocorticotropic deficiency was diagnosed by plasma basal cortisol values below 40 μg/L in neonates, and below 80 μg/L in older children, with no increase during hypoglycemia. Gonadotropin deficiency was diagnosed as the absence of clinical signs of puberty, undetectable plasma estradiol and testosterone concentrations, and no increase in gonadotropin level after a gonadotropin-releasing hormone test. The seasonal period evaluation was defined by the month of blood sampling, and we divided the patients into two groups: the sunny season, which was from June to September, and the cold season, which was from October to May.

Serum 25OHD and 1,25(OH)$_2$D concentrations were measured using immunochemiluminescent assays (Liaison XL, DiaSorin, Saluggia, Italy). The patients were stratified according to their serum 25OHD concentration: ≤ 12 ng/mL, 13–19 ng/mL, 20–30 ng/mL, and > 30 ng/mL. We considered that a concentration between 30 and 60 ng/mL to be an appropriate level [9, 24, 25].

Statistical analysis

Qualitative results are presented as percentages. Fisher's exact test was performed to detect differences between qualitative variables. Quantitative results are presented as the mean ± SD. Between-group differences were assessed with the non-parametric Mann-Whitney test in cases with two groups and with the Kruskal-Wallis test in cases with 3 or more groups. Correlations were assessed with the Spearman test. A p value < 0.05 was considered significant. One boy with an abnormally high 25OHD concentration was excluded from the analysis because of probable vitamin D treatment before blood collection.

Results

The mean serum 25OHD concentration was 33.2 ± 18.0 ng/mL. Two (4%), nine (18%), 15 (30%) and 24 (48%) patients had a 25OHD level ≤ 12 ng/mL, between 13 and 19 ng/mL, between 20 and 30 ng/mL, and above 30 ng/mL, respectively (Table 2). Among these, a concentration > 60 ng/mL was found for four patients. Sex and season were the two factors that significantly influenced 25OHD concentrations, with higher levels in boys than in girls and lower levels in the "cold" than in the "sunny" season (Tables 2 and 3). Conversely, no significant difference in 25OHD level was observed according to the isolated or multiple HP character deficiency, age, bone age, height, BMI, growth rate, GH peak level or IGF1 level.

The mean serum 1,25(OH)$_2$D concentration was 74.5 ± 40.7 ng/L (Table 3). No significant difference in 1,25(OH)$_2$D level was observed according to sex, isolated or multiple HP character deficiency, season, age, bone age, height, BMI and growth rate. However, we did observe a trend toward higher levels in those with multiple HP deficiency. No significant correlations were observed between serum 1,25 (OH)$_2$D concentration and age, bone age, height, BMI, growth rate, IGF1 level or 25 OHD level. Nonetheless, significant positive correlations were observed between the GH peak level and serum 1,25 (OH)$_2$D concentration (Rho = 0.35; p = 0.015) and the 1,25(OH)$_2$D/25OHD ratio (Rho = 0.29; p < 0.05).

Discussion

In the present study, we evaluated vitamin D status in a large series of children with GHD due to PSIS, as observed by a single endocrinologist. We performed this study because both GHD [26] and vitamin D deficiency [27] are associated with bone fragility, impaired growth, muscle weakness, cardiac outcomes and metabolic syndrome.

In our population, the mean 25OHD concentration was 33.2 ± 18.0 ng/mL, which appears to be a satisfactory level. As we did not include a control group, we

Table 2 Characteristics according to the serum 25OHD level subgroups

25OHD, ng/mL	25OHD ≤ 12		13 < 25OHD ≤ 19		20 < 25OHD ≤ 30		25OHD > 30		
	$n = 2$		$n = 9$		$n = 15$		$n = 24$		p
Boys	0	0%	3	33%	7	47%	18	75%	0.04
Girls	2	100%	6	67%	8	53%	6	25%	
Isolated GH deficiency	1	50%	6	67%	4	27%	11	46%	0.2
Multiple HP deficiency	1	50%	3	33%	11	73%	13	54%	
Sunny season	0	0%	0	0%	4	27%	11	46%	0.01
Cold season	2	100%	6	100%	11	73%	13	54%	
	Mean ± SD		Mean ± SD		Mean ± SD		Mean ± SD		
Age at diagnosis, years	13.5 ± 4.5		4.7 ± 5.1		6.5 ± 6.7		4.4 ± 2.8		0.1
Bone age, years	12 ± 5		3.6 ± 5.6		3.2 ± 3.5		2.5 ± 1.9		0.1
Height, SDS	−2.7 ± −2.7		−2.6 ± 0.6		−3 ± 1.2		−2.8 ± 1.5		0.9
BMI, SDS	1.3 ± 0.8		0.4 ± 1.6		0.3 ± 2.3		0 ± 1.6		0.6
Growth rate, SDS	− 2.6 ± 0		− 2.4 ± 0.6		− 2.7 ± 1.2		− 3 ± 1.2		NS
IGF1, SDS	−4.7 ± 0		−2.4 ± 1.8		−3.9 ± 0.8		−3.6 ± 1		NS

compared this level with published data for healthy French children/adolescents. Among 212 girls aged 11–16.9 years with Tanner stages of 4 and 5 and living in Normandy (northwest of France), which is at the same latitude as Paris, mean 25OHD concentrations were 20.0 ± 6.1 ng/mL at the end of summer and 15.9 ± 7.4 ng/mL between January and May [28]. Alarmingly, 41% of these otherwise healthy girls had a 25OHD < 12 ng/mL during winter, revealing a severe vitamin D deficiency. The European HELENA study evaluated the vitamin D status of 1006 adolescents with a mean age of 14.9 years living in 10 European cities [29]. The participating French city was Lille, which is located in the extreme north of France, and the mean 25OHD level was 20.4 ± 8.8 ng/mL in girls and 24.1 ± 10.8 ng/mL in boys. In a recent multicenter study of vitamin D status

Table 3 Serum 25OHD and 1,25(OH)$_2$D levels compared with the patient characteristics

	25OHD, ng/mL		1,25(OH)$_2$D, ng/mL	
	Mean ± SD	p	Mean ± SD	p
All PSIS (n = 50)	33.2 ± 18.0		74.5 ± 40.7	
Sex				
Boys ($n = 28$)	37.6 ± 18	0.04	70 ± 27	0.4
Girls ($n = 22$)	27.6 ± 17.3		75 ± 40	
Deficiency				
Isolated GH ($n = 22$)	32.4 ± 15	0.4	64 ± 11.9	0.1
Multiple HP ($n = 28$)	33.8 ± 20		83 ± 52	
Season				
Sunny (n = 15)	42 ± 18	0.03	71.5 ± 32	0.3
Cold ($n = 35$)	31 ± 13		73 ± 41	
Age, years				
≤ 1.5 years (n = 8)	31.4 ± 18	0.4	92 ± 17	0.5
1.5 < age ≤ 6 years ($n = 23$)	35.9 ± 19		73 ± 19	
6 < age ≤ 10 years ($n = 13$)	33.3 ± 17		74 ± 17	
10 < age ≤ 18 years ($n = 6$)	24.7 ± 9		58 ± 9	
BMI, SDS				
< 0 ($n = 21$)	33.2 ± 13	0.9	72 ± 36	0.8
≥ 0 ($n = 25$)	33 ± 20		69 ± 16	

in 326 healthy French children aged 6–10 years, it was found that 3.1% of the participants had a 25OHD concentration below 10 ng/mL and that 34.4% had a 25OHD concentration between 10 and 19.9 ng/mL [11]. Although the mean 25OHD values were not indicated in this article, it can be concluded that the vitamin D status of these children was quite similar to what we found in our children with PSIS. In our present study, female sex and winter season (from October to May) were significantly associated with lower serum 25OHD concentrations, which is consistent with other previous published studies in adult and pediatric healthy populations [9, 30].

We then compared the 25OHD concentration measured in the present study in our patients with PSIS to the values reported in recent studies on GHD patients from various countries prior to GH treatment. Saggese et al. evaluated 26 children with GHD [20] and found normal 25OHD concentrations but low 1,25 $(OH)_2D$ levels before GH treatment and a significant increase in 1,25 $(OH)_2D$ levels after 12 months of GH treatment. Ciresi et al. evaluated 80 Sicilian children with GHD [31]. These authors reported significantly higher values in the sunny season (31.1 ± 11.1 ng/mL in June–September) than in the cold season (17.3 ± 5.3 ng/mL in November–February), with 35% having vitamin D insufficiency and 40% vitamin D deficiency. Witkowska-Sedek et al. evaluated 84 children and adolescents with GHD and found low 25OHD concentrations (22.3 ± 6.9 ng/mL) [32], and Savanelli et al. evaluated 41 adult GHD patients and found mean 25OHD concentration of 21.3 ± 12.3 ng/mL, with vitamin D deficiency present in 51% of the patients compared to 14.6% of the controls [33]. In addition, Ameri et al. evaluated 69 adult GHD patients, most with postsurgical hypopituitarism [34], and found that only 6 patients (8.7%) had a serum 25OHD concentration above 30 ng/mL. These authors reported a positive association between vitamin D status and IGF1, and they also found a trend toward higher GH doses in patients with low vitamin D status (25OHD < 15 ng/mL), suggesting that a better vitamin D status may facilitate achieving normal IGF1 values in GHD patients. In a literature review, these authors proposed that assessment of vitamin D status might be an appropriate method of determining the dose of recombinant hGH for treatment of adult patients with GHD [34].

One possible explanation for the higher vitamin D status in our study may be related to the young age of the subjects (mean 5.4 years). Indeed, in France, the French Society of Paediatrics recommends systematic vitamin D supplementation of children up to five years of age. Unfortunately, no guidelines for older children have been implemented; an exception is adolescents, in whom winter supplementation is recommended but rarely performed [35]. Surprisingly, our patients of more than 5 years old, particularly those aged 6–9 years, had a mean 25OHD level similar to that of our younger patients. This may suggest that vitamin D supplementation had been offered to some of our older patients before evaluation in our unit. In support of this is the fact that although BMI is known to influence spontaneous vitamin D status with lower 25OHD concentrations in overweight subjects, we found no difference in 25OHD levels between patients with a BMI < 0 SDS and those with a higher BMI. If the hypothesis that some of our patients received vitamin D supplementation before their assessment is correct, the finding that they have a normal vitamin D status is likely independent of their GHD. However as no information on vitamin D supplementation before our evaluation was available in the medical charts of our patients, we were unable to confirm that their rather good vitamin D status was due to vitamin D supplementation.

As GH appears to increase the level of 1,25 $(OH)_2D$ [19, 20, 36, 37], albeit likely indirectly, through the effects of IGF1, it may be hypothesized that patients with GHD due to PSIS have a low 1,25 $(OH)\ _2D$ serum concentration. This was not the case in our patients who had normal levels. We, however, have no explanation for the higher 1,25(OH)2D level in those with multiple HP deficiencies. Regardless, we did find a significant positive correlation between the GH peak level obtained during a pharmacologic stimulation test and the 1,25 $(OH)\ _2D$ concentration as well as with the 1,25 $(OH)\ _2D$/25OHD ratio. These findings suggest that even in these patients who had severely impaired GH secretion and low IGF1 levels, an interplay between the GH/IGF1 axis and the vitamin D system still exists.

Our study has limitations: it was retrospective and did not include a control group. However, the strength of our study pertains to the large series of GHD patients with a homogenous diagnosis (i.e., PSIS) and the same protocol of exploration for years, as they were attended by the same endocrinologist. This design allowed avoiding the considerable selection biases that affect several studies on GH deficiency. The patients who were excluded because of unavailable plasma samples might have introduced a bias, but their similarities to the included patients limit this. Another limitation is the lack of information on vitamin D supplementation before the patients were evaluated.

Conclusions

We found quite an acceptable mean vitamin D status in our series of children with GHD due to PSIS.

There are currently no available data from a double-blind, placebo-controlled randomized trial of vitamin D supplementation in GH-treated GHD patients showing that vitamin D optimizes bone health, growth and possibly other outcomes. Despite this lack of high-level evidence, we believe that it is mandatory to maintain optimal vitamin D supplementation in GHD patients.

Abbreviations

$1,25(OH)_2D$: 1,25-dihydroxyvitamin D; 25OHD: 25-hydroxyvitamin D; BMI: Body mass index; GH: Growth hormone; GHD: Growth hormone deficiency; HP: Hypothalamic-pituitary; IGF1: Insulin-like growth factor 1; PSIS: Pituitary stalk interruption syndrome; SDS: Standard deviation score

Acknowledgements

Not applicable.

Funding

The study was self-funded.

Authors' contributions

CD drafted the manuscript, collected and analyzed the data; RB conceived the study and participated in its design and coordination and drafted the manuscript; JCS participated in the design of the study and drafted the manuscript. All the authors read and approved the final manuscript.

Ethics approval and consent to participate

All clinical investigations were conducted according to the principles expressed in the Declaration of Helsinki. Written informed consent for the clinical and biological evaluation was obtained from the parents of the children and included in their hospital medical records. No activity in addition to routine patient care was performed due to the study. The authors had no direct interaction with these patients, except for their medical follow-up, which was performed by R. Brauner. Each patient's information was anonymized by the medical secretary prior to analysis.

Competing interests

The authors declare that they have no competing interests.

Author details

[1]Fondation Ophtalmologique Adolphe de Rothschild and Université Paris Descartes, Paris, France. [2]Assistance Publique-Hôpitaux de Paris, Hôpital Necker-Enfants Malades, Service d'Explorations Fonctionnelles, Paris, France.

References

1. Argyropoulou M, Perignon F, Brauner R, Brunelle F. Magnetic resonance imaging in the diagnosis of growth hormone deficiency. J Pediatr. 1992;120:886–91.
2. Pham L-L, Lemaire P, Harroche A, Souberbielle J-C, Brauner R. Pituitary stalk interruption syndrome in 53 postpubertal patients: factors influencing the heterogeneity of its presentation. PLoS One. 2013;8:e53189.
3. Dupuis-Girod S, Gluckman E, Souberbielle JC, Brauner R. Growth hormone deficiency caused by pituitary stalk interruption in Fanconi's anemia. J Pediatr. 2001;138:129–33.
4. Leblanc T, Gluckman E, Brauner R. Growth hormone deficiency caused by pituitary stalk interruption in diamond-Blackfan anemia. J Pediatr. 2003;142:358.
5. Pinto G, Netchine I, Sobrier ML, Brunelle F, Souberbielle JC, Brauner R. Pituitary stalk interruption syndrome: a clinical-biological-genetic assessment of its pathogenesis. J Clin Endocrinol Metab. 1997;82:3450–4.
6. Reynaud R, Gueydan M, Saveanu A, Vallette-Kasic S, Enjalbert A, Brue T, et al. Genetic screening of combined pituitary hormone deficiency: experience in 195 patients. J Clin Endocrinol Metab. 2006;91:3329–36.
7. Bashamboo A, Bignon-Topalovic J, Moussi N, McElreavey K, Brauner R. Mutations in the human ROBO1 gene in pituitary stalk interruption syndrome. J Clin Endocrinol Metab. July 2017;102(7):2401–6.
8. Holick MF, Binkley NC, Bischoff-Ferrari HA, Gordon CM, Hanley DA, Heaney RP, et al. Evaluation, treatment, and prevention of vitamin D deficiency: an Endocrine Society clinical practice guideline. J Clin Endocrinol Metab. 2011; 96:1911–30.
9. Souberbielle J-C, Massart C, Brailly-Tabard S, Cavalier E, Chanson P. Prevalence and determinants of vitamin D deficiency in healthy French adults: the VARIETE study. Endocrine. 2016;53:543–50.
10. Whiting SJ, Langlois KA, Vatanparast H, Greene-Finestone LS. The vitamin D status of Canadians relative to the 2011 dietary reference intakes: an examination in children and adults with and without supplement use. Am J Clin Nutr. 2011;94:128–35.
11. Mallet E, Gaudelus J, Reinert P, Stagnara J, Benichou J, Basuyau J-P, et al. [vitamin D status in 6- to 10-year-old children: a French multicenter study in 326 children]. Arch. Pediatr. Organe off. Soc. Francaise Pediatr. 2014;21:1106–14.
12. Wacker M, Holick MF. Vitamin D - effects on skeletal and extraskeletal health and the need for supplementation. Nutrients. 2013;5:111–48.
13. Gilbert-Diamond D, Baylin A, Mora-Plazas M, Marin C, Arsenault JE, Hughes MD, et al. Vitamin D deficiency and anthropometric indicators of adiposity in school-age children: a prospective study. Am J Clin Nutr. 2010;92:1446–51.
14. Holick MF. Vitamin D deficiency. N Engl J Med. 2007;357:266–81.
15. Antico A, Tampoia M, Tozzoli R, Bizzaro N. Can supplementation with vitamin D reduce the risk or modify the course of autoimmune diseases? A systematic review of the literature. Autoimmun Rev. 2012;12:127–36.
16. Anderson JL, May HT, Horne BD, Bair TL, Hall NL, Carlquist JF, et al. Relation of vitamin D deficiency to cardiovascular risk factors, disease status, and incident events in a general healthcare population. Am J Cardiol. 2010;106:963–8.
17. Ameri P, Giusti A, Boschetti M, Murialdo G, Minuto F, Ferone D. Interactions between vitamin D and IGF-I: from physiology to clinical practice. Clin Endocrinol. 2013;79:457–63.
18. Soliman AT, Al Khalaf F, Alhemaidi N, Al Ali M, Al Zyoud M, Yakoot K. Linear growth in relation to the circulating concentrations of insulin-like growth factor I, parathyroid hormone, and 25-hydroxy vitamin D in children with nutritional rickets before and after treatment: endocrine adaptation to vitamin D deficiency. Metabolism. 2008;57:95–102.
19. Wei S, Tanaka H, Kubo T, Ono T, Kanzaki S, Seino Y. Growth hormone increases serum 1,25-dihydroxyvitamin D levels and decreases 24,25-dihydroxyvitamin D levels in children with growth hormone deficiency. Eur J Endocrinol Eur Fed Endocr Soc. 1997;136:45–51.
20. Saggese G, Baroncelli GI, Bertelloni S, Cinquanta L, Di Nero G. Effects of long-term treatment with growth hormone on bone and mineral metabolism in children with growth hormone deficiency. J Pediatr. 1993;122:37–45.
21. Sempé M, Pédron G, Roy-Pernot MP. Auxologie, méthode et séquence. Paris: Théraplix; 1979.
22. Rolland-Cachera MF, Cole TJ, Sempe M, Tichet J, Rossignol C, Charraud A. Body mass index variations: centiles from birth to 87 years. Eur J Clin Nutr. 1991;45:13–21.
23. Greulich W, Pyle S. Radiographic atlas of skeletal development of the hand and wrist. Stanford: University Press; 1959.
24. Vidailhet M, Mallet E. Vitamin D in childhood. Presse Medicale Paris Fr 1983. 2013;42:1383–90.
25. Saggese G, Vierucci F, Boot AM, Czech-Kowalska J, Weber G, CAJ C, et al. Vitamin D in childhood and adolescence: an expert position statement. Eur J Pediatr. 2015;174:565–76.
26. Molitch ME, Clemmons DR, Malozowski S, Merriam GR, Vance ML. Evaluation and treatment of adult growth hormone deficiency: an Endocrine Society clinical practice guideline. J Clin Endocrinol Metab. 2011;96:1587–609.
27. Souberbielle J-C, Body J-J, Lappe JM, Plebani M, Shoenfeld Y, Wang TJ, et al. Vitamin D and musculoskeletal health, cardiovascular disease, autoimmunity and cancer: recommendations for clinical practice. Autoimmun Rev. 2010;9:709–15.

28. Esterle L, Nguyen M, Walrant-Debray O, Sabatier J-P, Garabedian M. Adverse interaction of low-calcium diet and low 25(OH)D levels on lumbar spine mineralization in late-pubertal girls. J Bone Miner Res Off J Am Soc Bone Miner Res. 2010;25:2392–8.
29. Gonzalez-Gross M, Valtuena J, Breidenassel C, Moreno LA, Ferrari M, Kersting M, et al. Vitamin D status among adolescents in Europe: the healthy lifestyle in Europe by nutrition in adolescence study. Br J Nutr. 2012;107:755–64.
30. Valtuena J, Gonzalez-Gross M, Huybrechts I, Breidenassel C, Ferrari M, Mouratidou T, et al. Factors associated with vitamin D deficiency in European adolescents: the HELENA study. J Nutr Sci Vitaminol (Tokyo). 2013;59:161–71.
31. Ciresi A, Ciccio F, Giordano C. High prevalence of hypovitaminosis D in Sicilian children affected by growth hormone deficiency and its improvement after 12 months of replacement treatment. J Endocrinol Investig. 2014;37:631–8.
32. Witkowska-Sedek E, Kucharska A, Ruminska M, Pyrzak B. Relationship between 25(OH)D and IGF-I in children and adolescents with growth hormone deficiency. Adv Exp Med Biol. 2016;912:43–9.
33. Savanelli MC, Scarano E, Muscogiuri G, Barrea L, Vuolo L, Rubino M, et al. Cardiovascular risk in adult hypopituitaric patients with growth hormone deficiency: is there a role for vitamin D? Endocrine. 2016;52:111–9.
34. Ameri P, Giusti A, Boschetti M, Bovio M, Teti C, Leoncini G, et al. Vitamin D increases circulating IGF1 in adults: potential implication for the treatment of GH deficiency. Eur J Endocrinol. 2013;169:767–72.
35. Vidailhet M, Mallet E, Bocquet A, Bresson J-L, Briend A, Chouraqui J-P, et al. Vitamin D: still a topical matter in children and adolescents. A position paper by the committee on nutrition of the French Society of Paediatrics. Arch Pediatr Organe Off Soc Francaise Pediatr. 2012;19:316–28.
36. Condamine L, Menaa C, Vrtovsnik F, Friedlander G, Garabedian M. Local action of phosphate depletion and insulin-like growth factor 1 on in vitro production of 1,25-dihydroxyvitamin D by cultured mammalian kidney cells. J Clin Invest. 1994;94:1673–9.
37. Wei S, Tanaka H, Seino Y. Local action of exogenous growth hormone and insulin-like growth factor-I on dihydroxyvitamin D production in LLC-PK1 cells. Eur J Endocrinol. 1998;139:454–60.

3

Assessing retention in care after 12 months of the Pediatric Development Clinic implementation in rural Rwanda

Scheilla Bayitondere[1*†], Francois Biziyaremye[2†], Catherine M. Kirk[2], Hema Magge[2,3,4], Katrina Hann[5], Kim Wilson[4], Christine Mutaganzwa[2], Eric Ngabireyimana[1], Fulgence Nkikabahizi[1], Evelyne Shema[1], David B. Tugizimana[2] and Ann C. Miller[6]

Abstract

Background: In Africa, a high proportion of children are at risk for developmental delay. Early interventions are known to improve outcomes, but they are not routinely available. The Rwandan Ministry of Health with Partners In Health/Inshuti Mu Buzima created the Pediatric Development Clinic (PDC) model for providing interdisciplinary developmental care for high-risk infants in rural settings. As retention for chronic care has proven challenging in many settings, this study assesses factors related to retention to care after 12 months of clinic enrollment.

Methods: This study describes a retrospective cohort of children enrolled for 12 months in the PDC program in Southern Kayonza district between April 2014–March 2015. We reviewed routinely collected data from electronic medical records and patient charts. We described patient characteristics and the proportion of patients retained, died, transferred out or lost to follow up (LTFU) at 12 months. We used Fisher's exact test and multivariable logistic regression to identify factors associated with retention in care.

Results: 228 children enrolled in PDC from 1 April 2014–31 March 2015, with prematurity/low birth weight (62.2%) and hypoxic ischemic encephalopathy (34.5%) as the most frequent referral diagnoses. 64.5% of children were retained in care and 32.5% were LTFU after 12 months. In the unadjusted analysis, we found male sex ($p = 0.189$), having more children at home ($p = 0.027$), health facility of first visit ($p = 0.006$), having a PDC in the nearest health facility ($p = 0.136$), referral in second six months of PDC operation ($p = 0.006$), and social support to be associated (100%, $p < 0.001$) with retention after 12 months. In adjusted analysis, referral in second six months of PDC operation (Odds Ratio (OR) 2.56, 95% CI 1.36, 4.80) was associated with increased retention, and being diagnosed with more complex conditions (trisomy 21, cleft lip/palate, hydrocephalus, other developmental delay) was associated with LTFU (OR 0.34, 95% CI 0.15, 0.76). As 100% of those receiving social support were retained in care, this was not able to be assessed in adjusted analysis.

Conclusions: PDC retention in care is encouraging. Provision of social assistance and decentralization of the program are major components of the delivery of services related to retention in care.

Keywords: loss to follow-up, high-risk infants, kangaroo mother care, social support, early childhood development, prematurity, Rwanda, Sub-Saharan Africa

* Correspondence: bayitondere@gmail.com
†Equal contributors
[1]Ministry of Health, Rwinkwavu District Hospital, Rwinkwavu, Rwanda
Full list of author information is available at the end of the article

Background

In low- and middle-income countries, almost 250 million children under five years of age are estimated to be at risk for delay in intellectual, physical, psychological, or social abilities [1, 2]. Children born preterm, at low birth weight, or with other medical conditions at birth are at even greater risk for impaired growth and development [3, 4]. Early childhood interventions during the first years of life can play a major role in improving the future outcome for the child's development [5]. In addition, children who have higher participation in early intervention programs designed for at-risk children report greater benefits and longer lasting effects than those with less participation [6].

In an attempt to meet the child survival fourth Millennium Development Goal, many countries, including Rwanda, made significant progress in terms of improvement of child health, and subsequently, the reduction of child mortality [7]. With strong leadership and political will, Rwanda has made impressive improvements in maternal and child health with the decrease of under-five mortality from 152 per 1000 live births in 2005 to 50 per 1000 live births in 2014 [8, 9]. Additionally, Rwanda specifically emphasized improving the quality of care provided in the newborn period and developed a fully revised National Neonatal Protocol for hospital-based care in 2015 [10]. Despite these achievements, there was no systematic approach to follow and support vulnerable children who remained at developmental risk after surviving the early neonatal period, for example those born premature or at low birth weight [3, 11]. Children with such perinatal risk factors are at increased risk of medical complications, growth failure [12], developmental delay [3], and death [13]. Regular, systematic and ongoing monitoring allows early detection of health, growth, and developmental challenges and subsequently appropriate and timely intervention [14–16]. However, very few models for high-risk children have been tested in sub-Saharan Africa [17].

In 2014, the Rwandan Ministry of Health (MOH), in collaboration with Partners In Health/Inshuti Mu Buzima (PIH/IMB), launched Rwanda's first Pediatric Development Clinic (PDC) with the overall goal of providing interdisciplinary medical, nutritional, and developmental assessment and intervention in a non-specialist setting to infants and children at high risk for developmental delay [18]. The PDC serves children with premature birth and low birth weight or other perinatal complications, suspected genetic syndromes, and neurodevelopment impairments. However, retention in longitudinal care has proven challenging for health care services in rural African settings [19, 20]. In this study, we assessed PDC patient retention at 12 months post-referral into PDC and factors associated with retention in care.

Methods

Study setting and intervention:

We conducted a retrospective cohort study of children enrolled in PDC program between 1April 2014 and 31 March 2015, which was the PDCs first year of operation. Data on visits of children enrolled in this first year were extracted through 31 March 2016 to assess retention at 12 months. Each child was followed for his or her first 12 months in PDC care. This study was conducted in the Rwinkwavu District Hospital (RDH) catchment area in rural Kayonza District, Eastern Province, Rwanda. The catchment area includes eight health centers under RDH supervision, serving a population of about 200,000 [21]. RDH is a MOH public institution that has received support from PIH/IMB since 2005. The PDC was started in April 2014 at RDH and has since been decentralized to two of Southern Kayonza's eight health centers in August 2014 and two additional health centers in June 2015. During the study time period, an average of 450 deliveries per month occurred in RDH catchment area with about 39 newborns admitted to the neonatal unit each month – it is estimated that about half the these newborns would be eligible for PDC if discharged alive.

PDC aims to improve health outcomes for high-risk children under five years by providing medical, nutritional, and developmental support. The PDC clinic implementation is described in depth in Ngabireyimana et al. (2017), however, a brief description follows. At each visit, caregivers participate in a morning group education session followed by individual consultations with an assessment of the child's health status, including an assessment of danger signs and vitals, completed by a trained nurse under a General Practitioner's supervision. Children are treated or referred for specialist care according to the results of assessment. Nutritional support includes growth monitoring, feeding assessment and counseling on breastfeeding and nutrition. Food packages are provided to children whose mothers meet established criteria, including inability to produce sufficient breast milk or those whose social screening documents showed inability to provide adequate nutrition. Infant formula with teaching and safe preparation kits is provided for those infants meeting defined medical therapeutic criteria. Support to optimize child development, which includes regular developmental monitoring using the Ages and Stages Questionnaires [22], individual parent counseling and clinic-based group sessions on child developmental topics, is provided to all children at each visit. Play and communication counseling materials were developed for use in the clinic based on an expanded form of Care for Child Development materials [23]. Condition-specific follow-up is also provided as needed for each child, including kangaroo mother care follow-up for preterm and infants born under 2000 g. Transport reimbursements are provided in cash at each visit to eligible patients, based on nurse and social worker assessment of the caregiver's ability to pay, to reduce barriers to accessing care for those meeting pre-established criteria per social worker evaluation. Home visits for additional family counseling are conducted weekly by PDC staff to the most vulnerable children as identified by nurses and social workers in the weekly clinic assessments. In addition, community health workers are requested to conduct follow-up home visits with patients who are not making routine appointments.

Children are referred to the PDC either from RDH departments such as Neonatology, Maternity, and Pediatrics or a health center in RDH catchment area, with occasional cases referred from other health facilities outside the RDH catchment area or self-referrals from the community. Children are eligible to enroll in PDC if they have one or more of the following medical conditions: prematurity (< 37 weeks of gestational age or by clinician determination), birth weight under 2000 g, hypoxic ischemic encephalopathy (HIE), cleft lip/palate, hydrocephalus, significant developmental delays, suspected trisomy 21 and/or other suspected genetic syndromes. Eligibility is often determined by a doctor at the point of referral to PDC; in cases of developmental delay, there are no specific diagnostic criteria. However, children who are significantly behind on developmental milestones are often referred by hospital pediatrics wards, health centers, or by self-referral from the community. Referred children are enrolled at the nearest health facility with a PDC for regular follow-up. Follow-up visits are scheduled based on the child's age and specific medical condition. Individual patient data from each visit is recorded on a paper form and then entered into an Electronic Medical Record (EMR) system.

Data collection:

Data were extracted from PDC patient charts as well as the EMR for patients who enrolled between 1 April 2014 and 31 March 2015; data on these patient's visits were then extracted through 31 March 2016 to assess retention at 12 months. Data collected included baseline demographics on children and their primary caretakers, baseline clinical information, social supports received, details of PDC services delivered at each visit and retention outcomes at 12 months. Paper charts were reviewed by trained data collectors. Data quality audits and supervision of data validation were conducted by a research assistant. Crosschecking between EMR data and paper-based data was conducted for key indicators, and identified errors were corrected immediately with recommendations given to improve data quality.

Measures

Our primary outcome measure was retention in care, defined as a visit within 90 days before or after the 12 month date following the child's referral date into PDC. Children who were documented to have died or transferred out (discharged or relocated outside the catchment area) of the program were not considered lost to follow-up (LTFU). Period of referral to PDC was defined as a binary variable of two six-month periods (April–September 2014 and October 2014–March 2015).

Gestational age was categorized into four groups: term (37+ weeks), moderate/late preterm (32–37 weeks), very preterm (28–31 weeks) and extremely preterm (less than 28 weeks). Birth weight was collected as a continuous variable and divided into four categories: normal weight (≥2500 g), low birth weight (LBW, 1500–2499 g), very low birth weight (VLBW, 1000–1499 g) and extremely low birth weight (ELBW, < 1000 g).

Diagnosis or reason of referral included all PDC eligibility criteria in addition to children referred for other reasons. Children who were diagnosed with more than one condition were categorized as "diagnosed with multiple conditions" and also counted within each specific condition for which they were diagnosed. We defined a separate variable, "diagnosed with any other conditions", as any diagnosis that did not include preterm, low birth weight, or HIE due to the small number of children presenting with these other conditions. Socio-economic status was defined as binary variable of "qualifies for government support" to identify the poorest households in Rwanda versus "does not qualify" based on the Rwandan system of *Ubudehe*. *Ubudehe* is a measure of socio-economic status unique to Rwanda that serves as a community-based poverty ranking system; at the time of study there were six wealth categories in *Ubudehe* and the poorest two categories qualified for government support for free health insurance and other social protection services [24].

Social support was defined as provision of conditional cash transfers by the PDC to reimburse the costs of transport to the clinic, conditional food transfers in the form of food packages (either for breastfeeding mothers or as complementary feeding for children over age six months), or a follow-up home visit by community health workers for complicated cases. Infant formula with hygienic preparation kits were provided to infants who met defined medical therapeutic criteria.

Analysis

We provide descriptive analysis of the patient population, including frequencies, medians and interquartile ranges (IQR). We used Fisher's exact tests to identify factors associated with retention and LTFU. All factors significant in bivariate analysis at $p < 0.20$ were included in the multivariate analyses. Factors were assessed for collinearity prior to inclusion in the model. Multivariable logistic regression was used to build the final model

Table 1 Descriptive characteristics of Pediatric Development Clinic patients and caretakers

	Total (*N* = 228)	
	N	%
Child Characteristics		
Gender		
Female	132	57.9
Male	94	41.2
Missing	2	0.9
Age at the first visit (months)		
< 1	83	36.4
1–5	79	34.7
6–11	11	4.8
12+	21	9.2
Missing		
Gestational age at birth (weeks)		
Extremely preterm (< 28)	7	3.1
Very preterm (28–32)	18	7.9
Moderate/late (32–37)	63	27.6
Term (37+)	73	32.0
Missing	67	29.4
Birth weight (grams)		
Normal (> 2500)	66	29.0
Low (1500–2499)	75	32.9
Very Low (1000–1499)	35	15.4
Extremely Low (< 1000)	2	0.9
Missing	50	21.9
Diagnosis (Reason for referral)[1]		
PT/LBW (*N* = 227)	142	62.6
HIE (*N* = 226)	78	34.5
Trisomy 21 (*N* = 210)	6	2.9
Cleft palate (N = 210)	4	1.9
Hydrocephalus (N = 210)	3	1.4
Other delay (N = 210)	9	4.3
Other reasons (N = 210)	11	5.2
Diagnosed with multiple conditions (N = 227)	29	12.8
Caretaker Characteristics		
Age (years)		
15–19	12	5.3
20–24	67	29.4
25–34	86	37.7
35–44	39	17.1
44+	4	1.8
Missing	20	8.8
Relationship with the child		
Mother	161	70.6

Table 1 Descriptive characteristics of Pediatric Development Clinic patients and caretakers *(Continued)*

	Total (*N* = 228)	
	N	%
Father	2	0.9
Grandmother	2	0.9
Missing	63	27.6
Level of education completed		
No education	29	12.7
Some primary school	70	39.7
Primary school	69	30.3
Secondary or higher	8	3.5
Missing	52	22.8
Marital status		
Married or cohabitating	195	85.5
Single, widowed, or divorced	19	8.3
Missing	14	6.1
Socioeconomic status		
Does not qualify for government support	109	47.8
Qualifies for government support	21	9.2
Missing	98	43.0
Number of other dependents in home		
None	20	8.8
1–3 children	109	47.8
4–5 children	29	12.7
6+ children	16	7.0
Missing	54	23.7

PT/LBW preterm/low birth weight, *HIE* hypoxic ischemic encephalopathy
[1]Multiple diagnoses per patient were present

using backward stepwise procedures. All factors significant at $\alpha = 0.05$ were retained in the final model.

Results

From April 2014 to March 2015, 228 patients enrolled in the PDC program; 132 (57.9%) were female and 94 (41.2%) were male (Table 1). Prematurity/low birth weight (62.6%, $n = 142$ out of 227) and HIE (34.5%, $n = 78$ out of 226) were the most frequent reasons for referral. We found that 70.6% of primary caretakers were female ($n = 161$ out of 228), 85% were married or cohabitating ($n = 195$ of 228), and 12.7% had no formal education ($n = 29$ of 228).

Seventy-five percent of children were referred from the hospital ($n = 172$ of 228) and 60.1 % of children were enrolled during the first six months of implementing the PDC program ($n = 137$ of 228) (Table 2). The median days between referral and intake was 9 (IQR: 3–15) and the median number of visits per child in 12 months was 7 (IQR: 5–9). Almost half (47.0%, $n = 99$ of 211) of

Table 2 Pediatric Development Clinic visits in first 12 months of care

	Total ($N = 228$)	
	n	%
Source of referral		
Hospital	172	75.4
Health Centers	17	7.5
Other	6	2.6
Missing	33	14.5
Health Facility at first visit		
Rwinkwavu	133	58.3
Kabarondo	76	33.3
Ndego	19	8.3
Household's nearest health center has a PDC		
No	56	24.6
Yes	168	73.7
Missing	4	1.8
Period of referral to PDC		
April 2014–September 2014	137	60.1
October 2014 – March 2015	91	39.9
Patient mode of transport to PDC		
Walking	90	39.5
Motorbike	76	33.3
Mini bus	38	16.7
Other	15	6.6
Missing	9	4.0
Patient transferred between PDCs		
No	194	85.1
Yes	34	14.9
Number of visits in 12 months, median (IQR)	7	(5, 9)
Patient ever received food packages		
No	163	71.5
Yes	47	20.6
Missing	18	7.9
Patient ever received infant formula		
No	200	87.7
Yes	10	4.4
Missing	18	7.9
Patient ever received transport reimbursement		
No	118	51.8
Yes	93	40.8
Missing	17	7.5

Table 2 Pediatric Development Clinic visits in first 12 months of care *(Continued)*

	Total ($N = 228$)	
	n	%
Patient ever received a CHW home visit		
No	200	87.7
Yes	10	4.4
Missing	18	7.9

PDC Pediatric Development Clinic, *IQR* Interquartile range, *CHW* Community Health Worker

patients received some form of conditional cash or food transfer from the PDC (including therapeutic formula) in their first 12 months of care. Four percent of the children received an additional home visit by a community health worker ($n = 10$ of 228).

Out of 228 children, 147 (64.5%) were retained in care after one year, 74 (32.5%) were LTFU, four (1.8%) died and three (1.3%) were transferred out of the program (Table 3). In the unadjusted analysis, male sex ($p = 0.189$) and having more children at home ($p = 0.027$) were both socio-demographic factors associated with increased retention (Table 4). Having a diagnosis other than preterm/low birth weight or HIE ("other diagnosis" such as trisomy 21, cleft lip/palate, etc.) was associated with lower retention ($p = 0.024$). The health facility of first visit ($p = 0.006$), having a PDC in the nearest health facility ($p = 0.136$), and period of referral to PDC ($p = 0.006$) were associated with increased retention in care at 12 months. Social support was significantly associated with retention in care with 100% of children who received food packages ($n = 47$, $p < 0.001$), infant formula ($n = 10$, $p = 0.035$), transport fees ($n = 90$, $p < 0.001$), and community health worker home visits ($n = 10$, $p = 0.035$).

When adjusting for covariates, the period of referral (odds ratio (OR): 2.56; 95% confidence interval (CI): 1.36, 4.80, $p = 0.004$) was associated with increased retention in care (Table 5), and "other diagnosis" continued to be associated with decreased retention in care at 12 months (OR: 0.34, 95% CI: 0.15, 0.76, $p = 0.009$) compared to children who had either preterm/low birth weight or HIE. We were unable to assess social support in the adjusted model as receipt of support completely predicted retention in care; site of first visit was also not included in the full model due to collinearity with the period of referral to PDC.

Discussion

In our study, we found 64.5% retention for patients referred to PDC in the first 12 months, which is promising for a newly implemented program. However, studies on HIV treatment retention in infants in low- and middle-income countries show a higher retention [19, 25]. We also observed a low documented mortality rate for

Table 3 Patient retention status at 12 months by diagnosis

	In care		LTFU		Died		Transferred Out	
	N	%	*n*	%	*n*	%	*n*	%
All children (N = 228)	147	64.5	74	32.5	4	1.8	3	1.3
Diagnosed as PT/LBW (N = 142)	95	66.9	42	29.6	2	1.4	3	2.1
Diagnosed with HIE (N = 78)	54	69.2	22	28.2	1	1.3	1	1.3
Diagnosed with Trisomy 21 (*N* = 6)	1	16.7	5	83.3	0	0.0	0	0.0
Diagnosed with cleft lip/palate (N = 4)	2	50.0	2	50.0	0	0.0	0	0.0
Diagnosed with hydrocephalus (*N* = 3)	2	66.7	1	33.3	0	0.0	0	0.0
Diagnosed with other developmental delays (N = 9)	4	44.4	5	55.6	0	0.0	0	0.0
Diagnosed with other condition (*N* = 11)	6	54.6	4	36.4	1	9.1	0	0.0
Diagnosed with multiple conditions (N = 29)	19	65.5	9	31.0	1	3.5	0	0.0

LTFU lost to follow up, *PT/LBW* preterm/low-birth weight, *HIE* hypoxic ischemic encephalopathy

children enrolled in the PDC compared to other studies in developing countries for patient groups of a profile similar to the majority of PDC patients, including for children with very low birth weight [3] and birth asphyxia [26]. We assume that the PDC program was beneficial for these high-risk infants, however an evaluation comparing outcomes to a baseline conducted prior to the implementation of the program in the same population is still ongoing.

Our study showed that receipt of social support completely predicted retention in care. This result is unsurprising as the PDC serves a rural population with very limited resources with a quarter of the population living in poverty [27] and these supports may serve as a financial incentive for participation in the PDC program. The provided social support helps to remove financial barriers to participation in care, and we contend, is a critical component to support the health and development of these children. For example, provision of breastfeeding support, nutritional counseling, and infant formula when medically necessary is extremely important to the brain growth and development of premature children who have catch-up growth needs and may have feeding difficulties. Perceived (and actual) improvement in a child's growth would certainly provide encouragement to the child's caretakers to return to PDC. Social support was also found as predictor of good retention and good outcomes for an HIV clinic program for adults in a rural poor setting area [28]. In addition, partnering home visits with pediatric care as we have done has been shown to be a strong predictor of retention. In a study of a home visiting program in the United States, home-visited mothers kept pediatric appointments 10 times more than those who did not receive home visits [29].

The findings of an increase in retention in care in the second six-month period of referral in the PDC's first year of operation might be related to the increased awareness of the program importance over time; the more the population became aware of the PDC program, the more the retention in care increased. This finding might also be attributed to improved quality of care provision as providers gained more experience and iterative learning and improvement over time, particularly around identifying children who were missing visits. In addition, it was in the second six-month period of operation where the four decentralized health center clinics were all fully operational for the full time period, which may have eased access to care and contributed to greater retention.

Our analysis showed a relationship between less-common conditions such as Trisomy 21, cleft palate, hydrocephalus and other developmental delays and increased LTFU. This could be a result of a few different factors. First, stigma or misperceptions in the community of these conditions could deter care seeking and encourage a preference for keeping children with such conditions a secret [30]. Research in Malawi showed the caretakers of children with intellectual disability require supports to address mental health issues that arise due to elevated stress and stigma experienced when caring for these children [31]. Also, there could be some potential discouragement among caretakers as it may take more time to see change in children experiencing more pervasive developmental delays when compared to prematurity conditions that can develop quite normally with appropriate supports. This might also be related to the unique management of some of these conditions, which include surgical repair for cleft lip and palate. Once managed there may have been no need to continue with close follow up of these children. Further, conditions such as hydrocephalus require referrals for neurosurgery evaluation. LTFU may occur in the process of this transfer to a referral facility; better understanding of continuity of care following referrals is an important area for further investigation in this novel program. The sample size of those conditions is too small in the program to draw definitive conclusions and further studies

Table 4 Bivariate associations with retention to care at 12 months

	Retained ($n = 147$, 66.5%)		LTFU ($n = 74$, 33.5%)		*P* value
	n	%	*n*	%	
Gender ($N = 219$)					
Female	81	63.3	47	36.7	0.189
Male	66	72.5	25	27.5	
Age at the first visit (months) ($N = 203$)					
< 1	61	74.4	21	25.6	0.570
1–5	54	70.1	23	29.9	
6–11	6	54.6	5	45.5	
12+	23	69.7	10	30.3	
Gestational age in weeks at birth (weeks) ($N = 156$)					
Extremely preterm (< 28)	4	57.1	3	42.9	0.861
Very preterm (28–32)	12	75.0	4	25.0	
Moderate/late (32–37)	40	65.6	21	34.4	
Term (37+)	48	66.7	24	33.3	
Birth weight (grams) ($N = 171$)					
Normal (> 2500)	43	67.2	21	32.8	0.386
Low (1500–2499)	46	63.9	26	36.1	
Very Low (1000–1499)	26	78.8	7	21.2	
Extremely Low (< 1000)	1	50.0	1	50.0	
Diagnosed with PT/LBW ($N = 220$)					
No	52	62.7	31	37.4	0.376
Yes	95	69.3	42	30.7	
Diagnosed with HIE (N = 219)					
No	93	65.0	50	35.0	0.450
Yes	54	71.1	22	29.0	
Diagnosed with any other conditions ($N = 220$)					
No	132	69.8	57	30.2	0.024
Yes	15	48.4	16	51.6	
Diagnosed with multiple conditions (N = 220)					
No	128	66.7	64	33.3	> 0.999
Yes	19	67.9	9	32.1	
Age of the primary caretaker (years) ($N = 201$)					
15–19	9	81.8	2	18.2	0.595
20–24	45	70.3	19	29.7	
25–34	55	65.5	29	34.5	
35–44	22	57.9	16	42.1	
45+	3	75.0	1	25.0	
Caretakers relationship with the child ($N = 159$)					
Mother	104	67.1	51	32.9	> 0.999
Father	2	100.0	0	0.0	
Grandmother	1	50.0	1	50.0	
Caretaker's level of education (N = 172)					
No education	23	79.3	6	20.7	0.387
No formal education completed	48	68.6	21	30.4	

Table 4 Bivariate associations with retention to care at 12 months *(Continued)*

	Retained ($n = 147$, 66.5%)		LTFU ($n = 74$, 33.5%)		*P* value
	n	%	*n*	%	
Primary school completed	49	74.2	17	25.7	
Secondary or higher completed	4	50.0	4	50.0	
Caretaker's marital status ($N = 207$)					
Married or cohabitating	127	67.2	62	32.8	0.608
Single, widowed, or divorced	11	61.1	7	38.9	
Household socioeconomic status ($N = 128$)					
Does not qualify for government support	74	69.2	33	30.8	0.315
Qualifies for government support	12	57.1	9	42.9	
Number of other dependents in home ($N = 170$)					
None	10	50.0	10	50.0	0.027
1–3 children	81	75.0	27	25.0	
4–5 children	18	69.2	8	30.8	
6+ children	15	93.8	1	6.3	
Source of referral ($N = 190$)					
Hospital	107	64.1	60	35.9	0.416
Health Centers	13	76.5	4	23.5	
Other	5	83.3	1	16.7	
Health Facility of first visit ($N = 221$)					
Rwinkwavu	77	60.6	50	39.4	0.006
Kabarondo	52	69.3	23	30.7	
Ndego	18	94.7	1	5.3	
Household's nearest health center has a PDC ($N = 217$)					
No	32	58.2	23	41.8	0.136
Yes	113	69.8	49	30.3	
Period of referral to PDC (N = 221)					
April 2014–September 2014	79	59.4	54	40.6	0.006
October 2014 – March 2015	68	77.3	20	22.7	
Patient mode of transport to PDC ($N = 212$)					
Walking	58	67.4	28	32.6	0.832
Motorbike	47	63.5	27	36.5	
Minibus	26	70.3	11	29.7	
Other	9	60.0	6	40.0	
Patient transferred between PDCs (N = 221)					
No	121	64.7	66	35.3	0.236
Yes	26	76.5	8	23.5	
Patient ever received food packages ($N = 205$)					
No	97	61.4	61	38.6	< 0.001
Yes	47	100.0	0	0.0	
Patient ever received infant formula (N = 205)					
No	134	68.7	61	31.3	0.035
Yes	10	100.0	0	0.0	
Patient ever received transport fees ($N = 206$)					
No	55	47.4	61	52.6	< 0.001

Table 4 Bivariate associations with retention to care at 12 months *(Continued)*

	Retained (*n* = 147, 66.5%)		LTFU (*n* = 74, 33.5%)		*P* value
	n	%	*n*	%	
Yes	90	100.0	0	0.0	
Patient ever received a CHW home visit (N = 205)					
No	134	68.7	61	31.3	0.035
Yes	10	100.0	0	0.0	

LTFU lost to follow up, *PT/LBW* preterm/low-birth weight, *HIE* hypoxic ischemic encephalopathy, *PDC* Pediatric Development Clinic, *CHW* Community Health Worker

are needed to better understand the trajectory of these children in care.

The findings of our study need to be taken in context within some limitations. As our study used routinely collected data from patient charts and files, we found significant levels of missing data. Additionally, because we used routinely collected program data, information on some individual factors that might influence retention in care were not available. Respondents are not always able to provide information on variables such as gestational age due to challenges in determining gestational age [32] and *Ubudehe* status, which has been reported as unknown by a quarter of people in large national surveys [33] and further contributes to missing data. However, important information was provided despite these data limitations. Another limitation is generalizability of our findings; because PDC is a pilot program only operational at one district hospital and four health centers in rural Southern Kayonza District, the findings may not be generalizable to other settings. Nevertheless, this study can provide important information to program implementers to ensure high retention and help inform replication of the PDC program in other areas in Rwanda, other programs in rural African settings, or other countries with low resources.

The results from this study are heartening and highlight both the viability of providing longitudinal care through a program reaching a previously-underserved population of children in a rural, resource-limited African setting, as well as the importance of social support in retaining these at-risk children in care over the long term. While studies are underway to assess other factors related to feasibility of the PDC program like costs, acceptability and ability to self sustain as well as to understand the long-term impact of the PDC care on the health and developmental outcomes of these high-risk children, this program can serve as an example in other similar settings.

Conclusions

The PDC model implemented in rural Rwanda demonstrates promising retention rates at 12 months for a new clinic and low rates of documented mortality in this high-risk population of very young children. This model of integrated and holistic follow-up could contribute to strong retention in other early

Table 5 Multivariate analysis of predictors of retention in Pediatric Development Clinic at 12 months

	Full Model			Reduced Model		
	OR	95%CI	*P* value	OR	95%CI	*P* value
Child sex						
Female	Ref					
Male	1.48	(0.79, 2.74)	0.219			
Diagnosed with any other conditions[1]						
No	Ref			Ref		
Yes	0.31	(0.14, 0.70)	0.005	0.34	(0.15, 0.76)	0.009
Household's nearest health center has a PDC						
No	Ref					
Yes	1.70	(0.87, 3.31)	0.12			
Period of referral to PDC						
April 2014–September 2014	Ref			Ref		
October 2014 – March 2015	2.50	(1.32, 4.74)	0.005	2.56	(1.36, 4.80)	0.004

PDC Pediatric Development Clinic

[1]Diagnosed with any other condition includes diagnosis of Trisomy 21, cleft palate, hydrocephalus, other delay, or other reasons

childhood development programs and may improve future outcomes of children at high risk for development delay in resource-limited settings.

Abbreviations

HIE: hypoxic ischemic encephalopathy; LTFU: Loss to follow-up; MOH: Ministry of Health; PDC: Pediatric Development Clinic; PIH/IMB: Partners In Health/Inshuti Mu Buzima; RDH: Rwinkwavu District Hospital

Acknowledgements

We acknowledge Partners In Health/Inshuti Mu Buzima for the support of this work. This study was developed under the Partners In Health/Inshuti Mu Buzima Intermediate Operational Research Training Program, developed and facilitated by Bethany Hedt-Gauthier and Jackline Odhiambo. Ann Miller, Catherine Kirk and Katrina Hann provided direct mentorship to this paper as part of this training. We also acknowledge the contributions of Stephanie Bazubagira, Jean de Dieu Uwihaye, and Emmanuel Ndayishimiye for data collection. In addition, we are grateful for the data cleaning support from Kaya Hedt.

Availability of data

The data that support the findings of this study are available from Partners In Health/Inshuti Mu Buzima, but restrictions apply to the availability of these data which were used under license for the current study and are not publicly available. Data collected in Rwanda on Rwandan subjects may only be used in Rwanda. Data are however available from the authors upon reasonable request and with permission of Partners In Health/Inshuti Mu Buzima.

Author contributions

SB and FB led study design, analysis and interpretation of data, wrote and reviewed the first and all subsequent versions of the manuscript. CMK, HM. ACM, KW and KH provided inputs in study design, supported analysis and interpretation of data, and contributed to all versions of the manuscript. CM, EN, FN, DBT, and ES contributed in data interpretation and reviewed manuscript. CMK led data collection. HM, CMK, ACM and KH mentored manuscript development, analysis and manuscript development. All authors critically reviewed the manuscript and approved the final version for publication.

Funding

Data collection and training costs were covered by UNICEF Rwanda and Partners In Health/Inshuti Mu Buzima. Training costs were covered by the Harvard Global Health Initiative Burke Global Health Fellowship grant and by Partners In Health/Inshuti Mu Buzima. Some training facilitators and mentors are Rwanda Human Resources for Health faculty, funded with the support of the Government of Rwanda, the Global Fund to fight AIDS, Tuberculosis and Malaria and Centers for Disease Control and Prevention.

Competing interests

All authors declare that they have no competing interests.

Author details

[1]Ministry of Health, Rwinkwavu District Hospital, Rwinkwavu, Rwanda. [2]Partners In Health/Inshuti Mu Buzima, Rwinkwavu, Rwanda. [3]Boston Children's Hospital, Boston, MA, USA. [4]Brigham and Women's Hospital, Boston, MA, USA. [5]Partners In Health Sierra Leone, Freetown, Sierra Leone. [6]Harvard Medical School, Boston, MA, USA.

References

1. Lu C, Black MM, Richter LM. Risk of poor development in young children in low-income and middle-income countries: an estimation and analysis at the global, regional, and country level. Lancet Glob Health. 2016;4(12):e916-e22.
2. Grantham-McGregor S, Cheung YB, Cueto S, Glewwe P, Richter L, Strupp B, et al. Developmental potential in the first 5 years for children in developing countries. Lancet. 2007;369(9555):60–70.
3. Ballot DE, Potterton J, Chirwa T, Hilburn N, Cooper PA. Developmental Outcome of very low birth weight infants in a developing country. BMC Pediatr. 2012;12(11)
4. Yousafzai AK, Lynch P, Gladstone M. Moving beyond prevalence studies: screening and interventions for children with disabilities in low-income and middle-income countries. Arch Dis Child. 2014;
5. Engle PL, Fernald LCH, Alderman H, Behrman J, O'Gara C, Yousafzai A, et al. Strategies for reducing inequalities and improving developmental outcomes for young children in low-income and middle-income countries. Lancet. 2011;378(9799):1339–53.
6. Hill JL, Brooks-Gunn J, Waldfogel J. Sustained effects of high participation in an early intervention for low-birth-weight premature infants. Dev Psychol. 2003;39(4):730.
7. United Nations. The Millenium development goals report. New York: United Nations; 2015.
8. Farmer P, Nutt C, Wagner CM, Sekabaraga C, Nuthulanganti T, Weigel JL, et al. Reduced premature mortality in Rwanda: lessons from success. BMJ. 2013;346
9. National Institute of Statistics. Rwanda demographic and health survey 2014–15 final report. Kigali, Rwanda: Republic of Rwanda; 2016.
10. Hansen A, Magge H, Labrecque M, Munyaneza RBM, Nahimana E, Nyishime M, et al. The development and implementation of a newborn medicine program in a resource-limited setting. Public Health Action. 2015;5(1):17–22.
11. Walker SP, Wachs TD, Grantham-McGregor S, Black MM, Nelson CA, Huffman SL, et al. Inequality in early childhood: risk and protective factors for early child development. Lancet. 2011;378(9799):1325–38.
12. Mackay CA, Ballot DE, Cooper PA. Growth of a cohort of very low birth weight infants in Johannesburg, South Africa. BMC Pediatr. 2011;11(50)
13. Marchant T, Willey B, Katz J, Clarke S, Kariuki S, Kuile F, et al. Neonatal mortality risk associated with preterm birth in East Africa, adjusted by weight for gestational age: individual participant level meta-analysis. PLoS Med. 2012;9(8):e1001292.
14. American Academy of Pediatrics. Committee on children with disabilities. Developmental surveillance and screening of infants and young children. Pediatrics. 2001;101:192–5.
15. Frankenburg WK. Developmental surveillance and screening of infants and young children. Pediatrics. 2002;109(1):144–5.
16. Bright Futures Steering Committee, Medical Home Initiatives for Children With Special Needs Project Advisory Committee. Identifying infants and young children with developmental disorders in the medical home: an algorithm for developmental surveillance and screening. Pediatrics. 2006; 118(1):405–20.
17. Wallander JL, Bann CM, Biasini FJ, Goudar SS, Pasha O, Chomba E, et al. Development of children at risk for adverse outcomes participating in early intervention in developing countries: a randomized controlled trial. Journal of child psychology and psychiatry, and allied disciplines. 2014;55(11):1251–9.
18. Ngabireyimana E, Mutaganzwa C, Kirk CM, Miller AC, Wilson K, Dushimimana E, Bigirumwami O, Mukakabano ES, Nkikabahizi F, Magge H. A retrospective review of the pediatric development clinic implementation: a model to improve medical, nutritional and developmental outcomes of at-risk under-five children in rural Rwanda. Matern Health Neonatol Perinatol. 2017;3(13)
19. Fox MP, Rosen S. Systematic review of retention of pediatric patients on HIV treatment in low and middle-income countries 2008–2013. AIDS. 2015;29(4):493–502.
20. Chomba E, Carlo WA, McClure EM, Basini F, Wright LL, Mpabalwani E, et al. Feasibility of implementing an early intervention program in an urban low-income setting to improve neurodevelopmental outcome in survivors following birth asphyxia. Field Actions Science Reports. 2011;5
21. National Institute of Statistics. Fourth population and housing census, Rwanda, 2012: final results main indicators report. Kigali, Rwanda: Government of Rwanda; 2012.

22. Squires J, Twombly E, Bricker D, Potter L. ASQ-3 User's Guide. Baltimore: Paul H. Brookes Publishing Company; 2009.
23. UNICEF, World Health Organization. Care for child development: improving the care of young children. In. Geneva: World Health Organization; 2012.
24. Ministry of Finance and Economic Planning. Poverty reduction strategy paper. Kigali, Rwanda: Government of Rwanda; 2002.
25. Ekouevu KD, Azondekom A, Dicko F, Malateste K, Touré P, Eboua F, et al. 12-month mortality and loss-to-program in antiretroviral-treated children: the leDEA pediatric west African database to evaluate AIDS (pWADA), 2000-2008. BMC Public Health 2011;11(1):1.
26. Carlo WA, Goudar SS, Omrana P, Chomba E, McClure EM, Biasini FJ, et al. Neurodevelopmental outcomes in infants requiring resuscitation in developing countries. J Pediatr. 2012;160(5):781.
27. National Institute of Statistics. Rwanda poverty profile report: integrated household living conditions survey 2013/2014. Kigali, Rwanda: Government of Rwanda; 2015.
28. Rich ML, Miller AC, Niyigena P, Franke MF, Niyonzima JB, Socci A, et al. Excellent clinical outcomes and high retention in care among adults in a community-based HIV treatment program in rural Rwanda. J Acquir Immune Defic Syndr. 2012;59:e35-e42.
29. Radcliffe J, Schwarz D, Zhao H. The MOM program: home visiting in partnership with pediatric care. Pediatrics. 2013;132(Supp 2):S153–S9.
30. Tilahun D, Hanlon C, Fekadu A, Tekola B, Baheretibeb Y, Hoekstra RA. Stigma, Explanatory models and unmet needs of caregivers of children with developmental disorders in a low-income African country: a cross-sectional facility- based survey. BMC Health Serv Res. 2016;16(152)
31. Masulani-Mwale C, Mathanga D, Silungwe D, Kauye F, Gladstone M. Parenting children with intellectual disabilities in Malawi: the impact that reaches beyond coping. Child Care Health Dev. 2016;42(6):871–80.
32. Levin J, Gurau D, Levin D: One simple intervention begets another: Let's get the gestational age right first. Matern Child Health J 2016, 20:1767–1768.
33. National Institute of Statistics. Comprehensive food security and vulnerability analysis (CFSVA) and nutrition survey 2012. In. Kigali, Rwanda: Republic of Rwanda and UN world food. Program. 2013;

4

Comparison of accelerometer measured levels of physical activity and sedentary time between obese and non-obese children and adolescents

Rabha Elmesmari[1,4], Anne Martin[2], John J. Reilly[3] and James Y. Paton[1,5*]

Abstract

Background: Obesity has been hypothesized to be associated with reduced moderate-to-vigorous physical activity (MVPA) and increased sedentary time (ST). It is important to assess whether, and the extent to which, levels of MVPA and ST are suboptimal among children and adolescents with obesity. The primary objective of this study was to examine accelerometer-measured time spent in MVPA and ST of children and adolescents with obesity, compared with MVPA recommendations, and with non-obese peers.

Methods: An extensive search was carried out in Medline, Cochrane library, EMBASE, SPORTDiscus, and CINAHL, from 2000 to 2015. Study selection and appraisal: studies with accelerometer-measured MVPA and/or ST (at least 3 days and 6 h/day) in free-living obese children and adolescents (0 to 19 years) were included. Study quality was assessed formally. Meta-analyses were planned for all outcomes but were precluded due to the high levels of heterogeneity across studies. Therefore, narrative syntheses were employed for all the outcomes.

Results: Out of 1503 records, 26 studies were eligible ($n = 14{,}739$ participants; $n = 3523$ with obesity); 6/26 studies involved children aged 0 to 9 years and 18/26 involved adolescents aged 10.1 to19 years. In the participants with obesity, the time spent in MVPA was consistently below the recommended 60 min/day and ST was generally high regardless of the participant's age and gender. Comparison with controls suggested that the time spent in MVPA was significantly lower in children and adolescents with obesity, though differences were relatively small. Levels of MVPA in the obese and non-obese were consistently below recommendations. There were no marked differences in ST between obese and non-obese peers.

Conclusions: MVPA in children and adolescents with obesity tends to be well below international recommendations. Substantial effort is likely to be required to achieve the recommended levels of MVPA among obese individuals in obesity treatment interventions.
This systematic review has been registered on PROSPERO (International Database of Prospective Register Systematic Reviews; registration number CRD42015026882).

* Correspondence: James.Paton@glasgow.ac.uk
[1]School of Medicine, College of Medical, Veterinary, and Life Sciences, University of Glasgow, Glasgow G12 8 QQ, UK
[5]Office Block, Ground Floor, Zone 1 (Paediatrics) Royal Hospital for Children, 1345 Govan Road, Glasgow G51 4TF, UK
Full list of author information is available at the end of the article

Background

The prevalence of obesity among children and adolescents is now very high in both developing and developed countries [1, 2] and is a significant public health and clinical concern [3] that is attracting much research attention [4]. Obesity is known to have a significant impact on both physical and psychological health and children and adolescents with obesity face a number of health, social, and psychological problems [2, 5, 6]. Prevention of childhood obesity is a public health priority while treatment is becoming an increasingly important clinical issue.

A number of health behaviors have been associated with risk of obesity [7]. Poor diet, lack of physical activity (PA) and increased sedentary time (ST) have been linked to the development and maintenance of childhood and adolescent obesity [8–11]. Many evidence-based guidelines focusing on the amount of PA, particularly moderate–to-vigorous intensity physical activity (MVPA) required to produce health benefits, have been developed. These guidelines commonly recommend 60 min of MVPA as a daily minimum (7 days a week) for school-age children and adolescents [12–15].

Accelerometry currently represents the most accurate, inexpensive, and reliable method for objectively measuring both the amount and intensity of PA and amount of sedentary behavior (SB) [16, 17]. There have been many surveys and studies on the levels and adequacy of MVPA in healthy-weight children and adolescents [18, 19]. Since MVPA and ST are also important to health in those with obesity, and since obesity has been hypothesized to be associated with reduced MVPA [20] these variables need to be reviewed for children and adolescents with obesity. Whether and to what extent obesity in childhood and adolescence is associated with reduced objectively measured MVPA and ST/SB remains unclear, in part because of the lack of a synthesis of the evidence on this topic. Many studies have addressed the topic using subjective measurement methods, and/or considering the overweight as obese, and/or focusing on total volume of physical activity rather than MVPA. It is important to assess objectively measured time spent in MVPA and ST in children and adolescents with obesity. The primary aim of the present systematic review was therefore to determine obese children's and adolescents' habitual amount of time spent in MVPA, and examine whether those living with obesity met the current MVPA recommendation for health of a minimum of 60 min per day [14, 21]. Secondary aims were to examine time spent in accelerometer-measured SB by children and adolescents with obesity, and to determine whether MVPA and ST in obese children and adolescents were different from the non-obese peers.

Methods

Registration of systematic reviews

This systematic literature review was performed in accordance with the Preferred Reporting Items for Systematic Reviews (PRISMA) guidelines [22]. The review protocol was registered on PROSPERO (registration number CRD42015026882), the international prospective register for systematic reviews (http://www.crd.york.ac.uk/ NIHR_PROSPERO).

Literature search

The literature search was conducted searching for English language peer-reviewed studies using the five most relevant electronic databases from 2000 up to March 2015 (accelerometry became more widely used in research from the early 2000's): MEDLINE OVID; Cochrane library; EMBASE; SPORTSDiscus and CINAHL by AM. The literature search in the Cochrane Central Register of Controlled Trials is shown in Table 1, and was adapted as required for the other databases. Full literature search details are available from the corresponding author on request. The electronic search was complemented by reference citation tracking (forward and backward) of the included studies and of previous reviews.

Inclusion criteria

To be eligible for inclusion in the review, papers had to meet all of the following criteria as per the PICOS principles: Population: children and adolescents aged from 0 to 19 years as defined by the WHO; Intervention or exposure: children or adolescent classified as obese. Obesity had to be defined using an acceptable objective method, e.g. defined as having a body mass index (BMI) ≥ 95th percentile for children of the same sex and age, or defined as the equivalent of 30 kg/m^2 International Obesity Task Force (IOTF definition), or defined as obese relative to World Health Organization (WHO) BMI for age and sex charts; Comparison: habitual amount of time spent in MVPA and/or ST of non-obese children and adolescents; Outcomes: habitual amount of time spent in MVPA and/or ST measured by accelerometer and reported in the form of minutes/day of MVPA or ST; MVPA and its relationship to the 60 min/day recommended. All study designs were considered eligible: cross-sectional, longitudinal, case-control studies and intervention studies were eligible if pre-intervention data could be extracted.

Exclusion criteria

We excluded studies that included only overweight participants, combined overweight and obese groups, or included participants with any known barrier or limitation to physical activity (e.g. physical disability). Studies that

Table 1 Search strategy of Cochrane Central Register of Controlled Trials

. #1 MeSH descriptor: [Child] explode all trees
. #2 MeSH descriptor: [Adolescent] explode all trees
. #3 child* or adolesc* or teen* or boy* or girl* or youth:ti,ab,kw (Word variations have been searched)
. #4 young near/1 (person or people):ti,ab,kw (Word variations have been searched)
. #5 #1or#2or#3or#4
. #6 MeSH descriptor: [Motor Activity] this term only
. #7 MeSH descriptor: [Exercise] explode all trees
. #8 MeSH descriptor: [Sports] explode all trees
. #9 MeSH descriptor: [Sedentary Lifestyle] explode all trees
. #10 physical* activ*:ti,ab,kw (Word variations have been searched)
. #11 exercis* or sport*:ti,ab,kw (Word variations have been searched)
. #12 active near/2 (living or lifestyle):ti,ab,kw (Word variations have been searched)
. #13 sedentary behavi?r:ti,ab,kw (Word variations have been searched)
. #14 (screen or sedentary or sitting or TV or television or computer or PC or video games) near/2 time:ti,ab,kw (Word variations have been searched)
. #15 #6or#7or#8or#9or#10or#11or#12or#13or#14
. #16 MeSH descriptor: [Accelerometry] explode all trees
. #17 acceleromet*:ti,ab,kw (Word variations have been searched)
. #18 actigraph*:ti,ab,kw (Word variations have been searched)
. #19 activity near/1 monitor*.:ti,ab,kw (Word variations have been searched)
. #20 #16or#17or#18or#19
. #21 MeSH descriptor: [Overweight] explode all trees
. #22 overweight or obes*:ti,ab,kw (Word variations have been searched)
. #23 #21or#22
. #24 #5 and #15 and #20 and #23

used subjective methods, objective (e.g. doubly labelled water) or direct observation methods apart from accelerometer measurements were excluded.

Since the aim of the review was to examine habitual levels of MVPA and ST, studies that measured these variables for less than 6 h per day or over 2 days or less were excluded. Recommendations currently exist for habitual (overall) MVPA rather than MVPA during specific domains (e.g. the after school period) and so studies that focused only on specific periods of the day (e.g. school activity only, or outdoor activity only, or weekend activity only, or weekday activity only, or after-school only) were also excluded. A detailed description of the eligibility criteria is given in [Additional file 1].

Study selection

Titles, abstracts, and full-text articles were screened in duplicate for eligibility by RE and JYP and disagreements were resolved through discussions with other reviewers when required. Reference lists of eligible studies were examined for potentially eligible studies, and studies that cited eligible studies were identified and tested for eligibility. The reviewers were not blinded to authors or journal of publication. Reasons for exclusion are summarised in the study flow diagram (Fig. 1) and available in details from the corresponding author on request.

Data extraction

A standardised data extraction form was used to populate the evidence tables by RE and repeated by JJR and JYP. The extracted items were: first author, publication year, country, study design, sample group, comparison group-if applicable, accelerometer type, cut points for MVPA and ST, finding of MVPA (minutes/day) and ST (minutes/day or %) data, summary and author conclusions. International recommendations are usually for the achievement of at least 60 min of MVPA every day, but in the eligible studies the achievement of MVPA recommendations was never operationalised in this way. In most studies that referred to the achievement of MVPA recommendations, the mean or median daily MVPA (minutes/day) was provided, and so this was used as a proxy for achievement of recommendations in the present study.

Data analysis and synthesis

We considered the data for meta-analysis but identified a substantial level of statistical heterogeneity between the studies (I^2 statistic > 70%) that led to the decision not to present the combined results of individual studies. Hence, we performed a narrative synthesis of the data and present the findings in tabular, textual and graphical form. Data were synthesised by the age and sex of the subgroups as those are factors known to be strongly associated with both the exposure variable, obesity, and the outcomes, MVPA and ST, and so might explain some of the observed findings. The age subgroup was categorised according to the WHO definition of children and adolescence, i.e. as children aged 0 to 9.9 years old and adolescents aged 10.1 to 19 years old. Data for boys, girls and mixed-sex studies are reported separately where possible.

Quality assessment

Eligible articles were assessed for methodological quality using a 15-item quality assessment scale as shown in [Additional file 2], collapsed to 6 items for scoring, with higher scores suggesting higher study quality. Each eligible study was assessed by RE, and disagreements were resolved by discussion with JJR and JYP. The quality assessment scale was modified from the methodological quality assessment scale of Tooth et al. [23]. This is a

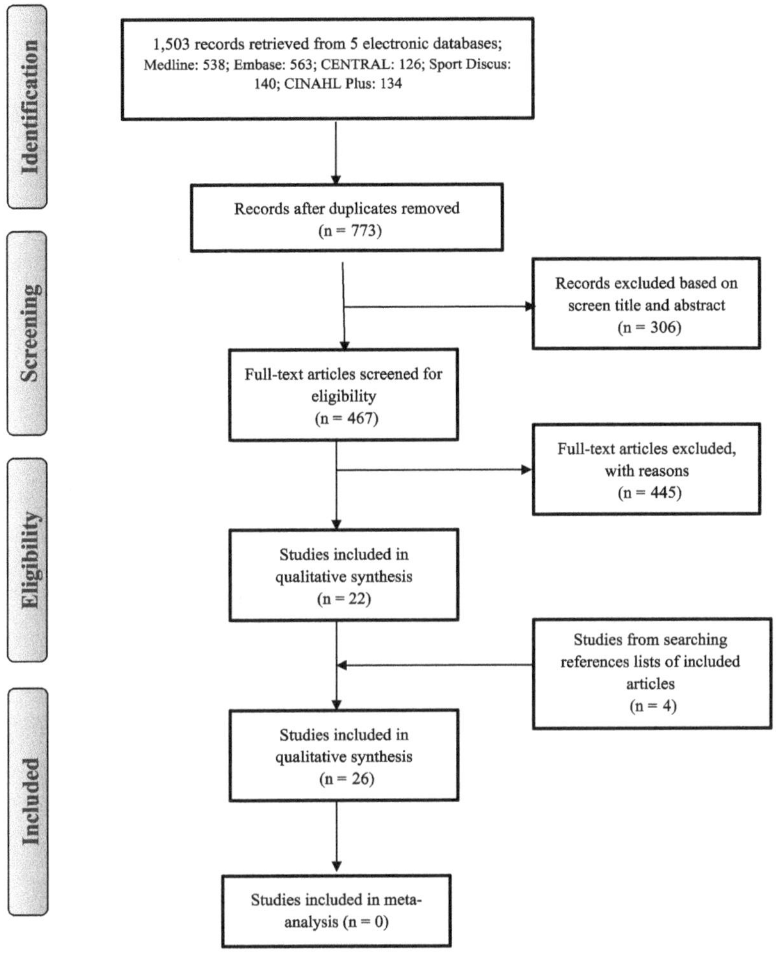

Fig. 1 The PRISMA flow diagram with numbers of included and excluded articles at each step of the review process

reliable and valid tool for assessing the quality of observational studies. It was considered initially for use in its original form, which consists of over 30 items. The modifications to the original scale were made to focus quality assessment on issues of particular importance to accelerometry measurement of physical activity. The modified Tooth et al. tool has been used in several recent systemic reviews of physical activity, all of which have reduced the number of items in the quality assessment to 8 to 17 items, which make up the quality score [24–28].

Results

Search results

The PRISMA flow diagram with the numbers of included and excluded articles at each step of the review process is provided in Fig 1. Tables 2 and 3 provide a brief summary of all studies included in this systematic review. Of 1503 papers identified in the initial review of the five databases, 467 were selected for full-text screening and of these, 22 met the inclusion criteria. A further four eligible studies were identified from searching reference of included studies and of previous reviews, giving a total of 26 studies which met the inclusion criteria.

Studies characteristics

Of the 26 included studies: six studies involved children, 18 studies involved adolescents and two studies involved both children and adolescents. Further, 22/26 compared MVPA data in those with obesity with a non-obese peers, while 13/26 studies also provided data on accelerometer measured ST; 10/13 studies compared ST data in those with obesity with non-obese peers.

Measurement protocol

The ActiGraph was the most common accelerometer type used to measure habitual MVPA and/or ST, used in 20/26 studies, though with a variety of different ActiGraph models and approaches to data collection and reduction. Of the remaining six studies: three used the Actical accelerometer [29–31]; two the Triaxial Research

Table 2 Overview of relevant characteristics and results of the included studies that involved child participants

Reference[a]	Place &time	Study design	Sample group	Comparison group	Measurement	Accelerometer cut off points	Findings	Meet 60 min/day of MVPA (%) and Author Conclusions
Chung et al. [36]	United States, 2012	Data of NHANES 2003–04 and 2005–06) surveys	n: 95 (47 boys, 48 girls) obese participants with BMI ≥95th to 99th centile	n: 514 (253 boys, 261 girls) participants with BMI ≥ 5th to 85th centile	Actigraph 7164 worn on the right hip for 7 consecutive days during waking hours	Epoch = 1 min	Obese group spent mean of (boys 118 (SD 6) and girls 83 (SD 10) min/day) on MVPA	97, 70% of obese boys and girls respectively achieved an average of 60 min/day of MVPA
			Age: range 6–8 years	Age: range 6–8 years		MVPA using Freedson cut-point (61)	Comparison group spent mean of (boys 129 (SD 4) and girls 104 (SD 4) min/day) on MVPA	98, 90% of the comparison boys and girls respectively achieved an average of 60 min/day MVPA. MVPA was significantly lower in obese than comparison group ($p < 0.05$)
Hughes et al. [39]	United Kingdom, 2006	Pairwise comparison study.	n: 53 (25 boys, 28 girls) obese participants with BMI ≥ 98th centile	n: 53 (25boys, 28 girls) participants with BMI < 85th centile.	CSA/MTI, 7164 worn on right hip for 7 consecutive days.	Epoch = 1 min	Obese group spent median of 16 (range 2–72) min/day on MVPA.	Obese participants failed t o achieve an average of 60 min/day of MVPA
			"Clinical sample"	Age: mean 8.7 (SD 2.1) years		MVPA > 3200 cpm	Comparison group spent median of 23 (range 7–77) min/day on MVPA.	MVPA was significantly lower in obese than comparison group ($p < 0.001$)
			Age: mean 8.6 (SD 2) years			Sedentary time < 1100 cpm	Obese group spent mean of 81 (SD 7) % of their waking time sedentary.	Sedentary time was similar in obese and comparison group
							Comparison group spent mean of 79 (SD 6) % of their waking time sedentary.	
Hussey et al. [32]	Dublin, 2007	Cross sectional study	n: 7/152 (3 boys, 4 girls) obese participants; with BMI > 97th centile.	n: 121/152 (43 boys, 78 girls) participants with BMI > 75th to 91th centile.	RT3Triaxial accelerometer, worn for 4 days.	Epoch = 1 min	Obese participants spent mean of (boys 14 (95%, CI- 11, 17) and girls 29 (95%, CI- 14, 43) min/day) on MVPA	Obese participants failed to achieve an average of 60 min/day of MVPA
			Age: range 7 to 10 years.	Age: range 7 to 10 years.		MVPA> 3500 cpm	Comparison group spent mean of (boys 39 (95%, CI-33, 45) and girls 24	MVPA was significantly lower in obese boys than comparison group ($p < 0.05$)

Table 2 Overview of relevant characteristics and results of the included studies that involved child participants *(Continued)*

Reference[a]	Place &time	Study design	Sample group	Comparison group	Measurement	Accelerometer cut off points	Findings	Meet 60 min/day of MVPA (%) and Author Conclusions
							(95%, CI- 22, 27) min/day) on MVPA	
						Sedentary time cut-points not clearly reported	Obese participants spent mean of (boys 1046 (95%, CI- 934, 1157) and girls 935 (95%, CI- 795, 1075) min/day) sedentary	Sedentary time was significantly higher in obese boys than comparison group ($p < 0.05$)
							Comparison group spent mean of (boys 928 (95%, CI-901, 955) and girls 963 (95%, CI- 941,985) min/day) sedentary	
Maggio et al. [64]	Switzerland, 2010	Cross-sectional study	n: 45/209 obese participants with BMI > 97th centile	n: 85 participants with BMI <90th centile	Actigraph 6471, worn on right hip for 7 consecutive days	Epoch not clearly reported	Obese group spent mean of 60 (SD 3) min/day on MVPA	52% of the obese participants achieved an average of 60 min/day of MVPA
			"Clinical sample"			MVPA > 2000 cpm	Comparison group spent mean of 71 (SD 5) min/day on MVPA	60% of the comparison group achieved an average of 60 min/day MVPA
			Age: mean 9.1 (SD 0.3) years	Age: mean 10 (SD 0.3) years		Sedentary time < 500 cpm	Obese participants spent mean of 71% of their waking time sedentary	MVPA was lower in obese than comparison group but not significantly ($p = 0.07$)
							Comparison group spent mean of 70% of their waking time sedentary	Sedentary time was significantly higher in obese than comparison group ($p < 0.01$)
Metallinos-Katsaras et al. [38]	United States, 2007	Cross sectional study	n: 21 obese children with BMI ≥ 95th centile	n: 35 children; BMI < 95th centile	CSA 7164, worn on the hip for 7 consecutive days	Epoch = 1 min	Obese group spent mean of 269 (SD not given) min/day on MVPA	Obese participants exceeded an average of 60 min/day of MVPA
			Age: range 2 to 5 years	Age: range 2 to 5 years		MVPA cut-points not clearly reported	Comparison group spent mean of 277 (SD not given) min/day on MVPA	MVPA was lower in obese than comparison group but this was not significant ($p > 0.05$)
	Canada, 2005		n: 112 (56 boys, 56 girls) obese	n: 341 (177 boys, 164 girls)	Actigraph 7164, worn on the hip	Epoch = 1 min	Obese group spent mean of (boys 172	

Table 2 Overview of relevant characteristics and results of the included studies that involved child participants *(Continued)*

Reference[a]	Place &time	Study design	Sample group	Comparison group	Measurement	Accelerometer cut off points	Findings	Meet 60 min/day of MVPA (%) and Author Conclusions
Thompson et al. [37]		Cross sectional study	participants with BMI ≥ 95th centile	participants with BMI ≤ 85th centile	for 7 consecutive days		(SD 58) and girls 157 (SD 52) min/day) on MVPA	Obese participants exceeded an average of 60 min/day of MVPA
			Age: mean 8 (SD 0.3) years	Age: 3, 7 and 11 years old		MVPA used Freedson cut-point (61)	Comparison group spent mean of (boys 179 (SD 63) and girls 165 (SD 51) min/day) on MVPA	Comparison group exceeded an average of 60 min/day of MVPA MVPA was similar in obese and comparison group
Vale et al. [41]	Portugal, 2013	Cross sectional study	n: 59/607 obese children with BMI defined according to the IOTF criteria	n: 425/607 children with BMI defined as non-overweight, non-obese according to the IOTF criteria	ActiGraph GT1M, worn on the hip for 7 consecutive days	Epoch = 5 s	Absolute MVPA not clearly given	MVPA was significantly lower in obese girls than comparison group ($p < 0.01$), but not in boys
			Age: mean 5.1 (SD 0.8) years	Age: range 4–6 years		MVPA ≥1680 cpm		
Wafa et al. [35].	Malaysia, 2014	Case control study.	n: 86 obese participants with BMI ≥ 95th centile	n: 86 participants with BMI < 85th centile matched for age and gender	ActiGraph GT1M, worn for 5 consecutive days	Epoch not reported	Obese group spent median 5 (IQR – 0, 32) min/day on MVPA	Obese participants failed to achieve an average of 60 min/day of MVPA
			Age: median 9.5 (IQR 8,11) years			MVA > 3200 cpm	Comparison group spent of median 9 (IQR – 0, 55) min/day on MVPA	Comparison group failed to achieve an average of 60 min/day of MVPA
						Sedentary time < 1100 cpm	Obese group spent an average of 90% of their waking time sedentary	MVPA was significantly lower in the obese than in the comparison group ($p < 0.001$)
							Comparison group spent an average of 88% of their waking time sedentary	Sedentary time was significantly higher in the obese group than in the comparison group ($p < 0.001$)

BMI: body mass index; *cpm*: counts per minutes; *IOTF*: International Obesity Task Force criteria; *MVPA*: moderate- vigorous physical activity; *n*: Number; *S*: Second, Data are expressed as mean, (*SD*) unless otherwise. Freedson *MVPA* cutpoint (61) using the following equation: *METS* = 2.757 + (0.0015 x counts/min) – (0.08957 x age (yr)) – (0.000038 x counts/min x age (yr)).[a] Studies are listed in alphabetic order

Table 3 Overview of relevant characteristics and results of the included studies that involved adolescent participants

Reference[a]	Place & time	Study design	Sample group	Comparison group	Measurement	Accelerometer cut off points	Findings	Meet 60 min/day of MVPA (%) and Author Conclusions
Butte et al. [34]	United States, 2007	Cross sectional study	n: 473 (247 boys, 226 girls) obese participants with BMI ≥ 95th centile	n: 424 (194 boys, 230 girls) participants with BMI <95th centile	Actiwatch, worn on the right hip for 24 h for 3 consecutive days	Epoch = 1 min	Obese spent mean of (boys 88 (SD 50) and girls 74 (SD 46) min/day) on MVPA	62% of all participants (obese and comparison group) achieved an average of 60 min/day of MVPA
			Age: mean 10.8 (SD 3.8) years	Age: mean 10.8 (SD 3.8) years		MVPA and sedentary time cut-points not clearly reported.	Comparison group spent mean of (boys 96 (SD 57) and girls 79 (SD 57) min/day) on MVPA	MVPA was lower in obese than comparison group but not significant
							Obese group spent mean of (boys 357 (SD 118) and girls 345 (SD 122) min/day) sedentary	Sedentary time was significantly higher in obese than comparison group ($P = 0.001$)
							Comparison group spent mean of (boys 305 (SD 121) and girls 308 (SD 131) min/day) sedentary	
Chung et al. [36]	United States, 2012	Data of NHANES 2003–04 and 2005–06) surveys	n: 185 (92 boys, 93 girls) obese participants with BMI ≥95th to 99th centile	n: 987 (489 boys, 498 girls) participants with BMI ≥ 5th to 85th centile	Actigraph 7164 worn on the right hip for 7 consecutive days during waking hours	Epoch = 1 min	Obese group spent mean of (boys 34 (SD 4) and girls 16 (SD 4) min/day) on MVPA	Obese participants failed to achieve an average of 60 min/day of MVPA
			Age: range 12 to 17 years	Age: range 12 to 17 years		MVPA used Freedson cut-point (61)	Comparison group spent mean of (boys 40 (SD 3) and girls 22 (SD 2) min/day) on MVPA	MVPA was significantly lower in obese than comparison group ($p < 0.05$)
Decelis et al. [47]	Malta, 2012	Cross sectional study	n: 34/187 (19 boys, 15 girls) obese participants with BMI defined according to the IOTF criteria	n: 106/187 (53 boys, 53 girls) participants with BMI defined as non-overweight and non-obese according to the IOTF criteria	Actigraph GT3X, worn on right hip for 5 days during waking hours	Epoch not defined	Obese group spent mean of (boys 30 (SD 13) and girls 19 (SD 8) min/day) on MVPA	Obese participants failed to achieve an average of 60 min/day of MVPA

Table 3 Overview of relevant characteristics and results of the included studies that involved adolescent participants *(Continued)*

Reference[a]	Place & time	Study design	Sample group	Comparison group	Measurement	Accelerometer cut off points	Findings	Meet 60 min/day of MVPA (%) and Author Conclusions
			Age: range 11 to 12 years	Age: range 11 to 12 years		MVPA ≥2912 cpm	Comparison group spent mean of (boys 44 (SD 16) and girls 26 (SD 9) min/day) on MVPA	11% of the comparison group achieved an average of 60 min/day MVPA
						Sedentary time ≤ 727 cpm	Obese group spent mean of (boys 638 (SD 95) and girls 619 (SD 106) min/day) sedentary	MVPA was significantly lower in obese than comparison group ($p < 0.05$)
							Comparison group spent mean of (boys 654 (SD 93) and girls 664 (SD 93) min/day) sedentary	Sedentary time was higher in obese than comparison group, but not significant
Decelis et al. [48]	Malta, 2014	Cross sectional study	n: 113/810 (59 boys, 54 girls) obese participants with BMI defined according to the IOTF criteria	n: 534/810 (254 boys, 280 girls) participants with BMI defined as non-overweight and non-obese according to the IOTF criteria	Actigraph GT3X, worn on right hip for 5 days during waking hours	Epoch = 10 s	Obese group spent mean of (boys 49 (SD 19) and girls 38 (SD 12) min/day) on MVPA	Obese participants failed to achieve an average of 60 min/day of MVPA
			Age: range 10 to 11 years	Age: range 10 to 11 years		MVPA > 2296 cpm	Comparison group spent mean of (boys 61 (SD 22) and girls 44 (SD 15) min/day) on MVPA	MVPA was significantly lower in obese than comparison group ($p < 0.05$)
						Sedentary time < 100 cpm	Obese group spent mean of (boys 553 (SD 94) and girls 610 (SD 125) min/day) sedentary	Sedentary time was higher in obese than comparison group, but not significant
							Comparison group spent mean of	

Table 3 Overview of relevant characteristics and results of the included studies that involved adolescent participants *(Continued)*

Reference[a]	Place & time	Study design	Sample group	Comparison group	Measurement	Accelerometer cut off points	Findings	Meet 60 min/day of MVPA (%) and Author Conclusions
							(boys 582 (SD 113) and girls 603 (SD 97) min/day) sedentary	
Ekelund et al. [45]	Sweden, 2002	Case control, cross sectional design study.	n: 18 (8 boys, 10 girls) obese participants with BMI defined according to the IOTF criteria	n: 18 (8 boys, 10 girls) participants with BMI defined as non-overweight and non-obese according to the IOTF criteria	CSA 7164, worn on lower part of the back (L 4–5) for 14 days	Epoch = 15 s	Obese group spent mean of (boys 58 (SD 30) and girls 60 (SD 28) min/day) on MVPA	MVPA was significantly lower in obese than comparison group ($p < 0.05$)
			Age: mean (boys 18.1 (SD 1.1), girls 17.3 (SD 1.9) years	Age: mean (boys 18.2 (SD 1.1), girls 17.3 (SD 1.9) years		MVPA cut-points not clearly reported	Comparison group spent mean of (boys 82 (SD 36) and girls 98 (SD 58) min/day) on MVPA	MVPA was similar in obese girls and boys ($p < 0.05$)
						Sedentary time < 100 cpm	Obese group spent mean of (boys 421 (SD 33) and girls 465 (SD 132) min/day) sedentary	Sedentary time was similar in obese and comparison group
							Comparison group spent mean of (boys 414 (SD 81) and girls 397 (SD 69) min/day) sedentary	
Gyllenham-mer et al. [65]	United States, 2013	Cross sectional study	n: 37 obese girls with BMI ≥ 95th centile	No comparison group	Actigraph GT1M, worn on the right hip for 7 consecutive days	Epoch = 1 min	Obese girls spent mean of 28 (SD 18) min/day on MVPA	Obese girls failed to achieve an average of 60 min/day of MVPA
			Age: mean 15.5 (SD 1.1) years			MVPA cut-points not clearly reported Sedentary time = 100 cpm	Obese participants spent 63% (SD 7) of their waking time sedentary	MVPA was lower in obese girls compared to published data from healthy adolescents

Table 3 Overview of relevant characteristics and results of the included studies that involved adolescent participants *(Continued)*

Reference[a]	Place & time	Study design	Sample group	Comparison group	Measurement	Accelerometer cut off points	Findings	Meet 60 min/day of MVPA (%) and Author Conclusions
Kitzman-Ulrich et al. [31]	United States, 2010	Randomized trial ACT (Active by Choice Today) data at baseline used here	n: 242/669 (98 boys, 144 girls) obese participants with BMI > 95th centile	n: 314/ 669 (138 boys, 176 girls) participants with BMI < 85th centile	Actical, worn on the right hip for 7 days all the day	Epoch = 1 min	Obese participants spent mean of (boys 46 (SD 20) and girls 36 (SD 15) min/day) on MVPA	Obese participants failed to achieve an average of 60 min/day of MVPA
			Age: mean 11.4 (SD 0.7) years	Age: mean 11.4 (SD 0.7) years		MVPA and sedentary time cut-points not clearly reported	Comparison group spent mean of (boys 65 (SD 27) and girls 46 (SD 20) min/day) on MVPA	MVPA level was significantly lower in obese than comparison group ($p < 0.05$)
Maggio et al. [64]	Switzerland, 2014	Case control study	n: 24 (12 boys, 12 girls) obese participants with BMI ≥ 97th centile. "Clinical sample"	n: 25 (12 boys, 13 girls) participants with BMI <90th centile	Actigraph GT1M, worn for at least 4 days	Epoch and MVPA cut-points not clearly reported	Obese participants spent mean of 43 (SD 19) min/day on MVPA	Obese participants failed to achieve an average of 60 min/day of MVPA
			Age: mean 13.9 (SD 1.2) years	Age: mean 13.2 (SD 1.7) years		Sedentary time < 500 cpm	Comparison group spent mean of 58 (SD 30) min/day on MVPA	MVPA was similar in obese girls and boys ($p < 0.05$)
								MVPA was significantly lower in obese than comparison group ($P = 0.01$)
Martins et al. [66]	Portugal, 2015	Cross sectional baseline study	n: 131 (48 boys, 83 girls) obese participants with BMI defined according to the IOTF criteria	No comparison group	Actigraph GT3x, worn for 7 consecutive days.	Epoch = 1 mim	Obese participants spent mean of (boys 65 (SD 28) and girls 51 (SD 22) min/day) on MVPA	Obese participants failed to achieve an average of 60 min/day of MVPA
			Age: mean 10.3 (SD 3.6) years			MVPA cut-points not clearly reported	Participants spent mean of (boys 575 (SD 108) and girls 562, (SD 82) min/day) sedentary	MVPA was significantly lower in obese girls than obese boys ($p < 0.05$)
						Sedentary time = 0–100 cpm		MVPA was lower in obese participants compared to published

Table 3 Overview of relevant characteristics and results of the included studies that involved adolescent participants *(Continued)*

Reference[a]	Place & time	Study design	Sample group	Comparison group	Measurement	Accelerometer cut off points	Findings	Meet 60 min/day of MVPA (%) and Author Conclusions
								data from healthy children and adolescents
McMurray et al. [67]	United States, 2008	Baseline data of Randomized controlled TAAG "Trial of Activity for Adolescent Girls"	n: 184/1021 obese girls with BMI ≥ 95th centile.	n: 645/1021 participants with BMI < 85th centile	Actigraph MTI, worn for 6 consecutive days	Epoch = 30 s	Obese girls spent mean of 21 (SD 2) min/day on MVPA	Obese participants failed to achieve an average of 60 min/day of MVPA
			Age: range 11 to 14 years	Age: range 11 to 14 years		MVPA cut-points not clearly reported.	Comparison group spent mean of 25 (SD 1) min/day on MVPA	MVPA was significantly lower in the obese than the comparison group (p = 0.01)
Page et al. [43]	United Kingdom, 2005	Cross sectional study	n: 25 (14 boys, 11 girls) obese participants with BMI ≥ 99th centile. "Clinical and non clinical sample"	n: 108 (54 boys, 54 girls) participants with BMI < 99th centile	Actigraph 7164, worn on the waist for 7 consecutive days	Epoch and MVPA cut-points not clearly reported.	Obese participants spent mean of (boys 140 (SD 47) and girls 105 (SD 48) min/day) on MVPA	Obese participants exceeded an average of 60 min/day of MVPA
			Age: mean 10.5 (SD 0.8) years				Comparison group spent mean of (boys 176 (SD 52) and girls 149 (SD 52) min/day) on MVPA.	MVPA was significantly lower in obese compared to comparison group ($p = 0.02$)
Peart et al. [68]	United States, 2011	Combined data of cross sectional NHANES (2003–04, 2005–06) surveys	n: 434/2368 (217 boys, 217 girls) obese participants with BMI ≥ 95 centile	n: 1469/ 2368 (749 boys, 720 girls) participants with BMI < 85th centile	Actigraph 7164, worn on hip over 7 day	Epoch = 1 min	Obese participants spent mean 28 (SD 35) min/day on MVPA	Obese participants failed to achieve an average of 60 min/day of MVPA
			Age: mean 15.4 (SD 2.2) years	Age: mean 15.4 (SD 2.2) years		MVPA≥1 500 cpm	Comparison group spent mean of 32 (SD 29) min/day on MVPA	MVPA was similar in obese boys and girls MVPA was lower in obese than comparison group but not significantly (p > 0.05)

Table 3 Overview of relevant characteristics and results of the included studies that involved adolescent participants *(Continued)*

Reference[a]	Place & time	Study design	Sample group	Comparison group	Measurement	Accelerometer cut off points	Findings	Meet 60 min/day of MVPA (%) and Author Conclusions
Ruiz et al. [46]	10 centers in 9 European countries, 2011	Cross sectional study	n: 104/2200 (45 boys, 59 girls) obese participants with BMI ≥ 95th centile	n: 1592/2200 (870 boys, 722 girls) participants with BMI < 85th centile	Actigraph GT1M, worn lower back for 7 consecutive days	Epoch = 15 s	Obese participants spent mean of (boys 60 (95%, CI- 53, 68) and girls 44 (95%, CI- 38,50) min/day) on MVPA	MVPA was significantly lower in obese boys than comparison boys group ($p = 0.002$)
			Age: median 14.9 (IQR 12.8 to 15.8) years	Age: median 14.9 (IQR 12.8 to 15.8) years		MVPA ≥2000 cpm	Comparison group spent mean of (boys 67, (95%, CI- 65, 69) and girls 51 (95%, CI- 49,52) min/day) on MVPA	Sedentary time was significantly higher in obese girls than comparison girls group ($p = 0.006$)
						Sedentary time < 100	Obese participants spent of (boys 68% and girls 71%) of their waking time sedentary	
							Comparison group spent mean of (boys 69% and girls 72%) of their waking time sedentary	
Shoup et al. [69]	United States, 2008	Cross sectional study	n: 85 obese participants; BMI ≥ 99th centile	n: 92 participants with BMI ≥85th and <95th centile matched for age	Actigraph 7164, worn on waist for 7 consecutive days.	Epoch and MVPA cut-points not clearly reported.	Obese participants spent mean of 54 (SD 22) min/day on MVPA.	40% ($n = 34$) of the obese group achieved an average of 60 min/day on MVPA
			"Clinical sample"				Comparison group spent mean of 59 (SD 30) min/day on MVPA.	40% (n = 35) of the comparison group achieved 60 min/day of MVPA
			Age: mean 10.6 (SD 1.4) years					MVPA was similar in obese and

Table 3 Overview of relevant characteristics and results of the included studies that involved adolescent participants *(Continued)*

Reference[a]	Place & time	Study design	Sample group	Comparison group	Measurement	Accelerometer cut off points	Findings	Meet 60 min/day of MVPA (%) and Author Conclusions
								comparison group
St George et al. [29].	United States, 2013	Baseline data of ACT Randomized trial (Active by Choice Today).	n: 484/1422 (203 boys, 281 girls) obese participants with BMI ≥ 95th centile.	n: 684/1422 (321 boys, 363 girls) participants with BMI < 85th centile.	Actical, worn on the right hip for 7 consecutive days.	Epoch = 1 min	Obese participants spent mean of 37 (SD 22) min/day on MVPA.	Obese participants failed to achieve an average of 60 min/day of MVPA
			Age: mean 11.3 (SD 0.6) years	Age: mean 11.4 (SD 0.6) years		MVPA used Puyau cut-point (66).	Comparison group spent mean of 47 (SD 28) min/day on MVPA.	MVPA was significantly lower in obese than comparison group ($p < 0.01$)
Starkoff et al [30].	United States, 2014	Cross sectional study.	n: 16 (5 boys, 11 girls) obese participants with BMI ≥ 95 centile.	No comparison group	Actical, worn on the right hip for 5 days during waking time	Epoch = 1 min	Obese participants spent mean of (boys 26 (SD 36) and girls 19 (SD 17) min/day) on MVPA	12.5% of the obese group achieved an average of 60 min/day of MVPA
			"Clinical sample" Age: mean 14.8 (SD 1.5) years.			Sedentary time and MVPA cut-points not clearly reported	Obese participants spent mean of (boys 731 (SD 110) and girls 726 (SD 98) min/day) on sedentary	MVPA was lower in obese participants compared to published data from healthy adolescents
Thompson et al. [36].	Canada, 2005	Cross sectional study.	n: 171 (93 boys, 78 girls) participants with BMI ≥ 95th centile.	n: 716 (327 boys, 389 girls) participants with BMI ≤ 85th centile.	Actigraph 7164, worn on the hip for 7 consecutive days.	Epoch = 1 min	Obese group spent mean of (boys 53 (SD 26) and girls 48 (SD 25) min/day) on MVPA.	Obese participants failed to achieve an average of 60 min/day of MVPA
			Age: range 12 to 16 years	Age: range 12 to 16 years		MVPA used Freedson cut-point (61)	Comparison group spent mean of (boys 58 (SD 30) and girls 47 (SD 24) min/day) on MVPA.	Comparison group failed to achieve an average of 60 min/day of MVPA MVPA was similar in obese

Table 3 Overview of relevant characteristics and results of the included studies that involved adolescent participants *(Continued)*

Reference[a]	Place & time	Study design	Sample group	Comparison group	Measurement	Accelerometer cut off points	Findings	Meet 60 min/day of MVPA (%) and Author Conclusions
								and comparison group
Trost et al. [44].	United States, 2001	Cross sectional study.	n: 54 obese participants with BMI ≥ 95th centile.	n: 133 non obese with	CSA 7164, worn on right hip for 7 consecutive days.	Epoch = 1 min	Obese participants spent mean of 70 (SD 6) min/day on MVPA.	Obese participants achieved an average of 60 min/day of MVPA
			Age: mean 11.4 (SD 0.6) years.	BMI < 95th centile.		MVPA used Freedson cut-point (61)	Comparison group spent mean of 82 (SD 4) min/day on MVPA.	Comparison group achieved an average of 60 min/day of MVPA
				Age: mean 11.4 (SD 0.6) years.				MVPA was significantly lower in obese than comparison group ($p < 0.001$)
Vanhelst et al. [33].	France, 2013	Cross sectional study.	n: 56 obese participants with BMI ≥ 97th centile.	No comparison group	RT3 worn on right hip up to 21 consecutive days.	Epoch = 1 min	Participants spent mean of 22 (SD 12) min/day on MVPA.	Obese participants failed to achieve an average of 60 min/day of MVPA
			"Clinical sample"			MVPA cut-points not clearly reported.		MVPA was lower in obese participants compared to published data from healthy children and adolescents
			Age: mean 12.8 (SD 2.9) years.			Sedentary time = 0–40 cpm		
Wang et al. [42]	Chine, 2013	Cross sectional "large-scale study"	n: 175/2163 (115 boys, 60 girls) obese participants with BMI defined according to the IOTF criteria.	n: 1709/2163; 808 boys; 901 girls with BMI defined as non-overweight, non-obese according to the IOTF criteria	ActiGraph GT3X, worn on right hip for 7 consecutive days	Epoch = 1 min	Obese group spent mean of (boys29 (SD 18) and girls 24 (SD 13) min/day) on MVPA	7% of the obese boys achieved an average of 60 min/day of MVPA
			Age: mean 13.41 (SD 2.25) years.	Age: mean 13.41 (SD 2.25) years.		MVPA cut-points not clearly reported	Comparison group spent mean of (boys 35(SD 19) and girls 22 (SD 14)	10%, 2% of the comparison boys and girls respectively

Table 3 Overview of relevant characteristics and results of the included studies that involved adolescent participants *(Continued)*

Reference[a]	Place & time	Study design	Sample group	Comparison group	Measurement	Accelerometer cut off points	Findings	Meet 60 min/day of MVPA (%) and Author Conclusions
							min/day) on MVPA	achieved an average of 60 min/day of MVPA
						Sedentary time < 100 cpm	Obese group spent mean of (boys 480 (SD 107) and girls 490 (SD 89) min/day) sedentary	MVPA was similar in obese and comparison groups
							Comparison group spent mean of (boys 521 (SD 113) and girls 533, (SD 103) min/day) sedentary	Sedentary time was similar in obese and comparison groups

BMI: body mass index; cpm: counts per minutes; *IOTF*: International Obesity Task Force criteria; *MVPA*: moderate- vigorous physical activity; *n*: Number; *S*: Second, Data are expressed as mean, (*SD*) unless otherwise. Freedson *MVPA* cutpoint (61) using the following equation: $METS = 2.757 + (0.0015 \times \text{counts/min}) - (0.08957 \times \text{age (yr)}) - (0.000038 \times \text{counts/min} \times \text{age (yr)})$. [a]Studies are listed in alphabetic order

Tracker (RT3) accelerometer [32, 33]; and one the Actiwatch accelerometer [34].

MVPA and ST in obese children

Eight eligible studies involved obese children, with a total sample size of 2138 children (478 with obesity; 131 boys, 136 girls and 211 no sex specified). Two of the eligible studies were clinical samples with study participants recruited from outpatient clinics. Eligible studies were from different nations with one study from Asia [35], three from Canada and USA [36–38] and four from Europe [32, 39–41], with the study characteristics summarized in Table 2. In four studies, MVPA data of boys and girls were reported separately while in the other four studies MVPA data were reported as mixed sex. 7/8 of eligible studies reported mean daily time spent in MVPA in minutes; in four studies mean time spent in MVPA was < 60 min/day. Furthermore, in 2/7 of the eligible studies, children with obesity reached or exceeded 60 min of MVPA per day [37, 38], while in one study they came close to a mean of 60 min/day of MVPA [36]. In all cases time spent in MVPA in the children who were obese was compared to the comparison group (non-obese peers). In only one study was the mean time spent in MVPA similar in both groups [37]; in three studies, time spent in MVPA was significant lower in children with obesity than in the comparison group [35, 36, 39], while in two studies time spent in MVPA of children with obesity was lower than the comparison group but differences were not significant [38, 40]. In the other 2 studies, time spent in MVPA of children with obesity was different in terms of gender compared to the comparison group: Hussey et al. reported that mean MVPA was significantly lower in boys with obesity but not in girls [32]; while Vale et al. reported that mean time spent in MVPA was significantly lower in girls with obesity but not in boys [41] compared to the comparison groups.

With respect to ST, 4/8 eligible studies reported on accelerometer-measured time spent in SB of children with obesity with a total sample size of 536 children (191 with obesity; 28 boys, 32 girls and 131 no sex specified). In one study, ST data of boys and girls was reported separately while in other the data were reported as mixed sex. Across all four eligible studies, mean time spent in SB was > 70% of waking time [32, 35, 39, 40]. In 3/4 of the studies ST was significantly higher in the obese than the non-obese groups, although, in one study it was significantly higher in boys with obesity but not in girls [32]. In one study ST was similar in both groups [39].

MVPA and ST in obese adolescents

Twenty of the eligible studies involved adolescents, with a total sample size of 12,601 adolescents (3045 with obesity; 1615 boys, 1575 girls and 195 no sex specified). Four of the eligible studies were clinical samples with participants recruited from outpatient clinics. Eligible studies were from different nations with one study from Asia [42], 11 from Canada and the USA, and eight from Europe, with the study characteristics summarized in Table 3. In 12/20 studies, MVPA data of boys and girls were reported separately; in 6/20 studies MVPA data were reported as mixed sex, while the other two studies involved only adolescent girls. All 20 eligible studies reported mean daily time spent in MVPA in minutes and in these studies it ranged from a low of 16 (SD 4) minutes/day [36] to a high of 140 (SD 47) minutes/day [43]. In only 2/ 20 studies did daily time spent in MVPA reach an average of at least 60 min [43, 44] in the adolescents who were obese. A total of 16/20 eligible studies compared time spent in MVPA of those with obesity with a comparison group: in 3/16 time spent in MVPA was similar between obese and non-obese groups, while in 10/16 mean time spent in MVPA was significantly lower in adolescents with obesity than in non-obese peers.

In regard to time spent in SB, nine out of the 20 eligible studies reported on accelerometer measured ST in adolescents with obesity with a total sample size of 5484 adolescents (1101 with obesity; 546 boys and 555 girls), as summarised in Table 3. In 8/9 studies, ST data of boys and girls were reported separately and 1/9 study involved only adolescent girls. In 7/9 studies, mean daily ST was reported in minutes and in these studies it ranged from a low of 345 (SD 122) minutes/day [34] to a high of 731 (SD 110) minutes/day [30]. In 6/9 studies there was a comparison group; in 2/6 studies mean daily ST was similar in obese and non-obese groups [42, 45]; in 2/6 studies ST was significantly higher in those with obesity than in the non-obese comparison groups [34, 46], while in the other 2/6 studies it was higher in the adolescents with obesity, but not significantly so [47, 48].

A graphical synthesis of the mean differences and 95% CI of time spent in MVPA by sex for both children and adolescents with obesity and non-obese groups, is shown in Fig. 2. A summary of the mean differences and 95% CI of time spent in SB by sex for both children and adolescents with obesity and non-obese groups, is shown in Fig. 3.

Study quality assessment

Study quality assessment summaries are given in [Additional file 3]. One study scored 4/6 12 studies scored 5/6 while 13 scored 6/6 on study quality.

Discussion

This systematic review provided clear evidence that children and adolescents with obesity have lower than the recommended levels of MVPA. In most of the eligible studies, daily time spent in MVPA averaged less than the

Study or Subgroup	Obese group Mean	SD	Total	Non-obese group Mean	SD	Total	Mean Difference 95% Confidence Interval
Girls							
Wang 2013	24	13	60	22	14	901	2.00 [-1.41, 5.41]
McMurray 2008	21	2	184	25	1	645	-4.00 [-4.30, -3.70]
Butte 2007	74	46	226	79	112	230	-5.00 [-20.67, 10.67]
Decelis 2014	38	12	54	44	15	280	-6.00 [-9.65, -2.35]
Decelis 2012	19	8	15	26	9	53	-7.00 [-11.72, -2.28]
Ruiz 2011	44	169	59	51	692	722	-7.00 [-73.39, 59.39]
Kitzman-Ulrich 2010	36	15	144	46	20	176	-10.00 [-13.84, -6.16]
Chung 2012	38	4	183	55	2	1022	-17.00 [-17.59, -16.41]
Ekelund 2002	60	28	10	98	58	10	-38.00 [-77.92, 1.92]
Page 2005	105	48	11	146	52	54	-41.00 [-72.57, -9.43]
Mixed sex							
Peart 2011	28	35	434	32	29	1469	-4.00 [-7.61, -0.39]
Shoup 2008	54	22	85	59	30	92	-5.00 [-12.71, 2.71]
Maggio 2010	60	3	45	71	5	85	-11.00 [-12.38, -9.62]
Trost 2001	70	6	45	82	4	133	-12.00 [-13.88, -10.12]
Maggio 2014	43	19	24	58	30	25	-15.00 [-29.00, -1.00]
Boys							
Wang 2013	29	18	115	35	19	808	-6.00 [-9.54, -2.46]
Ruiz 2011	60	201	45	67	1,008	870	-7.00 [-96.08, 82.08]
Butte 2007	88	50	247	96	57	194	-8.00 [-18.16, 2.16]
Decelis 2014	49	19	59	61	22	254	-12.00 [-17.55, -6.45]
Decelis 2012	30	13	19	44	16	53	-14.00 [-21.26, -6.74]
Chung 2012	57	4	191	74	3	1017	-17.00 [-17.60, -16.40]
Kitzman-Ulrich 2010	46	20	98	65	27	138	-19.00 [-25.00, -13.00]
Ekelund 2002	58	30	8	82	36	8	-24.00 [-56.47, 8.47]
Page 2005	140	47	14	176	52	54	-36.00 [-64.26, -7.74]

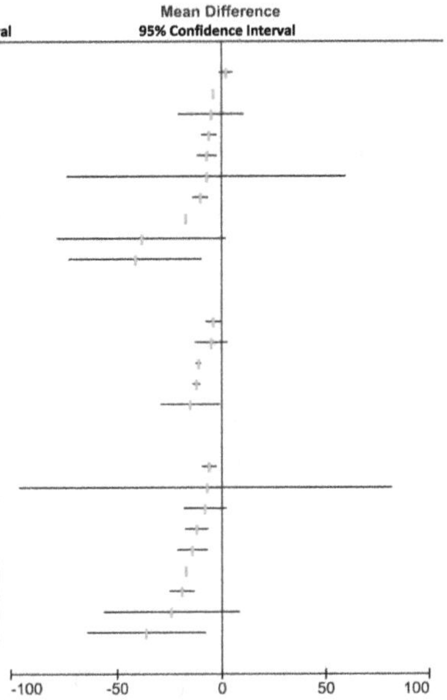

Fig. 2 Forest plot of the comparison of moderate-to-vigorous intensity physical activity between children and adolescents with obesity and non-obese participants by sex. SD: standard deviation; CI: 95% Confidence interval

60 min/day recommended in many guidelines. When comparing MVPA level between obese and non-obese peers, the findings indicated that daily MVPA was lower in children and adolescents with obesity.

In reviewing the methodology of the studies, it is noteworthy that the precise accelerometer methodology was often not stated clearly, or sometimes not stated at all, in the eligible studies particularly with respect to the cut-off used to define MVPA (Tables 2 and 3). However, mean time spent in MVPA was broadly similar within studies that employed comparable accelerometer methods. For example, in the two eligible Actigraph studies which used a cut-off of 2000 counts per minutes (cpm) to define MVPA (Maggio et al. [40], age 4–17 years old, and Ruiz et al. [46], age 12–17 year olds) mean daily time spent in MVPA was 60 min/day in the boys with obesity in the sample studied by Ruiz et al. [46], and 60 min/day in the boys with obesity studied by Maggio et al. [40]. Both of these studies might suggest the tentative conclusion that time spent in MVPA is relatively high in adolescents who are obese, possibly suggesting that adolescence and/or obesity do not present major barriers to MVPA. In contrast, three of the eligible Actigraph studies used higher MVPA cut-offs which ranged between 2912 cpm in 11–12 year olds: Decelis et al. [47] and 3200 cpm Hughes et al. [39] and Wafa et al. [35] in 8 and 9 year olds respectively. These studies found that mean daily time spent in MVPA was 30 min in boys and 19 min in girls with obesity [47] and a median of 16 min for both sexes combined in the study by Hughes et al. [39] and 5 min/day in the study by Wafa et al. [35]. The majority of children and adolescents with obesity achieved means of < 30 min of daily time spent in MVPA in studies with cut-offs of ≥2912 cpm [32, 38, 39, 43, 44].

Further, it should be noted that recommendations for MVPA state that 60 min per day is a minimum every day (e.g. usually operationalized as 7 days in a week)

Study or Subgroup	Obese group Mean	SD	Total	Non-obese group Mean	SD	Total	Mean Difference 95% Confidence Interval
Girls							
Decelis 2012	619	106	15	664	93	53	-45.00 [-104.20, 14.20]
Wang 2013	490	89	60	533	103	901	-43.00 [-66.50, -19.50]
Decelis 2014	610	125	54	603	97	280	7.00 [-28.22, 42.22]
Butte 2007	345	122	226	308	131	230	37.00 [13.77, 60.23]
Ekelund 2002	465	132	10	397	69	10	68.00 [-24.32, 160.32]
Boys							
Decelis 2014	553	94	59	582	113	254	-29.00 [-56.72, -1.28]
Decelis 2012	638	95	19	654	93	53	-16.00 [-65.51, 33.51]
Ekelund 2002	421	33	8	414	81	8	7.00 [-53.61, 67.61]
Butte 2007	357	118	247	305	121	194	52.00 [29.50, 74.50]

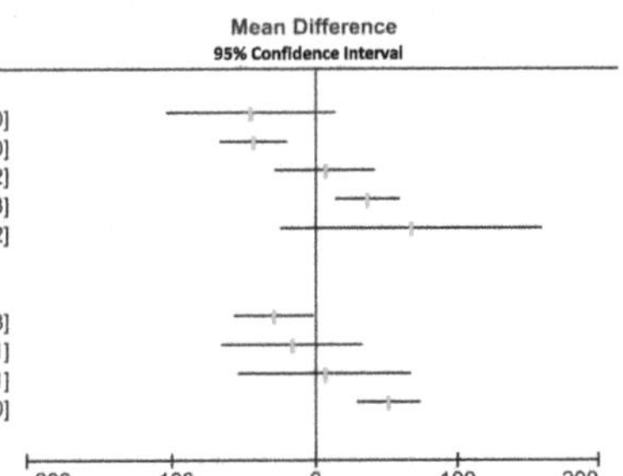

Fig. 3 Forest plot of the comparison of sedentary time between children and adolescents with obesity and non-obese participants by sex. SD: standard deviation; CI: 95% Confidence interval

[49–51], but adherence to recommendations was never operationalized in this way in any of the 26 eligible studies. We therefore used a mean or median daily MVPA of 60 min as a proxy for adherence, though this is conservative because in many individuals where 60 min MVPA/day was reached as an average, time spent in MVPA would have fallen below 60 min/day on at least one of the monitored days.

With respect to sedentary time, the present review found that studies fairly consistently reported that children and adolescents with obesity accumulated a high amount of ST during their waking hours, ranging typically between 65 and 90% of their waking monitoring time: 10 h was the mean daily ST in all 13/26 studies, which reaches or exceeds typical Actigraph measured levels of ST in North-American adults from surveys such as NHANES. All eligible studies, which had comparison groups, found ST was fairly consistent with no marked differences between obese and non-obese peers.

In the present systematic review, the level of heterogeneity between eligible studies made it impossible to combine data in a formal meta-analysis. The heterogeneity noted was due to differences in the location of the studies, differences in the way obesity was defined (different BMI cut-off points and different reference data), or differences in accelerometer models and methodology. Therefore, we narratively synthesized the differences in the time spent in MVPA and ST between obese and control groups by age and sex. Additionally, future research would benefit from an attempt to obtain the original study participant data and to reanalyse that with a common methodology, though this was beyond the scope of the present study.

Comparisons with other studies

We believe that the present study is the first systematic review to ask whether or not levels of accelerometer measured MVPA are adequate in children and adolescents with obesity, and whether time spent in MVPA and ST differed between obese and comparison groups based on accelerometer data. There are therefore no directly comparable studies. However, our findings are consistent with some studies on the correlates and determinants of objectively MVPA [52, 53], and consistent with a growing belief that obesity is associated with reduced MVPA and that low MVPA could be both a cause of obesity and a consequence of obesity, i.e., "bi-directional causation" [20, 54, 55].

Review and evidence strengths and weaknesses

The evidence considered by our review had a number of strengths. Firstly, it investigated the accelerometer-measured time spent in MVPA and ST of children and adolescents with obesity, with clear definitions of obesity so that samples included in the review were not contaminated by the inclusion of overweight but non-obese individuals. Secondly, there are several methodological strengths to this study. Studies were identified from an extensive search of the published literature conducted in a range of databases, over the last 15 years, covering the time when accelerometers started to become available and popular in PA research and, more recently, sedentary behavior research. The broad definition of search terms applied across multiple databases enabled the searching and identification across many potential studies with no limitations on place of publication, sample size or country of origin. Restricting eligibility to studies using accelerometry was important in increasing confidence in the measurement of MVPA [19, 56–58]. The included studies were in general rated as being of high or very high methodological quality with respect to their accelerometry methods. Also, in some cases the eligible studies were based on large nationally representative samples or surveys another strength in terms of generalizability.

There were some sources of weakness in our systematic review. Firstly, since studies had to be published in peer-reviewed journals in English, this may have excluded some relevant evidence. The generalisability of review results is subject to certain limitations; for instance, eligible studies in our systematic review were from high-income nations, and we lacked data from low-middle income countries. Most of the included studies were based on relatively small samples of obese children and adolescents with a total ($n = 14{,}739$ participants; $n = 3523$ with obesity) and their power to estimate habitual MVPA might have been limited, and thus the extent to which the results observed are generalizable to the general obese paediatric population is unclear. The method of quality assessment in our review, in which the original 15 items scale has been collapsed to 6 items, has been used in several accelerometry systematic reviews [24–28]. However, the process of collapsing 15 items to a six-item might have reduced the possibility of identifying differences in quality between studies.

Eligible studies generally obtained MVPA and ST data using the ActiGraph accelerometer, but methods used varied between studies. Methodological differences include: the definition of epoch, the number of hours and days of data constituting a valid/acceptable data set, MVPA and ST cut-points, and the choice of non-wear criteria. These methodological variation tends to produce meaningful differences in MVPA and ST estimates between studies [16] and also make it difficult to compare across studies. However, while there were multiple differences between studies in accelerometry methodology (e.g. in epochs, cut-points, handling of non-wear time, duration of accelerometry monitoring), in all cases the methods were the same within studies between the obese and non-obese comparison groups, so these methodological differences probably had limited effect on the ability of studies to identify differences in MVPA and ST between the obese and non-obese. Finally, the validity of accelerometry (in particular hip-worn accelerometry, the method in almost all eligible studies) to determine ST is less well established than the validity of this placement for measurement of MVPA [59]. Hip-worn accelerometers are not designed to measure posture, and devices such as inclinometers may provide improved measurement. Accelerometers are used widely to measure ST though, and there is some evidence of validity for group-comparisons as here (obese vs non-obese comparisons) [19, 16].

Conclusions

In summary, the data presented in our review demonstrated that a high percentage of obese children and adolescents did not achieve the minimum amount of 60 min per day MVPA that is recommended in guidelines and tended to spend what appeared to be the vast majority of their waking hours sedentary. Children and adolescents with obesity were generally slightly less physically active and slightly more sedentary compared to comparison groups, though the present review cannot test whether they were less active or more sedentary before becoming obese.

Given the many and varied health and non-health benefits of MVPA in children and youth [60, 61], and emerging evidence that ST influences health outcomes in children and adolescents [62, 63] the present review highlights the need to focus on increasing MVPA and reducing ST among children and adolescents with obesity, and the importance of raising these issues in clinical settings as part of treatment for obesity. Treatment of childhood and adolescent obesity should clearly involve a focus on increasing MVPA and reducing ST as recommended in multiple evidence based treatment and prevention guidelines published in recent years.

Additional files

Additional file 1: Inclusion and exclusion criteria for selection of studies. (XLSX 9 kb) MVPA: Moderate-to-Vigorous Intensity Physical Activity; PA: physical activity; SB: sedentary behavior.

Additional file 2: Study Quality Assessment Criteria, modified from Tooth et al. (22). MVPA: Moderate-to-Vigorous Intensity Physical Activity

Additional file 3: Methodological quality assessment of the included studies.

Abbreviations

BMI: Body mass index; MVPA: Moderate-to-vigorous physical activity; PA: Physical activity; SB: Sedentary behavior; ST: Sedentary Time

Acknowledgements

Not applicable.

Funding

no funding.

Authors' contributions

RE conceptualized and designed the study, performed screening, extracted the data, and assessed the methodological quality of included articles drafted the initial manuscript.AM conducted literature search, reviewed and revised the manuscript. JR conceptualized and designed the study, and coordinated and supervised data collection, critically reviewed and revised the manuscript. JP conceptualized and designed the study, screened shortlisted articles to ensure no missing articles, critically reviewed and revised the manuscript. All authors approved the final manuscript as submitted.

Competing interests

Statement for all authors: there is no potential Conflict of Interest to disclose and there are no financial relationships relevant to this article to disclose. The authors declare that they have no competing interests.

Author details

[1]School of Medicine, College of Medical, Veterinary, and Life Sciences, University of Glasgow, Glasgow G12 8 QQ, UK. [2]MRC/CSO Social and Public Health Sciences Unit University of Glasgow, Glasgow G12 8 QQ, UK. [3]Physical Activity for Health Group, University of Strathclyde, George Street, Glasgow G1 1XQ, UK. [4]Al-Fatah Hospital, Medical School, Benghazi University, Benghazi, Libya. [5]Office Block, Ground Floor, Zone 1 (Paediatrics) Royal Hospital for Children, 1345 Govan Road, Glasgow G51 4TF, UK.

References

1. Caballero B. The global epidemic of obesity: an overview. Epidemiol Rev. 2007;29:1–5.
2. Lobstein T, et al. Obesity in children and young people: a crisis in public health. Obes Rev. 2004;5(Suppl 1):4–104.
3. Dietz WH. Health consequences of obesity in youth: childhood predictors of adult disease. Pediatrics. 1998;101(3):518–25.
4. Waters E, et al. Interventions for preventing obesity in children. Sao Paulo Med J. 2014;132(2):128–9.
5. Hardy LL, et al. Co-occurrence of obesogenic risk factors among adolescents. J Adolesc Health. 2012;51(3):265–71.
6. Eissa MA, Gunner KB, University of Texas-Houston Health Science center. Evaluation and management of obesity in children and adolescents. J Pediatr Health Care. 2004;18(1):35–8.
7. Leech RM, McNaughton SA, Timperio A. The clustering of diet, physical activity and sedentary behavior in children and adolescents: a review. Int J Behav Nutr Phys Act. 2014;11(4). doi:https://doi.org/10.1186/1479-5868-11-4.
8. Rippe JM, Hess S. The role of physical activity in the prevention and management of obesity. J Am Diet Assoc. 1998;98(10):S31–8.
9. Mitchell JA, Byun W. Sedentary behavior and health outcomes in children and adolescents. Am J Lifestyle Med. 2014;8(3):173–99.
10. Simon C, et al. Successful overweight prevention in adolescents by increasing physical activity: a 4-year randomized controlled intervention. Int J Obes. 2008;32(10):1489–98.
11. Stroebele N, Hill JO, Willich SN. Identifying the energy gap in the German population using results from representative national health surveys (1985–2002). Public Health Nutr. 2011;14(01):44–8.
12. Lau DC, et al. 2006 Canadian clinical practice guidelines on the management and prevention of obesity in adults and children [summary]. CMAJ. 2007;176(8):S1–13.
13. Organization WH. Global recommendations on physical activity for health; 2010.
14. Tremblay MS, et al. Canadian sedentary behaviour guidelines for children and youth. Appl Physiol Nutr Metab. 2011;36(1):59–64.

15. Tremblay MS, et al. New Canadian physical activity guidelines. App Phys Nut Meta-Phys Appli Nutr Et Meta. 2011;36(1):36–46.
16. Reilly JJ, et al. Objective measurement of physical activity and sedentary behaviour: review with new data. Arch Dis Child. 2008;93(7):614–9.
17. Riddoch CJ, et al. Objective measurement of levels and patterns of physical activity. Arch Dis Child. 2007;92(11):963–9.
18. Reilly JJ. Low levels of objectively measured physical activity in preschoolers in child care. Med Sci Sports Exerc. 2010;42(3):502–7.
19. Pate RR, O'Neill JR, Mitchell J. Measurement of physical activity in preschool children. Med Sci Sports Exerc. 2010;42(3):508–12.
20. Bauman AE, et al. Correlates of physical activity: why are some people physically active and others not? Lancet. 2012;380(9838):258–71.
21. Pate RR, et al. Physical activity and public health. A recommendation from the Centers for Disease Control and Prevention and the American College of Sports Medicine. JAMA. 1995;273(5):402–7.
22. Moher D, et al. Preferred reporting items for systematic reviews and meta-analyses: the PRISMA statement. Open Med. 2009;3(3):e123–30.
23. Tooth L, et al. Quality of reporting of observational longitudinal research. Am J Epidemiol. 2005;161(3):280–8.
24. Reilly JJ, et al. Contribution of school recess to daily physical aactivity: systematic review. Health Behav Pol Rev. 2016;3(6):581–589(9).
25. Martin A, et al. Contribution of walking to school to individual and population moderate-vigorous intensity physical activity: systematic review and meta-analysis. Pediatr Exerc Sci. 2016;28(3):353–63.
26. Jones RA, et al. Tracking physical activity and sedentary behavior in childhood a systematic review. Am J Prev Med. 2013;44(6):651–8.
27. Tanaka C, Reilly JJ, Huang WY. Longitudinal changes in objectively measured sedentary behaviour and their relationship with adiposity in children and adolescents: systematic review and evidence appraisal. Obes Rev. 2014;15(10):791–803.
28. Elmesmari R, et al. Accelerometer measured levels of moderate-to-vigorous intensity physical activity and sedentary time in children and adolescents with chronic disease: a systematic review and meta-analysis. PLoS One. 2017;12(6):e0179429.
29. St George SM, et al. Weight status as a moderator of the relationship between motivation, emotional social support, and physical activity in underserved adolescents. J Pediatr Psychol. 2013;38(4):387–97.
30. Starkoff BE, et al. Sedentary and physical activity habits of obese adolescents. Am J Health Educ. 2014;45(6):335–41.
31. Kitzman-Ulrich H, et al. Relationship of body mass index and psychosocial factors on physical activity in underserved adolescent boys and girls. Health Psychol. 2010;29(5):506–13.
32. Hussey J, et al. Relationship between the intensity of physical activity, inactivity, cardiorespiratory fitness and body composition in 7-10-year-old Dublin children. Br J Sports Med. 2007;41(5):311–6.
33. Vanhelst J, et al. Concurrent validity of the modified international physical activity questionnaire for French obese adolescents. Percept Motor Skills. 2013;116(1):123–31.
34. Butte NF, et al. Physical activity in nonoverweight and overweight Hispanic children and adolescents. Med Sci Sports Exerc. 2007;39(8):1257–66.
35. Wafa SW, et al. Objectively measured habitual physical activity and sedentary behaviour in obese and non-obese Malaysian children. J Trop Pediatr. 2014;60(2):161–3.
36. Chung AE, et al. Physical activity and BMI in a nationally representative sample of children and adolescents. Clin Pediatr. 2012;51(2):122–9.
37. Thompson AM, et al. Are overweight students in grades 3, 7, and 11 less physically active than their healthy weight counterparts? Int J Pediatr Obes. 2009;4(1):28–35.
38. Metallinos-Katsaras ES, et al. The association between an objective measure of physical activity and weight status in preschoolers. Obes. 2007;15(3):686–94.
39. Hughes AR, et al. Habitual physical activity and sedentary behaviour in a clinical sample of obese children. Int J Obes. 2006;30(10):1494–500.
40. Maggio AB, et al. Reduced physical activity level and cardiorespiratory fitness in children with chronic diseases. Eur J Pediatr. 2010;169(10):1187–93.
41. Vale S, et al. Physical activity guidelines and preschooler's obesity status. Int J Obes. 2013;37(10):1352–5.
42. Wang C, Chen P, Zhuang J. A national survey of physical activity and sedentary behavior of Chinese city children and youth using accelerometers. Res Quar Exer S. 2013;84(Suppl 2):S12–28.
43. Page A, et al. Physical activity patterns in nonobese and obese children assessed using minute-by-minute accelerometry. Int J Obes. 2005;29(9): 1070–6.
44. Trost SG, et al. Physical activity and determinants of physical activity in obese and non-obese children. Int J Obes Rel Met Dis J Int Assoc Stud Obes. 2001;25(6):822–9.
45. Ekelund U, et al. Physical activity but not energy expenditure is reduced in obese adolescents: a case-control study. Am J Clin Nutr. 2002;76(5):935–41.
46. Ruiz JR, et al. Objectively measured physical activity and sedentary time in European adolescents the HELENA study. Am J Epidemiol. 2011; 174(2):173–84.
47. Decelis A, Jago R, Fox KR. Objectively assessed physical activity and weight status in Maltese 11-12 year-olds. Euro J Sport Sci EJSS : Offic J Euro Col Sport Sci. 2014;14(Suppl 1):S257–66.
48. Decelis A, Jago R, Fox KR. Physical activity, screen time and obesity status in a nationally representative sample of Maltese youth with international comparisons. BMC Public Health. 2014;14:664.
49. Organization, W.H., Global recommendations on physical activity for health. 2010.
50. Twisk JW. Physical activity guidelines for children and adolescents: a critical review. Sports Med. 2001;31(8):617–27.
51. Barlow SE, Dietz WH. Obesity evaluation and treatment: expert committee recommendations. Mater Child Health Bureau, Health Res Ser Admin Dep Health Human Ser Pediatrics. 1998;102(3):E29.
52. Ekelund U, et al. Moderate to vigorous physical activity and sedentary time and Cardiometabolic risk factors in children and adolescents. Jama-J Am Med Assoc. 2012;307(7):704–12.
53. Jimenez-Pavon D, Kelly J, Reilly JJ. Associations between objectively measured habitual physical activity and adiposity in children and adolescents: systematic review. Int J Pediatr Obes. 2010;5(1):3–18.
54. Must A, Tybor DJ. Physical activity and sedentary behavior: a review of longitudinal studies of weight and adiposity in youth. Int J Obes. 2005;29: S84–96.
55. Richmond RC, et al. Assessing causality in the association between child adiposity and physical activity levels: a Mendelian randomization analysis. PLoS Med. 2014;11(3):e1001618.
56. Toschke JA, et al. Reliability of physical activity measures from accelerometry among preschoolers in free-living conditions. Clin Nutr. 2007;26(4):416–20.
57. Nyberg G, Ekelund U, Marcus C. Physical activity in children measured by accelerometry: stability over time. Scand J Med Sci Sports. 2009;19(1):30–5.
58. Bender JM, et al. Children's physical activity: using accelerometers to validate a parent proxy record. Med Sci Sports Exerc. 2005;37(8):1409–13.
59. van Nassau F, et al. Validity and responsiveness of four measures of occupational sitting and standing. Int J Behav Nutr Phys Act. 2015;12(1):144.
60. Janssen I, LeBlanc AG. Systematic review of the health benefits of physical activity and fitness in school-aged children and youth. Int J Behav Nutr Phys Act. 2010;7(40). doi:https://doi.org/10.1186/1479-5868-7-40.
61. Strong WB, et al. Evidence based physical activity for school-age youth. J Pediatr. 2005;146(6):732–7.
62. Mann K, et al. Longitudinal study of the associations between change in sedentary behavior and change in adiposity during childhood and adolescence: Gateshead millennium study. Int J Obes (2005). 2017; 41(7):1042.
63. Belcher BR, et al. Effects of interrupting children's sedentary behaviors with activity on metabolic function: a randomized trial. J Clin Endocrin Metabol. 2015;100(10):3735–43.
64. Maggio ABR, et al. High bone density in adolescents with obesity is related to fat mass and serum leptin concentrations. J Pediatr Gastroenterol Nutr. 2014;58(6):723–8.

5

Parental separation and behaviours that influence the health of infants aged 28 to 32 months

Nadine Kacenelenbogen[1*], Michèle Dramaix-Wilmet[2], M. Schetgen[1], M. Roland[1] and Isabelle Godin[3]

Abstract

Background: In Western countries, many children are affected by the separation of their parents. The study's main objective was to analyse the parental behaviours potentially influential for preschool children's health by family structure (parents together or separated).

Methods: We conducted a cross-sectional study based on data collected from examinations as part of free preventive medical consultations in the French Community of Belgium. During the assessment of 30,769 infants aged 28 to 32 months, information was collected on the parents' use of tobacco, brushing of the infant's teeth, being monitored by a dentist, and receiving vision screening. The chi^2 test was applied and the odds ratios were derived to compare the two groups of children (exposed/not exposed to parental separation). Multivariate logistic regression analyses were used to adjust the effect of exposure.

Results: Nearly one in ten (9.8%) did not live with both parents under the same roof. Taking into account the social and cultural environment and other potential confounders at our disposal, we found that in the event of parental separation, behaviours differ in comparison with situations where parents live together; the adjusted odds ratios (ORs) (95% confidence interval) for the infant's exposure to tobacco, absence of teeth brushing, lack of monitoring by a dentist and absence of visual screening, were respectively 1.7 (1.2–2.0), 1.1 (0.9–1.2), 1.3 (1.1–1.6), 1.2 (1.1–1.2), and 1.2 (1.1–1.4).

Conclusions: This study confirms the suspicion that parental separation is an independent risk factor for parental behaviours that negatively influence the infant's health. If these results are confirmed, this it could affect the work of the family doctors and paediatricians, especially in terms of family support and information to parents.

Keywords: Preschool children, Parental separation, Passive smoking, Prevention and screening

Background

In Belgium in 2011, the crude divorce rate was 2.9 per 1000 inhabitants, which is in line with in the rest of Europe, despite some North/South disparities. This rate is similar in a number of other countries in Europe (e.g. Denmark and Germany) [1] and in other continents (United States, Canada and Australia) [2–4]. Again in Belgium, in 2013, almost 80,000 people registered for legal cohabitation, the Belgian equivalent of registered or civil partnership, compared with 36,000 who declared the dissolution of their legal cohabitation (or 450 per 1000) [5]. Therefore, in Western countries, parental separation affects many minors. In Canada in 2011, 20% of people aged under 15 years were living with a single parent [6]. In the United Kingdom (UK) in 2001, 20% of people aged under 18 years did not live with both of their parents living as a couple [7]. According to a longitudinal study of 3000 households, 20% of children aged 0 to 16 years were living in a single-parent family or stepfamily in Belgium in 2002 [8].

* Correspondence: nkacenel@ulb.ac.be
[1]Université Libre de Bruxelles, General Medicine Department, Campus Facultaire Erasme, Route de Lennik 808/612, 1070 Brussels, Belgium

In Flanders, a cross-sectional study carried out in 2013 showed that 10% of children under 2 years of age had experienced parental separation: this figure rises to 26% for all children aged 0 to 17 [9]. It is indeed expected that the older children become, the more likely they are to experience the separation of their parents. In Belgium in 2009, in the French-speaking community, 6.4% of children aged 7 to 11 months monitored by the *Office de la naissance et de l'enfance (ONE – Office for Births and Childhood – see 'Methods' section)* [10], did not live with two biological parents who were together as a couple, with the figure rising to 9% in children aged 28 to 32 months [11]. Lastly, a 2010 survey of more than 10,000 young Belgian French-speakers showed that more than 23% of children aged 10 to 12 years lived in either a stepfamily (10%) or a single-parent family (13%). That figure rises to 34% when children were aged between 13 and 19 years [12].' [13]

Thus, using cumulative frequency, we estimate that parental separation affects more than 25% of young people aged under 18 years in Belgium. If we take into account the annual number of births for the last 17 years [14], at least 500,000 minors (of a total population of 11 million inhabitants) experience an officially recorded parental separation. Some authors describe a link between a child not living with parents who are together as a couple and a greater frequency of somatic, psychological, behavioural and academic problems. For instance, a cross-sectional American study that surveyed 102,000 families between 2002 and 2003 observed that, after adjusting for socio-economic levels, children presented significantly more oral, respiratory, trauma-related, behavioural and academic problems, as well as using specialised care more often, in the event of parental break-up [15]. In Spain, recent studies have indicated that for children and adolescents, parental separation represents a risk factor for their physical health, particularly genito-urinary, gastrointestinal, dermatological and neurological, in addition to exposure to violence and emotional or psychopathological disorders [16].' [17] A national survey conducted in Belgium between 1992 and 2002 of 27,500 families confirmed this increase in risk factors when parents separated, such as the loss of contact with one of the parents, parental psychopathology, passive smoking or a materially less-advantaged environment. In that survey, the children of separated couples were more often absent from school or had fallen behind [8]. In 2006, a focus group-based qualitative study described the issues that hindered the work of Belgian general practitioners (GPs) while monitoring the children of separated parents. These included difficulties communicating with parents about the children's health and barriers to monitoring the children medically, particularly for chronic diseases, or adherence to the immunisation schedule. Those GPs also described somatic and psycho-behavioural repercussions in the children following separation [18].

To our knowledge, little research has been specifically carried out on the association between separation or divorce and parental behaviour that may influence child health. We hypothesise that the behaviour of parents with regard to their child's health may be different when they are separated compared with when they are together. A cross-sectional study of nearly 80,000 Belgian infants aged 7 to 11 months has already shown a significant association between a child not living with both parents and passive smoking, absence of breastfeeding and non-adherence to the immunisation schedule [19].

Objectives

Our study's primary objective was to assess parental behaviour regarding children's health according to family structure (parents separated or together) in a cohort of preschool children (28 to 32 months). The secondary objective was to identify other factors of use to primary care medical practitioners that were associated with parental behaviours detrimental to child development. Our study is of use to primary care practice, as it makes it possible to better tailor informative and preventive action in families.

Methods

Study population

In the French-speaking community of Belgium, the ONE [20] offers free preventive monitoring of pregnant women and children up to the age of 6 years. Data collected during assessments is centralised in a computerised database. For children aged under 3 years, data is collected at birth in the maternity hospital, on arrival home, and, for those who are seen at the ONE, between 7 and 11 months, 16 and 20 months, and 28 and 32 months. For each encounter, social and demographic data, along with parenting behaviours, are recorded by a nurse, midwife or social worker. Specially trained paediatricians or GPs assess the child's health status (including psychomotor development). Once filled in, the anonymised sheets are entered into the central database. This system makes it possible to evaluate and adapt medico-social policy during the perinatal period and early childhood. We studied the data from 30,769 children recorded in the ONE database between 2006 and 2012 for whom there existed a preventive health assessment at 28 to 32 months after birth.

Assessment of main exposure

Family structure was divided into six categories: the two parents together, parents separated, child only sees one parent, the child is in a children's home/ foster home, other situations (with grandparents or other parents) and unknown. A summary of the study sample, comprising 30,769 children, is provided in Table 5 (Appendix). For subsequent analyses, only parents who were together or separated ($n = 28{,}871$) were retained, with children who see only one parent falling under the second category; the parents of 2835 children (9.8%) were separated and those of 26,036 children (90.2%) lived together. Table 1 compares the socio-demographic characteristics of the two types of family structure.

Assessment of other covariates

Using a 'ready-made' database (issued by the ONE), we selected the dependent variables that shed light on parental behaviour that is likely to influence the health of young children. However, the choice was limited as we could select only the variables that were available in this database. Therefore, the other independent variables retained for analysis were the mother's age at childbirth, her level of education, her occupation and family income. The mother's occupation and family income were mainly analysed to describe our sample, but they were not retained for creating the regression models because, as categories, they were ill suited to our research question. We placed stay-at-home mothers and those on benefits into as single occupational category, and those on early retirement or who had disabilities in another. Family income did not describe the level of earnings in euros but the type of income: for instance, families with one or two incomes from employment were in the same group, which partly covered the 'couple' variable (one or two parents) (Table 5 – Appendix). Our univariate analyses showed that the mother's level of education was a good indicator of socio-economic status. This means that the higher the mother's level of education, the more often they worked and had income from employment. Regarding language, two variables were available: the mother's level of French (very good, a little, none) and the language spoken in the family (French, other language). Based on these two variables, we created the 'first language' variable (French, other language). We broke down the mother's age, separating very young mothers (≤ 17 years) and older mothers (≥ 38 years) in particular. In addition, the child's gender, birth weight and body mass index (BMI) were also analysed. 'Unknown' responses were eliminated for each of the variables taken into account: however, before doing this, we noted that the distributions of the variables relating to socio-economic status did not significantly differ among these 'unknowns'. For multivariate analysis, the independent variable categories were grouped together according to the categories presented in the tables (Table 5 – Appendix).

Outcome ascertainment

Dependent variables that were available and bore a relation to our research question were children's being exposed to smoking on a daily basis between 2006 and 2009, brushing their teeth daily between 2006 and 2012, regularly seeing a dentist, and undergoing vision screening between 2010 and 2012. It ought to be noted that this vision-screening test has been made available since 2003 for all children monitored by the ONE at the 28–32-month examination. The aim is to detect functional amblyopia, which is the most common cause of unilateral visual impairment in children in Europe and the United States [21].

When treated between the ages of 2 and 3 years, amblyopia is curable, whereas it becomes permanent from the age of 6 years. Screening is performed using refractometry. It should be noted that, to take advantage of this free screening test by an orthoptist, parents must bring their child by appointment to a centre located at a different address to where the basic assessment takes place [22].

Statistical analysis

The chi^2 test was applied and the odds ratios (ORs) were derived to compare the two groups of children aged 28 to 32 months (exposed/not exposed to parental separation). Multivariate logistic regression analyses were used to adjust the effect of exposure. The models were designed using a backwards elimination method for potential confounders, and the variable of parental situation was automatically included in the models. Interactions between this variable and the other predictors were tested. The only interaction observed was for passive smoking, and it was between family structure and first language. The Hosmer–Lemeshow test was also used to check model fit. The absence of collinearity between the predictors included in the model was verified by means of variance inflation factors. The analyses were conducted using the STATA 12.0 software (http://www.stata.com).

Results

In the 30,769 children, there were slightly more boys (51.3%) than girls (48.7%) and 7% of the children weighed less than 2500 g at birth (Table 5 – Appendix). In our sample, 1% of mothers were aged under 18 years at childbirth and 7% were aged 38 or over. Of the

Table 1 Sample description

Initial variable	%	New categories (*without *unknowns*)	%
Gender $n = 30{,}769$			
Boy	51.3	–	–
Girl	48.7		
Child's age $n = 30{,}707$		–	
≤27 mo	7.3		
28–32 mo	88.9		
≥33 mo	3.8		
Birthweight $n = 30{,}757$		$n = 30{,}757$	
< 1000 g	0.1		
1000–1499 g	0.6		
1500–1999 g	1.2		
2000–2499 g	5.1	< 2500 g	7.0
2500–2999 g	19.6	≥2500 g	
3000–3499 g	39.9		93.0
3500–3999 g	25.0		
4000–4499 g	5.5		
≥4500 g	3.0		
BMI (kg/m^2) at examination	percentiles	$n = 29{,}120$	
$n = 29{,}120$			
< 13.1	1.0		
< 13.9	5.0		
< 14.4	10.0		
< 15.2	25.0	p3-p97	91.8
< 16.0	50.0	>p97	6.3
< 17.0	75.0	<p3	1.9
< 18.0	90.0		
< 18.7	95.0		
< 20.9	99.0		
Mother's age in years at childbirth $n = 29{,}883$		n = 29,883	
9–15	0.2		
16–17	0.7	< 18	0.9
18–24	18.3	18/30	59.0
25–30	40.8	31/37	33.0
31–37	32.9	≥38	7.1
38–44	6.9		
45–53	0.2		
Mother's level of education $n = 30{,}769$		$n = 24{,}530$	
Did not complete primary school/no schooling	2.3		22.4
Completed primary school/did not complete lower secondary	4.3	< Upper secondary school	30.8
Completed lower secondary school	11.2	Completed upper secondary school	46.8
Completed upper secondary school	24.6	Completed third-level/university or not	
Completed third-level/university or not	37.3		
Unknown	20.3		

Table 1 Sample description *(Continued)*

Initial variable	%	New categories (*without *unknowns*)	%
Mother's occupation $n = 15{,}038$ (2006–9)		$n = 7293$	
Unemployed/stay-at-home	18.5	Unemployed/stay-at-home	
Part time	9.9		
Early retirement/invalidity/work incapacity	1.0	Early retirement/work incapacity/invalidity	38.1
On full-time career break/parental leave or similar	1.2	Student	2.1
Student	0.1	Works full time or part time/career break/parental leave	0.3
Works full time	17.7		59.5
Unknown	51.6		
Family income $n = 15{,}038$ (2006–9)		$n = 7285$	
No stable income	0.6		
1 or 2 incomes from benefits	5.5	No stable income	1.2
1 income from employment	16.3	1or 2 incomes from benefits	11.4
1 income from employment + 1	0.1	1 income from employment	33.6
income from benefits	0.3	2 incomes, of which ≥1 income from employment	53.8
Other (specify)	26.0		
2 incomes from employment	51.2		
Unknown			
Mother's standard of French $n = 16{,}990$ (2006–9)			
None	1.8		
A little	8.1		
Very good	86.9		
Unknown	3.2	First language $n = 28{,}582$ (2006–12)	
Language spoken at home $n = 13{,}783$ (2010–12)			
Language other than French	34.3	French	77.6
French	53.8	Other	22.4
Unknown	11.9		
Goes to a nursery $n = 13{,}783$ (2010–12)		$n = 12{,}040$	
Yes	48.8		
No	38.5	Yes	55.9
Unknown	12.7	No	44.1
Family environment $n = 30{,}769$		$n = 28{,}871$	
Parents separated	7.5		
Only sees one parent	1.3		
Stepfamily	0.4	Parents separated/only sees one parent/stepfamily	9.8
Children's home/home/foster home	0.6	Parents together	90.2
Grandparents, uncles/aunts, others	0.6		
Parents together	84.6		
Unknown	5.0		

mothers, 22% had not completed secondary education. The percentage of mothers who did not have a job was 38%. French was not the first language in more than one in five families (Table 5 – Appendix). It should be noted that 9.8% of children did not live with both of their parents under the same roof (Table 5 – Appendix). The study of socio-demographic characteristics revealed significant differences between both types of families (Table 1). When parents did not live under the same roof, compared to non-separated parents, the mothers were more often younger than 18 years of age at childbirth (3.9% versus 0.5%) and less frequently had a higher level of education (28.9% versus 48.9%). We also noted that mothers who were separated from the child's father were less likely to be French native speakers (18.1% versus 23.0%).

Between 2006 and 2009, 36% of children were exposed to smoking every day if the parents were separated compared with 20.7% when the parents were together ($p < 0.001$) (Table 2). Between 2006 and 2012, 9.3% of children did not have their teeth brushed daily when the parents were separated, compared with 7.7% when the parents lived together ($p = 0.007$). Regardless of family situation, between 2010 and 2012, more than 81% of the children had never had a check-up with a dentist (80.8% in couples living together), but the figure rose to 84.8% when the parents did not live together ($p = 0.002$). Lastly, again between 2010 and 2012, 48.2% of the children had not undergone vision screening when the parents were separated, compared with 40.7% when the parents were still together ($p < 0.001$) (Table 2). After adjusting for socio-economic and cultural factors, we observed that parental separation remained significantly associated with the variables having a potential impact on children's health that were considered in this study, except for the absence of tooth brushing, the OR for which was no longer significant (OR 1.1–95% CI 0.9–1.2) (Table 3). Adjusted ORs were generally a little lower than the crude ORs, the highest observed being for passive smoking (OR 1.7–95% CI 1.5–2.0) (Table 3).

The mother not having undergone higher education and young age (under 18 at childbirth) were significantly associated with exposure to smoking in children. However, when accounting for socio-economic status, passive smoking appeared to be rarer in families in which French was not the first language. A significant interaction was noted between family structure and first language: when French was the language spoken at home, parental separation became more strongly associated with exposure to smoking in children compare with parents living together (OR 1.9–95% CI 1.6–2.2), whereas family structure mattered little in non-French-speaking families (OR 0.7–95% CI 0.4–1.3) (Table 4). In addition, exposure to smoking was significantly associated with low birthweight (OR 1.4–95% CI 1.2–1.8). We also observed that the more parents suffered from allergic symptoms, the more smoking there was at home. Conversely, when a child suffered from eczema, there was less often exposure to smoking (Table 3).

Regarding oral hygiene (tooth brushing and regular check-ups with a dentist), it seems that the more educated the mother was, and when French was the mother's first language, the better oral hygiene was. We found a similar pattern with screening for amblyopia: the lower the mother's level of education, and when French was not the first language, the less frequently children underwent screening (Table 3). Of course, the older a child was, the more they had had the opportunity to take advantage of dental and visual preventive check-ups. Also as expected, when a child attended a nursery accredited by the same organisation that manages vision screening (the ONE), they were more likely to undergo vision screening (Table 3).

Discussion

Thus, adjusting for socio-economic and cultural factors as well as for the mother's age at childbirth and certain characteristics of the children, we observed certain factors that were detrimental to children's health more frequently when the parents did not live together under the one roof compared with when the parents were together.

Passive smoking

Generally, smoking remains the primary risk factor of morbidity and mortality in Western countries; [23] in

Table 2 Parental behaviour influencing the health of children aged 28 to 32 months

Variables of behaviour	Total	Parents together	Parentsseparated	P
≥ 1 person smokes in the home daily –2006-09 (n = 13,667)	(*n* = 2962)	(*n* = 2473)	(*n* = 489)	
% yes	22.2	20.7	36.1	
Crude OR (95% CI)		1	2.2 (1.9–2.4)	< 0.001
Daily tooth brushing –2006-12 (*n* = 25,976)	(*n* = 2046)	(*n* = 1851)	(*n* = 195)	0.007
% No	7.9	7.7	9.3	
Crude OR (95% CI)		1	1.2 (1.1–1.4)	
Sees the dentist –2010-12 (*n* = 10,686)	(*n* = 7826)	(*n* = 7054)	(*n* = 772)	0.002
% No	81.2	80.8	84.8	
Crude OR (95% CI)		1	1.3 (1.1–1.6)	
Vision screening –2010-12 (n = 12,725)	(*n* = 4923)	(n=	(*n* = 527)	< 0.001
% No	41.4	4396)	48.2	
Crude OR (95% CI)		40.7	1.4 (1.2–1.5)	

Table 3 Behaviour of parents of children aged 28 to 32 months: adjusted ORs

	≥ 1 person smokes at home daily (2006–09)	Child does not brush his or her teeth daily (2006–12)	Child doesnot have a dentist (2010–12)	No vision screening (2010–12)
Variable	OR (95% CI)	OR (95% CI)	OR (95% CI)	OR (95% CI)
Family structure				
Parents together	1	1	1	1
Parents separated	1.7 (1.5–2.0)	1.1 (0.9–1.2)	1.3 (1.1–1.6)	1.2 (1.1–1.4)
P	< 0.001	0.8	0.03	0.005
Mother's level of education				
Third-level	1	1	1	1
Completed upper secondary	2.6 (2.3–2.9)	2.0 (1.7–2.3)	1.5 (1.3–1.7)	1.6 (1.4–1.8)
< Upper secondary	4.9 (4.3–5.6)	4.1 (3.6–4.7)	1.6 (1.4–1.9)	2.1 (1.8–2.4)
P	< 0.001	< 0.001	< 0.001	< 0.001
Mother's age at childbirth				
< 18 years	1.7 (1.1–2.7)	0.9 (0.5–1.4)		
18/30 years	1	1		
31/37 years	0.9 (0.8–1.0)	1.1 (1.0–1.3)		
38 years and more	1.1 (0.9–1.3)	1.3 (1.1–1.6)		
P	0.03	0.02		
Mother speaks French				
Yes	1	1	1	1
No	0.7 (0.6–0.9)	1.5 (1.3–1.7)	1.2 (1.1–1.3)	1.5 (1.4–1.7)
P	< 0.001	< 0.001	0.02	< 0.001
≥ 1 parent allergic				
No	1			
Yes	1.2 (1.1–1.4)			
P	< 0.001			
Nursery attendance				
Yes			1	1
No			0.8 (0.7–0.9)	2.0 (1.8–2.3)
P			0.006	< 0.001
Birthweight				
≥2500 g	1		1	
< 2500 g	1.4 (1.2–1.8)		1.3 (1.1–1.7)	
P	< 0.001		0.02	
Age of the child				
≥33 mo		1	1	1
28–32 mo		0.9 (0.7–1.1)	1.4 (1.1–1.9)	1.3 (1.0–1.6)
≤ 27 mo		1.2 (0.9–1.6)	1.7 (1.2–2.5)	1.9 (1.4–2.6)
P		0.002	0.01	< 0.001
Grommets				
Yes				1
No				0.7 (0.5–0.9)
P				< 0.001

Table 3 Behaviour of parents of children aged 28 to 32 months: adjusted ORs *(Continued)*

	≥ 1 person smokes at home daily (2006–09)	Child does not brush his or her teeth daily (2006–12)	Child doesnot have a dentist (2010–12)	No vision screening (2010–12)
The child has eczema				
No	1			
Yes	0.9 (0.7–1.0)			
P	0.04			

Belgium, we attribute 20,000 premature deaths (< 69 years) to smoking every year [24]. The health problems in children that are linked in the short term to smoking in their environment are well documented, including, besides the increased risk of sudden infant death syndrome [25], increased risk at all ages of upper [26] and lower [27] respiratory tract infections, as well as allergy symptoms [22]. In children aged 4 to 16 years, a correlation has also been described between cotinine levels and absenteeism from school, reduced respiratory function and wheezing [28]. In the longer term, nearly 17% of lung cancers in non-smokers may be attributable to high levels of passive smoking during childhood and adolescence [22, 29, 30]. Furthermore, in Belgium, parents who smoke double the rate of active smoking in their children [31]. Therefore, the main result of our study is that, regardless of the mother's age or level of education, children were exposed to passive smoking significantly more often when their parents were separated than when their parents were together. From a public health perspective, we estimated at the community level the impact of family structure on smoking at home by assessing the population attributable fraction, which amounted to 14.9%. This is far from being negligible for a relatively commonplace situation. These observations are similar to those made in a cross-sectional study that analysed a large sample of Belgian infants aged 7 to 11 months: [19] between 2010 and 2012, exposure to smoking was more frequent in children when the parents were separated, with an OR of 1.5 (95% CI 1.3–1.7) adjusting for the mother's age, occupation, and level of education. That confirms what has been said by Belgian GPs, who indeed offered an explanation for their observations: that separated parents exhibited more risky behaviours, including smoking, because of their anxiety [18]. Indeed, we find the link between separation, psychopathology,and parental smoking in other Belgian [8] and international [32, 33] studies. Consequently, our adjusted results that revealed more passive smoking in children when their parents did not live together appear to be consistent with those found in the literature. The association between passive smoking in children and parental separation seems particularly strong in families in which French was the first language, as we obtained an OR of approximately 2. In contrast, the risk was lower for children when French was not the language spoken at home, where the association between family structure and smoking disappeared (Tables 3 and 4). In the Wallonia-Brussels Federation, most non-Belgian families whose first language is not French are Muslim, and so come from a culture in which smoking habits are not necessarily comparable with those in the general population [34]. A recent systematic review has shown that smoking among immigrants coming from non-Western to Western countries was associated in men with a low level of education and with following their original way of life, but in women, conversely, the consumption of tobacco was associated with a high level of education and acculturation [35]. In our sample, 71% of women whose first language was not French had not finished or gone beyond secondary education (versus 18% of French-speaking mothers), which, according to the preceding study, is associated with a lower smoking rate in these foreign-born women.

Table 4 Interactions

Smoking at home*		
Family structure	First language: FR Adjusted OR (95% CI)	First language: ≠FR Adjusted OR (95% CI)
Parents together	1	1
Parents separated	1.9 (1.6–2.2)	0.7 (0.4–1.3)
P	< 0.001	0.3

*Adjusted for mother's level of education, child's birthweight, child's age on examination, and family's allergy status

Oral hygiene

To a lesser extent than passive smoking, when parents were separated, we observed less optimal behaviour in children in terms of oral hygiene, namely less regular brushing of teeth (non-significant adjusted OR), but in particular less frequent visits to the dentist. We should point out that the ONE recommends a first visit to the dentist between the eruption of the first tooth and the age of 2 years at the latest, when most primary teeth are in place. This is consistent with the guidelines of the American Academy of Pediatrics, for example [36]. In our sample, there existed a positive association between the mother's level of education and oral hygiene. The literature likewise associates social status and oral health [37, 38], but rarely family structure. In Brazil, not living with biological parents under the same roof may be more associated with poorer dental health, including cavities [39, 40]. The same observation has been made in the United States [15].

Vision screening

We obtained similar results with vision screening as we did with oral hygiene. There exists a positive association between the mother's level of education and children's taking receiving this preventive service. That being said, children who did not live with parents who were still together received this screening less often. For vision screening and oral hygiene, it seems reasonable to interpret these results in light of the research (in Belgium, for example) that shows health differences according to economic, social and family status, particularly where access to preventive services is concerned [41].

Strengths and weaknesses of the study

This study has a cross-sectional design, so the direction of the associations calculated between family structure and parental behaviour is unknown to us. Nevertheless, the fact that our analysis shows a statistical association between family structure and parental behaviour, and comparison with results provided by the literature, confirms for us that parents not living together constitutes at the very least an indicator of risk for the suboptimal behaviours studied here that influence children's health. All socio-cultural strata were represented in our sample, thereby allowing us to build our regression models. However there was at least one selection bias. Families who bring their children to preventive check-ups at the ONE between 28 and 32 months are generally socially advantaged: 46% of the mothers had obtained a higher education qualification, whereas the figure does not exceed 30% in the general population [42] (Table 5 – Appendix). As national statistics in Belgium describe financial income in terms of euros per year, it is more difficult to compare the family incomes reported in our sample with those of the general population. However, the Brussels-Capital Health and Social Observatory [43], Wallonia Region [44], and the social integration services [45] report that benefits (unemployment or social protection benefits) are the only source of income for around 20% of the general population, which may be very cautiously compared with the 11% of families in our sample. This bias cannot be due to how the ONE operates, as it offers its services free of charge to all families, Belgian or foreign, regardless of immigration status. The positive association that persists in Belgium [41] between social status and use of preventive services is, in contrast, a possible explanation. This bias does not necessarily invalidate our results. The study population was relatively advantaged and, therefore, more likely to use preventive services, and so this confirms that the association between family structure (parents living together or not) and parental behaviour is independent of social status. We could even hypothesise that the selection bias minimised the ORs calculated. Lastly, our analysis arrived at expected conclusions, namely that the mother's level of education and age at childbirth are predictors of behaviour in relation to health, which corroborates the other results found in our sample.

Conclusion

Implications for GPs

In French-speaking Belgium, in terms of prevention targeting children under three, our results reveal that, whatever the social environment, information work is necessary for all families regarding passive smoking, oral hygiene and vision screening. Our work confirms, however, that among the most precarious families, parental behaviour is less optimal. Here the role of the GP is essential; our statistics show that contacts with the family doctor increase with the level of poverty [46]. Moreover, our study shows that when parents are separated, parental behaviour is significantly poorer concerning the health of children aged under 3 years (passive smoking, oral hygiene and amblyopic screening) regardless of the level of maternal education or cultural environment. These results are echoed in other studies, which also show a greater risk of exposure to smoking, suboptimal nutrition and lower adherence to the immunisation schedule when infants did not live with two parents who were together [19]. In the event of parental separation, family doctors or paediatricians should be more focused on parental behaviour that may affect the health of their children such as interruption of contraception, pregnancy plans and/or postnatal follow-up. These are examples of situations where the GP could inform his patients at this level. The aim is not to stigmatize some families, but rather to better target health promotion work. Other studies, including prospective studies, should be conducted to better understand these public health challenges.

Appendix

Table 5 Sociodemographic characteristics and family structure

Variable	Parents living together n (%)	Separated parents n (%)	P
Gender			0.240
Boy	13,271 (51.4)	1411 (50.2)	
Girl	12,549 (48.6)	1398 (49.8)	
Child's age			0.006
≤27 mo	1805 (6.9)	238 (8.4)	
28–32 mo	23,223 (89.4)	2474 (87.5)	
≥33 mo	962 (3.7)	117 (4.1)	
Birth weight (g)			< 0.001
< 2500	1697 (6.5)	293 (10.3)	
≥2500	24,330 (93.5)	2542 (89.7)	
BMI – percentiles			0.797
p3-p97	22,687 (92.0)	2481 (92.0)	
>p97	1513 (6.1)	171 (6.3)	
<p3	457 (1.9)	46 (1.7)	
Mother's age in years at childbirth			< 0.001
< 18	131 (0.5)	108 (3.9)	
18–30	14,964 (59.0)	1670 (60.7)	
31–37	8549 (33.7)	739 (26.8)	
≥38	1729 (6.8)	236 (8.6)	
Mother's level of education			< 0.001
< Upper secondary school	4497 (20.5)	836 (36.3)	
Completed upper secondary school	6697 (30.6)	801 (34.8)	
Completed third-level/university or not	10,714 (48.9)	666 (28.9)	
Mother's occupation (2006–9)			< 0.001
Unemployed/stay-at-home	2343 (36.6)	380 (50.7)	
Early retirement/work incapacity/invalidity	101 (1.6)	36 (4.8)	
Student	17 (0.3)	8 (1.1)	
Works full time or part time/career break/parental leave	3948 (61.6)	325 (43.4)	
Family income (2006–9)			< 0.001
No stable income	63 (1.0)	20 (2.6)	
1or 2 incomes from benefits	503 (7.9)	303 (40.0)	
1 income from employment	2000 (31.3)	395 (52.1)	
2 incomes, of which ≥1 income from employment	3834 (59.9)	40 (5.3)	
First language (2006–12)			< 0.001
French	19,412 (77.0)	2255 (81.9)	
Other	5813 (23.0)	499 (18.1)	
Goes to a nursery (2010–12)			0.927
Yes	5977 (55.8)	610 (56.0)	
No	4731 (44.2)	480 (44.0)	

Abbreviations

BMI: Body mass index; ONE: Office of Birth and Childhood; OR: Odds ratio

Acknowledgments

The authors would like to thank the entire staff of the *Conseil Scientifique et de la Direction Etudes et Stratégies de l'Office de la Naissance et de l'Enfance* (ONE-Office of Birth and Childhood) for graciously providing the data used in this study. The authors thank Dr. Gabrielle Cremer from Cremer Consulting SARL and ISO Translation & Publishing sprl for expert English editing. They also extend their thanks to the Department of general medicine at the *Université Libre de Bruxelles,* Belgium, for providing logistic support to the project. Lastly, the first author extends her thanks to the School of Public Health, Brussels, where she attended a training course in biostatistics.

Funding

The Department of General Medicine of the Université Libre de Bruxelles, Belgium, provided logistical support to the project.

Author's contributions

NK: Author who made the research question-Contributions to the conception and design of the work-Main author who analyzed and interpreted the data-Who wrote the article. MD-W: Substantial contributions to the conception and design of the work, analysis and interpretation of data for the work-Drafting the work and revising it critically for important intellectual content-Final approval of the version to be published-Agreement to be accountable for all aspects of the work in ensuring that questions related to the accuracy or integrity of any part of the work are appropriately investigated and resolved. MS: Substantial contributions to the conception of the work-Revising the work critically for important intellectual content-Final approval of the version to be published-Agreement to be accountable for all aspects of the work in ensuring that questions related to the accuracy or integrity of any part of the work are appropriately investigated and resolved. MR: Substantial contributions to the conception of the work-Revising the work critically for important intellectual content-Final approval of the version to be published-Agreement to be accountable for all aspects of the work in ensuring that questions related to the accuracy or integrity of any part of the work are appropriately investigated and resolved. IG: Substantial contributions to the conception of the work-Revising the work critically for important intellectual content-Final approval of the version to be published-Agreement to be accountable for all aspects of the work in ensuring that questions related to the accuracy or integrity of any part of the work are appropriately investigated and resolved. All authors read and approved the final manuscript.

Author's information

NK is a general practitioner and has a PhD in Medical Sciences. She is Professor in charge of lectures on applied paediatrics in first-line general medicine at the Medical Faculty of the *Université libre de Bruxelles* and in charge of a lecture on initiation to general practice and Evidence Based medicine at the Medical Faculty of the *Université de Mons.* She is also actively involved in research pertaining to the family domain, infant health, intra-family violence, and parental separation. M D-W has a PhD in public health, is Professor of biostatistics, and Director of the *Centre de Recherche en Epidémiologie, Biostatistique et Recherche Clinique, Ecole de santé publique,Université Libre de Bruxelles,* Belgium. MS is a general practitioner (MD) and Professor, in charge of a lecture on initiation to general practice. He is involved in research on prevention. Associate Dean of the Medical Faculty of the *Université libre de Bruxelles,* Belgium. MR has a PhD in public health, is a general practitioner (MD) and a researcher, and in charge of lectures on public and community-based health issues at the Medical Faculty of the *Université libre de Bruxelles,* Belgium. IG is a sociologist and has a PhD in public health; she is a researcher notably concerning determinants of health regarding children and youth. She is Director of the *Service communautaire en promotion de la santé (SIPES), Ecole de santé publique, Université Libre de Bruxelles,* Belgium.

Competing interests

All authors declare: no support from any organisation for the submitted work; no financial relationships with any organisations that might have an interest in the submitted work in the previous 3 years; no other relationships or activities that could appear to have influenced the submitted work.

Author details

[1]Université Libre de Bruxelles, General Medicine Department, Campus Facultaire Erasme, Route de Lennik 808/612, 1070 Brussels, Belgium. [2]Université Libre de Bruxelles, Centre for Research in Epidemiology, Biostatistics and Clinical Research, School of Public Health, Campus Erasme CP598, Route de Lennik 808, 1070 Brussels, Belgium. [3]Université Libre de Bruxelles, Department of Health Information Promotion Education (SIPES), School of Public Health, Campus Erasme CP598, Route de Lennik 808, 1070 Brussels, Belgium.

References

1. Europa statistics explained. File: crude divorce rate, selected years, 1960–2011. http://ec.europa.eu/eurostat/statistics-explained/index.php?title=Special:ListFiles&user=Marcumc Accessed 17 Feb 2018.
2. United States Census Bureau. The 2012 statistical abstract. Births, deaths, marriages, & divorces: marriages and divorces. https://www.census.gov/prod/2011pubs/12statab/vitstat.pdf. Accessed 17 Feb 2018.
3. Statistics Canada. Description for Chart 8. Divorce and suicide rates, per 100,000, Canada, 1950 to 2008. http://www.statcan.gc.ca/pub/82-624-x/2012001/article/chart/11696-02-chart8-eng.htm. Accessed 17 Feb 2018.
4. Australian Bureau of Statistics. Marriages and Divorces, Australia. 2013. http://www.abs.gov.au/ausstats/abs@.nsf/mf/3310.0. Accessed 17 Feb 2018.
5. Statistics Belgium. Cohabitations légales.http://www.ibz.rrn.fgov.be/fr/registre-national/statistiques-de-population/. Accessed 17 Feb 2018.
6. Statistique Canada. Portrait des familles et situation des cas particuliers dans les ménages au Canada. 2011. http://www12.statcan.gc.ca/census-recensement/2011/as-sa/98-312-x/98-312-x2011001-fra.cfm. Accessed 17 Feb 2018.
7. Babb P, Bird C, Bradford B, Burtenshaw S, Gardener D, Howell S, et al. Social focus in brief: children 2002. National. Statistics. 2002; http://www.fairplayforchildren.org/pdf/1228009730.pdf. Accessed 17 Feb 2018.
8. Petit S, Casman MT. Utilisation des données du PSBH pour mieux connaître les familles recomposées en Belgique: rapport de recherche. Fondation Baudouin. 2008. https://pure.fundp.ac.be/ws/files/12627193/pub2008_1839_l_enfantdanslafamillerecomposee.pdf. Accessed 17 Feb 2018.
9. Vanassche S, Corijn M, Sodermans A K, Matthijs K. Gezinstrajecten van ouders en kinderen na een (echt) scheiding. 2013. https://lirias.kuleuven.be/bitstream/123456789/394469/2/Gezinstransities.pdf. Accessed 17 Feb 2018.
10. Office de la naissance et de l'enfance. http://www.one.be/presentation/about-us/. Accessed 17 Feb 2018.
11. Fontaine L, Goetghebuer T, Liégeois M, Mauroy MC, Morales I, Ndame Ebongue S. Rapport 2010; Banque de Données médico-sociales. Office de la naissance et de de l'enfance. Fédération Wallonie-Bruxelles. 2012. http://www.one.be/uploads/tx_ttproducts/datasheet/Rapport_BDMS_2012_BD.pdf. Accessed 17 Feb 2018.
12. Decant P, de Smet P, Favresse D, Godin I. la sante des Élèves de 5e et 6e années primaires. 2013. Résultats de l'enquête HBSC 2010 en Fédération Wallonie-Bruxelles. https://dipot.ulb.ac.be/dspace/bitstream/2013/142427/1/HBSC_primaire_2013.pdf. Accessed 17 Feb 2018.
13. Moreau N, Favresse D, de Smet P, Godin I. la sante des Élèves de l'enseignement secondaire. 2013. Résultats de l'enquête HBSC 2010 en Fédération Wallonie-Bruxelles. http://sipes.ulb.ac.be/index.php?option=com_mtree&task=att_download&link_id=165&cf_id=24. Accessed 17 Feb 2018.
14. Statistics Belgium. Naissances et fécondité. Evolution du nombre de naissances en Belgique. 1830–2012. https://statbel.fgov.be/fr/themes/population/naissances-et-fecondite#figures. Accessed 17 Feb 2018.
15. Bramlett MD, Blumberg SJ. Family structure and Children's physical and mental health. Health Aff. 2007;26(2):549–58.
16. Seijo D, Fariña F, Corras T, Novo M, Arce R. Estimating the epidemiology and quantifying the damages of parental separation in children and adolescents. Front Psychol. 2016;7:1611.
17. Martinón JM, Fariña F, Corras T, Seijo D, Souto A, Novo M. Impacto de la ruptura de los progenitores en el estado de salud física de los hijos. European Journal of Education and Psychology. 2017;10(1):9–14.
18. Kacenelenbogen N, Roland M, Schetgen M, Dusart AF. The general practitioner and 510 children of separated parents in Belgium: a qualitative study and its implications. J Gen Pract. 2013;1:133.
19. Kacenelenbogen N, Dramaix-Wilmet M, Schetgen M, Roland M. Parental separation and behaviours that influence the health of infants aged 7-11

months: a cross-sectional study. BMJ Open. 2014 Jul;4(7):e005183. https://doi.org/10.1136/bmjopen-2014-005183.
20. Office de la Naissance et de l'Enfance. Consultations pour enfants. http://www.one.be/index.php?id=2391. Accessed 17 Feb 2018.
21. Levi DM, Knill DC, Bavelier D. Stereopsis and amblyopia: a mini-review. Vis Res. 2015;114:17–30.
22. Indicateurs de suivi des enfants à l'ONE. http://www.one.be/uploads/tx_ttproducts/datasheet/RA_BDMS_2002-2003_03.pdf. Accessed 17 Feb 2018.
23. World Health Organization. GLOBAL HEALTH RISKS GLOBAL HEALTH RISKS WHO mortality and burden of disease attributable to selected major risks. 2009. http://www.who.int/healthinfo/global_burden_disease/GlobalHealthRisks_report_full.pdf. Accessed 17 Feb 2018.
24. Peto R, Lopez A D, Boreham, Thun M. Mortality from smoking in developed countries 1950–2000. 2nd edition, revised June 2006. http://gas.ndph.ox.ac.uk/deathsfromsmoking/download%20files/Country%20presentations/Malta/Malta%20data.pdf. Accessed 17 Feb 2018.
25. Carmona RH, Moritsugu KP, Williams RC, Near KA, Schoenfeld R, Gerberding JL, et al. The health consequences of involuntary exposure to tobacco smoke: a report of the surgeon general. US Department Of Health And human Services Public Health Service Office of the Surgeon General. 2006;709.
26. Lieu JE, Feinstein AR. Effect of gestational and passive smoke exposure on ear infections in children. Arch Pediatr Adolesc Med. 2002;156(2):147.
27. Oberg M, Jaakkola MS, Woodward A, et al. Worldwide burden of disease from exposure tosecond-hand smoke: a retrospective analysis of data from 192 countries. Lancet. 2011;377(9760):139.
28. Mannino DM, Moorman JE, Kingsley B, et al. Health effects related to environmental tobacco smoke exposure in children in the United States: data from the third National Health and nutrition examination survey. Arch Pediatr Adolesc Med. 2001;155(1):36.
29. Pang D, McNally R, Birch JM. Parental smoking and childhood cancer: results from the United Kingdom childhood cancer study. Br J Cancer. 2003;88(3):373.
30. Boffetta P, Trédaniel J, Greco A. Risk of childhood cancer and adult lung cancer after 558 childhood exposure to passive smoke: a meta-analysis. Environ Health Perspect. 2000;108(1):73.
31. Favresse D., De Smet P., Tabac, alcool, drogues et multimédias chez les jeunes en Communauté française de Belgique. Résultats de l'enquête HBSC 2006. Service d'Information Promotion Education Santé (SIPES), ESP-ULB, Bruxelles, 2008. http://sipes.ulb.ac.be/index.php?option=com_mtree&task=att_download&link_id=13&cf_id=24. Accessed 17 Feb 2018.
32. Clancy N, Zwar N, Depression RR. Smoking and smoking cessation: a qualitative study. Fam Pract. 2013;30(5):587–92.
33. Lawrence D, Hafekost J, Hull P, Mitrou F, Zubrick SR. Smoking, mental illness and socioeconomic disadvantage: analysis of the Australian National Survey of mental health and wellbeing. BMC Public Health. 2013;11(13):462.
34. Philippe H, Lucchini S. "Diversité sociolinguistique et ressources partagées. Regards critiques sur les politiques d'intégration linguistique en Belgique'." Revista de Sociolingüística. 2005. https://www.researchgate.net/profile/Silvia_Lucchini2/publication/28087857_Diversite_sociolinguistique_et_ressources_partagees_Regards_critiques_sur_les_politiques_d'integration_linguistique_en_Belgique/. Accessed 17 Feb 2018.
35. Reiss K, Lehnhard J, Razum O. Factors associated with smoking in immigrants from non579 western to western countries – what role does acculturation play? A systematic review. Tob Induc Dis. 2015;13(1):11.
36. Hale KJ, American Academy of Pediatrics, Section on Pediatric. Dentistry oral health risk assessment timing and establishment of the dental home. Pediatrics. 2003;111(5 Pt 1):1113–6.
37. Piovesan C, Antunes JL, Guedes RS, Ardenghi TM. Impact of socioeconomic and clinical factors on child oral health-related quality of life (COHRQoL). Qual Life Res. 2010;19(9):1359–66.
38. Petersen PE. Sociobehavioural risk factors in dental caries - international perspectives. Community Dent Oral Epidemiol. 2005;33(4):274–9.
39. Paula JS, Leite ICG, Almeida AB, Ambrosano GMB. 590 Pereira AC, Mialhe F L the influence of oral health conditions, socioeconomic status and home environment factors on schoolchildren's self-perception of quality of life. Health Qual Life Outcomes. 2012;10:6.
40. Paula JS, Leite IC, de Almeida AB, Ambrosano GM, Mialhe FL. The impact of socioenvironmental characteristics on domains of oral health-related quality of life in Brazilian schoolchildren. BMC Oral Health. 2013 Jan 28;13:10.
41. Bossuyt N, Van Oyen H. Rapport de santé: Différences socio-économiques en santé. Institut Scientifique de la Santé Publique Service d'Epidémiologie IPH/EPI REPORTS N° 2001–013. https://www.wiv-isp.be/epidemio/epifr/santefr/sociofr.pdf. Accessed 17 Feb 2018.
42. Stabel. La belgique en Chiffre. Census 2011 - Age, Situation sur le marché de l'emploi, Pays de citoyenneté, Niveau d'instruction, Lieu de résidence, Sexe, Sexe. https://statbel.fgov.be/fr/open-data/census-2011-age-situation-sur-le-marche-de-lemploi-pays-de-citoyennete-niveau-1. Accessed 17 Feb 2018.
43. Observatoire de la santé et du Social Bruxelles. Baromètre social. Rapport bruxellois sur l'état de La pauvreté 2013 .http://www.ccc-ggc.irisnet.be/sites/default/files/documents/graphics/rapport-pauvrete/barometre_social_2013.pdf. Accessed 17 Feb 2018.
44. Statistics Belgium. Taux d'emploi, taux de chômage, taux d'activité par sexe pour la Belgique et les régions, derniers 4 trimestres. https://statbel.fgov.be/fr/themes/emploi-formation/marche-du-travail/emploi-et-chomage. Accessed 17 Feb 2018.
45. SPP Intégration Sociale. Bulletin statistique 2013.2. https://www.mi-is.be/sites/default/files/documents/bulletin_2013_septembre.pdf. Accessed 17 Feb 2018.
46. Drieskens S, Gisle L. Enquête de Santé 2013 Rapport 3 : Utilisation des services de soins de santé et des services sociaux. Institut Scientifique de Santé Publique. Direction Opérationnelle Santé publique et surveillance. 2013. https://his.wiv-isp.be/fr/Documents%20partages/Summ_HC_FR_2013.pdf. Accessed 9 July 2017. Accessed 17 Feb 2018.

6

Health care quality measures for children and adolescents in Foster Care: feasibility testing in electronic records

Katherine J. Deans[1], Peter C. Minneci[1], Kristine M. Nacion[2], Karen Leonhart[1], Jennifer N. Cooper[1], Sarah Hudson Scholle[3] and Kelly J. Kelleher[1*]

Abstract

Background: Preventive quality measures for the foster care population are largely untested. The objective of the study is to identify healthcare quality measures for young children and adolescents in foster care and to test whether the data required to calculate these measures can be feasibly extracted and interpreted within an electronic health records or within the Statewide Automated Child Welfare Information System.

Methods: The AAP *Recommendations for Preventive Pediatric Health Care* served as the guideline for determining quality measures. Quality measures related to well child visits, developmental screenings, immunizations, trauma-related care, BMI measurements, sexually transmitted infections and depression were defined. Retrospective chart reviews were performed on a cohort of children in foster care from a single large pediatric institution and related county. Data available in the Ohio Statewide Automated Child Welfare Information System was compared to the same population studied in the electronic health record review. Quality measures were calculated as observed (received) to expected (recommended) ratios (O/E ratios) to describe the actual quantity of recommended health care that was received by individual children.

Results: Electronic health records and the Statewide Automated Child Welfare Information System data frequently lacked important information on foster care youth essential for calculating the measures. Although electronic health records were rich in encounter specific clinical data, they often lacked custodial information such as the dates of entry into and exit from foster care. In contrast, Statewide Automated Child Welfare Information System included robust data on custodial arrangements, but lacked detailed medical information. Despite these limitations, several quality measures were devised that attempted to accommodate these limitations.

Conclusions: In this feasibility testing, neither the electronic health records at a single institution nor the county level Statewide Automated Child Welfare Information System was able to independently serve as a reliable source of data for health care quality measures for foster care youth. However, the ability to leverage both sources by matching them at an individual level may provide the complement of data necessary to assess the quality of healthcare.

Keywords: Foster care, Quality measures, Electronic health record, Statewide automated child welfare information system

* Correspondence: Kelly.kelleher@nationwidechildrens.org
[1]The Research Institute at Nationwide Children's Hospital, 700 Children's Drive, FB3145, Columbus, OH 43205, USA
Full list of author information is available at the end of the article

Background

Demands for information on the quality of pediatric preventive care have spurred investment in the development of quality measures designed to access the current state of children's health care and ultimately define areas for improvement [1]. Specific quality measures for the foster care population, though, are largely untested [2, 3], even though youth entering foster care have greater physical, developmental, and mental health needs than their peers in the general population [4, 5]. Although children in foster care are known to have higher rates of social and medical morbidity, guidelines for the care of foster children are rarely adhered to in routine practice and may be difficult to measure [6–10]. One of the most important ways to improve care and reduce poor long term health outcomes is through the development and testing of reliable quality measures for these high risk youth. To date, measurement has largely been dependent on labor-intensive chart reviews. Two other possible sources of quality data that might be extracted electronically exist for foster care children [11]. A clinical electronic health record (EHR) has potential to provide comprehensive and detailed patient-level data with electronic extraction on a large population. In addition, the Statewide Automated Child Welfare Information System (SACWIS) is a database used by protective services agencies to hold the official case records of children in care. Many states hold health data in their SACWIS records.

In order for these datasets to be useful, each of them would have to contain sufficient detail on health services to compare them against recommended guidelines, entry and exit dates for foster care to calculate eligibility, and demographic data for stratification. The primary objectives of this study were to identify quality measures, such as the appropriate number of well care visits, vaccinations and developmental screening for young children (ages 0–3) and adolescents (ages 12–18) in foster care and test whether the data required to calculate these measures can be feasibly interpreted within an EHR or within SACWIS. These two age groups were chosen because of the diversity of well care measures available for testing in both groups.

Methods

This work was performed as part of the Children's Health Insurance Program Reauthorization Act (CHIPRA) Pediatric Quality Measures Program (PQMP), specifically as part of the National Collaborative for Innovation in Quality Measurement (NCINQ). Our approach considered three time periods of child welfare engagement: (1) entry into foster care, (2) ongoing foster care, and (3) foster home change or exit. [12–24] We gathered input from a national advisory panel representing foster care alumni, national policy makers, state child welfare and Medicaid officials, health plan staff, and academic researchers.

Retrospective chart reviews were performed at Nationwide Children's Hospital (NCH). For the study of children aged 0 to 3 years, we abstracted data from the time period of January 1, 2007- February 28, 2013 from children who met inclusion criteria: 1) In foster care (not including kinship care) within Franklin County, Ohio, and 2) at least one comprehensive well-care visit at a primary care physician (PCP) clinic or foster care specialty clinic at NCH. For the study of children aged 12–18 years, we abstracted data from the time period of January 1, 2009- October 31, 2013 with the same criteria. All extracted data was for care that occurred while the child was in foster care. We defined foster care as full-time care provided by an approved foster care family or group home and excluded any care provided by kin or close family friends (Table 1).

Chart reviews were performed by two staff members familiar with EHR data abstraction (Epic Systems Corporation, Wisconsin). An instruction document outlining the data elements and their common locations was created and used by both reviewers. Inter-rater reliability analyses were performed on the first 41 reviewed records of children within each age group to ensure reproducibility between data abstractors with excellent reproducibility [25, 26]. Study data were managed using REDCap data tool [27]. This study was approved by the NCH Institutional Review Board.

Because exact entry and exit dates for out of home care were often missing from EHRs, entry and exit dates were calculated in three different ways depending on the availability of data: 1) exact entry or exit dates were recorded whenever available, 2) the midpoint of an available date range (dates between health care visits wherein a child was documented to have entered/exited foster care) was used for entry or exit dates, and finally 3) the first well-care visit (or other documented healthcare encounter for adolescents) after entry was considered the entry date and the last well-care visit (or other documented healthcare encounter for adolescents) was considered the exit date when an exact date or date range was unavailable.

SACWIS is a "comprehensive automated case management tool that supports foster care and adoptions assistance case management practice." [28] This system is intended to hold the official case record of all children currently or previously in out-of-home care in a state. Not all states use SACWIS, and there is substantial heterogeneity across states in the contents of SACWIS [28]. This study used data available in the Franklin County, Ohio SACWIS system in order to reflect the

Table 1 Calculation of Proposed Quality Measures for Children in Foster Care within an EHR: Proportion Measures

Measure	Numerator	Denominator	Guideline(s) Referenced	Notes
Young children (age 0–3 years)				
1st well-care visit within 30 days of initial entry into foster care	Children with a first well-care visit within 30 days of entry	All children with an exact date or date range of entry into foster care	Health Care of Young Children in Foster Care [23]	Only children with an exact date or date range of initial entry into foster care are included in the denominator
Appropriate number of well care visits for their age during foster care	Children who received all recommended well-care visits for their age during foster care	All children	Recommendations for Preventive Pediatric Health Care [24]	Well-care visits were not required to occur within any particular window of time around the exact ages of recommended well-care visits
Appropriate number of vaccinations by age 1	Children with all recommended vaccinations received by 1 year of age, whether received while in foster care or not	All children who turned 1 year of age while in foster care	CDC 2013 Immunization Schedules [32] HEDIS Childhood Immunization Status [29]	HEDIS requirements for the appropriate timing of vaccines as specified for their Combination #2 measure were followed. Only those vaccinations that are supposed to occur by age 1 were included (i.e. DTaP, IPV, HiB and HepB)).
Appropriate number of vaccinations by age 2	Children with all recommended vaccinations received by 2 years of age, whether received while in foster care or not	All children who turned 2 years of age while in foster care	CDC 2013 Immunization Schedules [32] HEDIS Childhood Immunization Status [29]	HEDIS requirements for the appropriate timing of vaccines as specified for their Combination #2 measure were followed. Only those vaccinations that are supposed to occur by age 2 were included (i.e. DTaP, IPV, HiB, HepB, MMR and VZV)
Appropriate number of lead screenings for their age during foster care	Children who received the appropriate number of lead screenings while in foster care	All children who turned 1 year and/ or 2 years of age while in foster care	Guidelines for Medicaid Lead Testing [33]	Screenings had to occur during the following age periods, if the child was in foster care at age 1 year and 2 years respectively: 9–21 months of age and 22–36 months of age
Appropriate number of developmental screenings for their age during foster care	Children who received all recommended developmental screenings for their age during foster care	All children	Recommendations for Preventive Pediatric Health Care [24]	Screenings were not required to occur within any particular window of time around the exact ages of recommended screenings. Documentation that a specific standardized tool used was not necessary; any mention of a developmental screening was included.
Developmental screening during foster care within 3 months after documentation of traumatic brain injury (TBI)	Children who received a developmental screening within 3 months after documentation of TBI	All children diagnosed with a TBI prior to entry into foster care	Evaluation of suspected child physical abuse [21] Head Injury. Triage, Assessment, Investigation and Early Management of Head Injury in Infants, Children and Adults [13]	A 3 month window was used based on professional medical opinion
Follow up skeletal survey after receiving an initial skeletal survey	Children who received a follow up skeletal survey	All children who received an initial skeletal survey	Evaluation of suspected child physical abuse [21]	The follow up skeletal survey was not required to occur within any certain period of time after the initial skeletal survey
Care coordination letters at foster home changes	Instances of foster home changes that had evidence of a care coordination letter	All documented foster home changes	Health Care of Young Children in Foster Care [23]	

Table 1 Calculation of Proposed Quality Measures for Children in Foster Care within an EHR: Proportion Measures *(Continued)*

Measure	Numerator	Denominator	Guideline(s) Referenced	Notes
Adolescents (age 12–18 years)				
Appropriate number of well care visits during foster care	Adolescents who received all recommended annual well-care visits during foster care	All adolescents	Recommendations for Preventive Pediatric Health Care [24]	For every portion of a year that a child spent in foster care, whether that time was continuous or not, at least one well care visit should have occurred
Appropriate adolescent immunizations	Adolescents who received at least one TdaP vaccination on or after their 10th birthday but before their 19th birthday and at least one Meningococcal vaccination on or after their 11th birthday but before their 19th birthday, whether received while in foster care or not	All adolescents	CDC 2013 Immunization Schedules [32] HEDIS Adolescent Immunization Measure [29]	TdaP or Td vaccinations both counted towards this measure
Three Human Papilloma Virus (HPV) vaccinations in females	Three Human Papilloma Virus (HPV) vaccinations on or after the 9th birthday but before the 13th birthday, whether received while in foster care or not	Females only	HEDIS Human Papillomavirus Vaccine for Female Adolescents Measure [29]	
Appropriate number of BMI measurements	Adolescents who received all recommended annual BMI measurements during foster care	All adolescents	Recommendations for Preventive Pediatric Health Care [24]	For every portion of a year that a child spent in foster care, whether that time was continuous or not, at least one BMI measurement should have occurred
Appropriate number of drug use assessments	Adolescents who received all recommended annual drug use assessments during foster care	All adolescents	Recommendations for Preventive Pediatric Health Care [24]	For every portion of a year that a child spent in foster care, whether that time was continuous or not, at least one drug use assessment should have occurred
Appropriate number of alcohol use assessments	Adolescents who received all recommended annual alcohol use assessments during foster care	All adolescents	Recommendations for Preventive Pediatric Health Care [24]	For every portion of a year that a child spent in foster care, whether that time was continuous or not, at least one alcohol use assessment should have occurred
Appropriate number of sexually transmitted infection screenings	Adolescents who received all recommended annual chlamydia and gonorrhea screenings during foster care	All adolescents	Recommendations for Preventive Pediatric Health Care [24]	For every portion of a year that a child spent in foster care, whether that time was continuous or not, at least one chlamydia and at least one gonorrhea screening should have occurred
Appropriate number of depression screenings	Adolescents who received all recommended annual depression screenings during foster care	All adolescents	Recommendations for Preventive Pediatric Health Care [24]	For every portion of a year that a child spent in foster care, whether that time was continuous or not, at least one depression screening should have occurred

same population studied in the EHR review. A data extract from SACWIS was sent to the investigators containing the records of all children who were in custody during the study period and met inclusion criteria. Inclusion criteria were identical to those used for the EHR review, with the one exception that documentation of a well-care visit was not required. To determine whether data from the EHR and SACWIS could be reliably combined for analyses, we performed matching, using social security numbers when these were available in both the EHR and in SACWIS. As social security numbers were unavailable in one or both databases for approximately 70% of patients, when this number was unavailable we also considered records to be from the same child if they matched on all four of the following criteria: last name, first name, date of birth, and gender. A last name in the EHR was considered to match a last name in SACWIS if the first four characters were identical. Both the primary name and alias listed in SACWIS were considered. A first name in the EHR was considered to match a first name in SACWIS if the first four characters, either with or without symbols, were identical. Again, both the primary name and alias listed in SACWIS were considered.

Continuous variables were described with medians and interquartile ranges (IQR) as none were normally distributed. Categorical variables were described using frequencies and percentages. Quality measures were calculated in either the entire young child or the entire adolescent study cohort. We chose to review a sample of 400 EHRs for both the young child and adolescent EHR studies. The medical record numbers of all included children were sorted randomly such that the children whose charts were reviewed were a random sample of all children who could have been included.

In order to provide the most flexible information on the feasibility of obtaining the proposed quality measures from our data sources, two methods were used to calculate the proposed quality measures: proportions and observed-to-expected ratios. Most quality measures of pediatric healthcare focus on the former. Unfortunately, calculations of such often require steady denominators with fixed lengths of follow-up such as the number of children screened over the number of children eligible who were tracked for a full year. Because foster children cycle in and out of care, the denominator calculations may be ineffective in describing this unstable population.

Several quality measures were calculated as observed (received) to expected (recommended) ratios (O/E ratios) to better describe the actual quantity of recommended health care that was received by individual children, whereas the proportion measures indicate the percentage of children in the study cohort that received all recommended care. Weighted mean O/E ratios were calculated wherein each child's individual O/E ratio was weighted by his or her total time spent in foster care during the study period. This weighting was performed because it enabled children who spent more time in foster care to contribute more to the calculated O/E measures. We used the AAP *Recommendations for Preventive Pediatric Health Care* as the guideline for determining the expected, or recommended, number of well-care visits and developmental screenings in the young children and the recommended number of well-care visits, BMI measurements, drug use assessments, alcohol use assessments, sexually transmitted infection screenings, and depression screenings in the adolescents [24]. For each measure, an individual O/E ratio was calculated for each child and then a weighted average of these individual O/E ratios was calculated to provide an appropriate average O/E for the entire cohort.

Continuous variables were described with medians and interquartile ranges (IQR). Categorical variables were described using frequencies and percentages. We also attempted to extract data on the same types of health care encounters that were examined in the chart reviews. SAS version 9.3 (SAS Institute Inc., NC) was used to analyze all data.

Results

Study of EHR data of children age 0–3 years

A total of 400 charts were reviewed. Twenty-five children were excluded from analyses because they did not meet inclusion criteria; 8 were without any well-care visits and 17 entered foster care prior to January 1, 2007. This left 375 patients to be included in analyses (Table 2). Overall, the median duration of time spent in foster care during the study period of 9.2 months (IQR 3.0–17.9) (Table 2). Around 76% of children had exact dates of entry but only 44.8% of children had both exact entry and exact exit dates recorded in their EHR. A quarter of the study population lacked documentation in their EHR of the reason for their first entry into foster care.

Table 3 illustrates the performance of the proposed health care quality measures for young children within our EHR. Among 341 children in the study cohort with an exact date or date range of initial entry into foster care, we observed that 78.6% received a well-care visit within 30 days of entry. Over 79% of all children included in this study received the appropriate number of lead screenings, and 100% with traumatic brain injury (TBI) had a developmental screening within 3 months of their diagnosis. More than half of all children in foster care received the appropriate number of well-care visits (59.2%) and developmental screenings (57.9%) during foster care, and 83% received all of the recommended diphtheria, tetanus, pertussis vaccine (TDap), inactivated poliomyelitis (IPV), Haemophilus Influenzae Type b (HiB), and hepatitis b (HepB) vaccinations by age 1. Over 70% of children received the appropriate number of recommended vaccinations by age 2. Only about 1 in 5 children suspected of physical abuse received a follow-up skeletal survey after one was initially performed, and only 3.2% of transitions from foster home to foster home showed any evidence of a care coordination letter. Data from children who had exact dates of entry and exit revealed similar results for all quality measures (data not shown).

O/E ratios were calculated for the well-child visit and developmental screening measures (Table 3). On average, children received 90% of their recommended well care visits while in foster care and 94% of their recommended developmental screenings while in foster care. These O/E measures, for the reasons already discussed, are higher than their analogous proportion measures.

SACWIS data of children age 0–3 years

A total of 1887 children age 0–3 years with records in SACWIS met our inclusion criteria. (Table 2) Demographic,

Table 2 Demographic, Entry, and Exit Related Characteristics of 0–3 Year Olds

	EHR $N = 375$	SACWIS $N = 1887$
Age in months at first entry into foster care	6 (0, 16)	6 (0, 19)
Number of months in foster care from birth through age 3 years or Feb 28, 2013[a]	9.2 (3.0, 17.9)	8.4 (1.9, 17.0)
Exact dates for all entries into and exits from foster care	168 (44.8)	1887 (100)
Exact dates of all entries into foster care during study period	287 (76.5)	1887 (100)
Male	193 (51.5)	984 (52.2)
Race/Ethnicity		
White	129 (34.4)	713 (37.8)
Black/African-American	152 (40.5)	772 (40.9)
≥ 2 Races	39 (10.4)	223 (11.8)
Other	30 (8.0)	4 (2.1)
Unknown/Not documented	25 (6.7)	39 (2.1)
Hispanic	13 (3.5)	136 (7.2)
Reason for first entry into foster care[b]		
Neglect[c]	N/A	550 (29.2)
Dependency[d]	N/A	368 (19.5)
Parental drug or alcohol abuse	122 (32.5)	358 (19.0)
Physical abuse	37 (9.9)	311 (16.5)
Caretaker's inability to cope	N/A	99 (5.3)
Incarceration of parents	15 (4.0)	49 (2.6)
Other	138 (36.8)	152 (8.1)
Not documented	96 (25.6)	0 (0)
Number of entries into foster care		
1	353 (94.1)	1734 (91.9)
2	22 (5.9)	138 (7.3)
3	0 (0)	15 (0.8)
Foster home changes during all foster care episodes		
None	322 (85.9)	1091 (57.8)
1	46 (12.3)	490 (26.0)
2	4 (1.1)	210 (11.1)
> 2	3 (0.8)	96 (5.1)
Still in foster care as of 3rd birthday or Feb 28, 2013		
Yes	114 (30.4)	219(11.61)
No, reunited	76 (20.3)	813 (43.1)
No, entered kinship care	63 (16.8)	336 (17.8)
No, adopted	44 (11.7)	314 (16.6)
Other	N/A	193 (10.2)
Unknown/Not documented	78 (20.8)	12 (0.6)

Data are shown as median (interquartile range) or frequency (%). [a]Unknown dates of entry and exit in the EHR study cohort were estimated as described in the methods. For the calculation of months spent in foster care, a 30 day period was treated as a month. [b]Some patients had multiple reasons for entry into foster care, all of which were extracted. However, only the primary reason for removal is available in a structured field in SACWIS. [c]Neglect was not captured as a reason for entry into foster care in the EHR study. Rather, particular types of neglect or reasons for neglect were captured such as parental drug and alcohol abuse, abandonment, and parental developmental disability or mental illness. [d]Dependency removals were for reasons not related to abuse or neglect, or in cases when parents could not care for their children but were not neglecting or abusing them (e.g. homelessness or death of parents in a car accident). This type of reason for entry was also not captured as a distinct category in the EHR study, but rather is incorporated within the "Other category"

Table 3 Quality Measures in all Children Aged 0–3 Years

Proportion Measures			
	Numerator	Denominator	%
1st well-care visit within 30 days of initial entry into foster care[a]	268	341	78.6
Appropriate number of well care visits for their age during foster care[b]	190	321	59.2
Appropriate number of vaccinations by age 1 year[c]	112	135	83.0
Appropriate number of vaccinations by age 2 years[c]	82	114	71.9
Appropriate number of lead screenings for their age during foster care	153	193	79.3
Appropriate number of developmental screenings for their age during foster care[b]	186	321	57.9
Developmental screening during foster care within 3 months after documentation of TBI	4	4	100.0
Follow up skeletal survey after receiving an initial skeletal survey	7	33	21.2
Care coordination letters at foster home changes	2	63	3.2
Observed to Expected Ratio Measures			
	# of children contributing to the weighted average[d]	Weighted Average Observed/ Expected Ratio	
Appropriate number of well care visits for their age during foster care[b]	321	0.90	
Appropriate number of developmental screenings for their age during foster care[b]	321	0.94	

[a]Only children who had an exact date of entry or a date range for entry were included in this measure
[b]54 children who had zero expected well-care visits for their age while in foster care (per AAP Bright Futures Guidelines) are not included in these measures
[c]Vaccinations included DTaP, IPV, HiB, and HepB for age 1 and DTaP, IPV, HiB, HepB, MMR, and VZV vaccinations for age 2
[d]The denominator of the O/E measures indicates how many individuals' O/E ratios were included in the calculation of the overall weighted average O/E ratio

entry and exit characteristics were similar between the EHR and SACWIS study cohorts, but one key difference between data sources is the consistent documentation of entry and exit dates in SACWIS (100% in SACWIS vs. 44.8% in the EHRs). In addition, SACWIS contains a greater amount of detail regarding foster care history compared to data from the EHR. Unfortunately, SACWIS contains far less detail on the health care provided to children in foster care than EHRs. After reviewing the SACWIS records of a matched sample of the EHR study cohort, it was found that SACWIS was not a viable resource for medical data (data not shown).In addition, only approximately 50% (198/375) of patients with EHR data could be matched across the two data sources.

EHR data of adolescents

A total of 401 charts were reviewed. Two were excluded because they did not have any well-care visits while in foster care during the study period. This left 399 patients. Table 4 depicts the demographic and entry and exit related characteristics of both the EHR and SACWIS study populations. Overall, the median duration of time spent in foster care during the study period was 10.1 months (IQR 2.5–21.0) (Table 4). Almost 75% of children had exact dates of entry but only 21.8% of children had both exact entry and exact exit dates recorded in their EHR. The most frequently cited reason for first entry into foster care was a child's behavior problem (30.3%). However, almost 40% lacked documentation in their EHR of the reason for their first entry into foster care.

Table 5 illustrates the performance of the proposed adolescent health care quality measures within our EHR. More than 3/4ths received the appropriate number of annual well-care visits and recommended TdaP and Meningococcal vaccinations. However, less than 1 in 10 girls had documentation in their EHR of having received a full 3-dose course of the human papillomavirus (HPV) vaccine. Over 90% of adolescents had documentation of an annual BMI. Over 75% had documentation of annual drug use assessments, but only 33.8% had documentation of annual alcohol use assessments. Less than half of adolescents were screened annually for both chlamydia and gonorrhea, and less than 25% were screened annually for depression.

O/E ratios were calculated for all of the same events for which proportion measures were calculated, with the exception of the immunization measures (Table 5). On average, adolescents received 96% of their recommended well care visits while in foster care. On average, they received 89% of the recommended number of drug use assessments for the time they spent in foster care, but the rates of screening for alcohol use, sexually transmitted infections, and depression were considerably lower.

SACWIS data of adolescents

A total of 3674 adolescents aged 12–18 years with records in SACWIS met our inclusion criteria (Table 4). Demographic, entry and exit characteristics were similar between the EHR and SACWIS study cohorts, though the proportion of adolescents with undocumented reasons

Table 4 Demographic, Entry, and Exit Related Characteristics of Adolescents Aged 12–18 Years

	EHR	SACWIS
	$N = 399$	$N = 3674$
Age in years at entry into the first period in foster care that overlapped with or occurred entirely during the study period	15 (13, 16)	15 (14, 16)
Number of months in foster care while aged 12–18 years during the study period[a]	10.1 (2.5, 21.0)	7.0 (2.3, 14.0)
Exact dates for all entries into and exits from foster care	87 (21.8)	3674 (100)
Exact dates of all entries into foster care during study period	299 (74.9)	3674 (100)
Male	205 (51.4)	2097 (51.7)
Race/Ethnicity		
White	119 (29.8)	1272 (34.6)
Black/African-American	240 (60.2)	1952 (52.4)
≥ 2 Races	18 (4.5)	288 (7.8)
Other	17 (4.3)	223 (11.8)
Unknown/Not documented	5 (1.3)	22 (0.6)
Hispanic	20 (5.0)	152 (4.1)
Primary reason for entry into the first period in foster care that overlapped with or occurred entirely during the study period[b]		
Child Behavior Problem	121 (30.3)	1073 (29.2)
Delinquency[c]	N/A	1056 (28.7)
Dependency[d]	N/A	275 (7.5)
Neglect	23 (5.8)	272 (7.4)
Physical abuse	28 (7.0)	205 (5.6)
Sexual abuse	29 (7.3)	82 (2.2)
Other	45 (11.3)	711 (19.4)
Not documented	153 (38.3)	0 (0)
Number of distinct episodes in foster care during study period		
1	369 (92.5)	2890 (78.7)
2	26 (6.5)	590 (16.1)
3	4 (1.0)	152 (4.1)
> 3	0 (0)	42 (1.1)
Foster home changes during all foster care episodes[e]		
None	258 (64.7)	1554 (42.3)
1–2	118 (29.6)	1307 (35.6)
3–4	18 (4.5)	437 (11.9)
> 4	5 (1.3)	376 (10.2)
Still in foster care as of 19th birthday or Oct 31, 2013 (whichever came first)		
Yes	66 (16.5)	163 (4.4)
No, reunited	49 (12.3)	2033 (55.3)
No, entered kinship care	13 (3.3)	353 (9.6)
No, adopted	10 (2.5)	41 (1.1)
No, aged out, living independently, or emancipated	13 (3.3)	650 (17.7)
No, runaway	2 (0.5)	243 (6.6)

Table 4 Demographic, Entry, and Exit Related Characteristics of Adolescents Aged 12–18 Years *(Continued)*

	EHR $N = 399$	SACWIS $N = 3674$
Other	0 (0)	191 (5.2)
Unknown/Not documented	246 (61.7)	12 (0.6)

Data are shown as median (interquartile range) or frequency (%). [a]Unknown dates of entry and exit in the EHR study cohort were estimated as described in the methods. For the calculation of months spent in foster care, a 30 day period was treated as a month. [b]Only the primary reason for removal was recorded in both the EHR and SACWIS data. [c]Delinquency was not captured as a reason for entry into foster care in the EHR study. [d]Dependency removals were for reasons not related to abuse or neglect, or in cases when parents could not care for their children but were not neglecting or abusing them (e.g. homelessness or death of parents in a car accident). This type of reason for entry was also not captured as a distinct category in the EHR study, but rather is incorporated within the "Other category". [e]Only transitions into or out of standard foster homes or group homes were included. Transitions into and out of other placement settings were not included

for entry into and exit from foster care in their EHR makes it challenging to compare these characteristics between cohorts. SACWIS contains minimal detail on the health care provided to children in foster care when compared to EHRs.

Discussion

Documentation of data important to the tracking and optimization of the health care of children and adolescents in foster care is frequently incomplete and difficult to find in either EHRs or SACWIS in our patient population. However, despite their limitations, EHRs and SACWIS can be useful data sources for the calculation of some important measures of quality of care in the foster care population, and would be even more useful if certain important data elements were more consistently available and easily extractable from each database. Alternatively, individual level matching across platforms may allow for the optimal methods by which to assess these measures.

Manual review to calculate our proposed foster care quality measures was laborious. The majority of information was located in free text fields and scanned documents rather than structured fields. Many important data elements, specifically the reasons for initial entry into foster case and the entry and exit dates from foster care, were often missing, and this lack of documentation proved to be limiting factors in data abstraction. The accuracy of nearly all of our proposed health care quality measures is contingent upon this critical information. Similar issues were identified for SACWIS data. While demographics and entry and exit characteristics were found in discrete fields, all other information of interest to this study was

Table 5 Quality Measures in Adolescents Aged 12–18 Years

Proportion Measures			
	Numerator	Denominator	%
Appropriate number of well care visits for their age during foster care	329	399	82.5
Appropriate adolescent immunizations[a]	311	399	77.9
Three HPV vaccinations in females	26	194	13.4
Appropriate number of BMI measurements	368	399	92.2
Appropriate number of drug use assessments	300	399	75.2
Appropriate number of alcohol use assessments	135	399	33.8
Appropriate number of sexually transmitted infection screenings	161	399	40.4
Appropriate number of depression screenings	94	399	23.6
Observed to Expected Ratio Measures			
	# of children contributing to the weighted average[b]	Weighted Average Observed/ Expected Ratio	
Appropriate number of well care visits for their age during foster care	399	0.96	
Appropriate number of BMI measurements	399	1.82	
Appropriate number of drug use assessments	399	0.89	
Appropriate number of alcohol use assessments	399	0.40	
Appropriate number of sexually transmitted infection screenings	399	0.67	
Appropriate number of depression screenings	399	0.28	

[a]Vaccinations included TdaP and meningococcal vaccinations. [b]The denominator of the O/E measures indicates how many individuals' O/E ratios were included in the calculation of the overall weighted average O/E ratio

located in free text fields. This required study investigators to visually examine text notes. Even after this task was performed, it was found that the quantity of information and detail on medical care in SACWIS was far less than from the EHRs.

Identifying the best method to calculate the proposed quality measures revealed the complexity of EHR data abstraction and quality measure development for children in foster care. For example, the Healthcare Effectiveness Data and Information Set (HEDIS) Well-Child Visit measure at 15 months of age would have minimal utility in the foster care population as it requires continuous enrollment for 12 months prior to age 15 months as an inclusion criteria [29]. The O/E ratios examined in this study seemed to be a viable option for the calculation of quality of care measures in the foster care population, primarily because every child can be included in the calculation of these measures regardless of their length of stay or number of episodes in foster care. In addition, children who spend more time in foster care appropriately contribute more to these measures than children who spend less time in foster care. The results in Tables 3 and 5 indicate that select quality measures appear better when calculated using O/E ratios rather than proportions, namely because all health care events contribute to the O/E measures whereas with the proportion measures, a child is counted in the numerator only if the ideal number of events of interest occurred. Admittedly however, the greater mathematical complexity of the weighted average O/E measures, compared to simple proportions, may limit their widespread use.

Considering the challenges we encountered in this study, modification of current EHRs, the use of another data source, or combination of data sources may improve the feasibility of foster care quality measures. An ideal EHR format specific to children was recently proposed [30]. The format provides specific elements and requirements that could be added to current EHRs to enhance the care of children, especially those enrolled in Medicaid and in the care of child welfare [30]. These recommendations include system capacity to store and display 1) whether the child has ever been in out-of home care 2) information about the dates of the out-of-home care and 3) information on the child's history of abuse or neglect. In addition, the SACWIS data system used by child welfare agencies could also be useful. Although its current use varies by state, it is intended to be a comprehensive database that supports the efforts of case workers to assist children in out of home care [28]. The availability of exact dates of entry into foster care and exit from foster care in SACWIS and the availability of accurate data on health care received in the EHR could, together in a combined database, enable the calculation of more accurate health care quality measures than those presented here. However, a higher match rate than we found would be necessary to make such a combined database useful.

Conclusion

Extraction of data to test foster care quality measures is not currently feasible in a single institution EHR, even though we conducted this study at a large, free-standing children's hospital with a longstanding commitment to electronic health records, nor is it feasible in a metropolitan county's SACWIS data. Most proposed quality measures tested did not achieve high adherence as recommended by current guidelines, but it is difficult to tell to what extent missing data elements such as entry and exit dates contributed to these results. Because the quality of information is important to improve patient care, testing foster care quality measures in SACWIS or an augmented EHR that utilizes the children's EHR format may be a better alternative, and subsequently may yield more reliable results [31].

Abbreviations

BMI: Body mass index; CHIPRA: Children's Health Insurance Program Reauthorization Act; EHR: Electronic health record; HEDIS: Healthcare effectiveness data and information set; HepB: Hepatitis b vaccine; HiB: Haemophilus Influenzae Type b vaccine; HPV: Human papillomavirus; IPV: Inactivated Poliomyelitis vaccine; IQR: Interquartile ranges; NCH: Nationwide Children's Hospital; NCINQ: National Collaborative for Innovation in Quality Measurement; O/E ratios: Observed to expected ratios; PCP: Primary care physician; PQMP: Pediatric Quality Measures Program; SACWIS: Statewide Automated Child Welfare Information System; TBI: Traumatic brain injury; TdaP: Tetanus,Diphtheria, Pertussis vaccine

Acknowledgements

We acknowledge Mr. Don Peasley, Director of Evaluation at Franklin County Children Services, who provided us with SACWIS data and whose knowledge of SACWIS informed our interpretation and analysis of the data.

Funding

This project was supported by grant number U18HS020503 from the Agency for Healthcare Research and Quality (AHRQ) and Centers for Medicare & Medicaid Services and, by Award Number Grant UL1TR001070 from the National Center For Advancing Translational Sciences.

The funding sources had no role in the design and conduct of this study; collection, management, analysis and interpretation of the data; preparation, review, or approval of the manuscript; or in the decision to submit the manuscript for publication.

Disclaimer

The content is the responsibility of the authors and does not necessarily represent the official views of AHRQ or of the National Center for Advancing Translational Sciences or the National Institutes of Health.

Authors' contributions

KD - participated in study design and coordination, helped to draft and revise the manuscript. PM - participated in study design and coordination, helped to revise the manuscript. KN – Acquisition of data, helped to draft and revise the manuscript. KL – Database design, acquisition of data, and revised manuscript.

JC – Analysis and interpretation of data, helped to draft and revise the manuscript. SS - conceived of the study, and participated in its design, helped to draft and revise the manuscript. KK - conceived of the study, and participated in its design, helped to draft and revise the manuscript. All authors read and approved the final manuscript.

Competing interests
The authors declare that they have no competing interests.

Author details
[1]The Research Institute at Nationwide Children's Hospital, 700 Children's Drive, FB3145, Columbus, OH 43205, USA. [2]National Quality Forum, 1030 15th Street NW, Suite 800, Washington, DC 20005, USA. [3]National Committee for Quality Assurance, 1100 13th St, NW, Suite 1000, Washington, DC 20005, USA.

References
1. Mangione-Smith R, McGlynn EA. Assessing the quality of healthcare provided to children. Health Serv Res. 1998;33(4 Pt 2):1059–90.
2. Beal AC, Co JP, Dougherty D, et al. Quality measures for children's health care. Pediatrics. 2004;113(1 Pt 2):199–209.
3. Centers for Medicare and Medicaid. Children's Health Insurance Program Reauthorization Act (CHIPRA). Childrens Health Insurance Program CHIP https://www.medicaid.gov/medicaid/quality-of-care/performance-measurement/child-core-set/index.html. Accessed 4 Jan 2013.
4. Chernoff R, Combs-Orme T, Risley-Curtiss C, Heisler A. Assessing the health status of children entering foster care. Pediatrics. 1994;93(4):594–601.
5. Steele JS, Buchi KF. Medical and mental health of children entering the utah foster care system. Pediatrics. 2008;122(3):e703–9.
6. U.S. Government Accountability Office. Foster Care: Health needs of many young children are unknown and unmet. 1995; http://www.gao.gov/products/HEHS-95-114. Accessed 3 Jan 2013.
7. Ritchie B. "Children's use of health care services while in Foster Care: common themes" memorandum to Susan Orr, associate commissioner for the Children's Bureau, Administration for Childen and Families, and Dennis G. Smith, director of Centers for Medicare and Medicaid Services. OEI-07-00-00645 ed. Washington, DC: U.S. Department of Health and Human Services, Office of the Inspector General; 2005.
8. Levinson DR. Most Medicaid children in nine states are not receiving all required preventive screening services. OEI-05-08-00520 ed. Washington, DC: U.S. Department of Health and Human Services, Office of Inspector General; 2010.
9. Leslie LK, Hurlburt MS, Landsverk J, Rolls JA, Wood PA, Kelleher KJ. Comprehensive assessments for children entering foster care: a national perspective. Pediatrics. 2003;112(1 Pt 1):134–42.
10. Hakim RB, Bye BV. Effectiveness of compliance with pediatric preventive care guidelines among Medicaid beneficiaries. Pediatrics. 2001;108(1):90–7.
11. Lewandowski RE, Acri MC, Hoagwood KE, et al. Evidence for the Management of Adolescent Depression. Pediatrics. 2013;132(4):e996–e1009.
12. American Academy of Child and Adolescent Psychiatry, Child Welfare League of America. AACAP/CWLA Policy Statement on Mental Health and Use of Alcohol and Other Drugs, Screening and Assessment of Children in Foster Care. 2003; http://www.aacap.org/. Accessed 18 Dec 2012.
13. National Collaborating Centre for Acute Care. Head injury. Triage, assessment, investigation and early Management of Head Injury in infants, children and adults. London, UK: National Institute for Health and Clinical Excellence (NICE); 2007. p. 54.
14. Pringsheim T, Panagiotopoulos C, Davidson J, Ho J. Evidence-based recommendations for monitoring safety of second generation antipsychotics in children and youth. J Can Acad Child Adolesc Psychiatry. 2011;20(3):218.
15. American Academy of Child and Adolescent Psychiatry. Practice parameter on the use of psychotropic medication in children and adolescents. J Am Acad Child Adolesc Psychiatry. 2009;48(9):961–73.
16. American Academy of Child and Adolescent Psychiatry. Practice parameter for the assessment and treatment of children and adolescents with schizophrenia. American Academy of Child and Adolescent Psychiatry. J Am Acad Child Adolesc Psychiatry. 2001;40(7 Suppl):4S–23S.
17. American Academy of Pediatrics Committee on Early Childhood and Adoption and Dependent Care. Developmental issues for young children in foster care. Pediatrics. 2000;106(5):1145–50.
18. Section on Radiology, American Academy of Pediatrics. Diagnostic imaging of child abuse. Pediatrics. 2009;123(5):1430–5.
19. Lahoti SL, McClain N, Girardet R, McNeese M, Cheung K. Evaluating the child for sexual abuse. Am Fam Physician. 2001;63(5):883–92.
20. Jenny C, Crawford-Jakubiak JE, Committee on Child Abuse and Neglect. The evaluation of children in the primary care setting when sexual abuse is suspected. Pediatrics. 2013;132(2):e558–67.
21. Kellogg ND, American Academy of Pediatrics Committee on Child Abuse and Neglect. Evaluation of suspected child physical abuse. Pediatrics. 2007;119(6):1232–41.
22. Kellogg N, American Academy of Pediatrics Committee on Child A, Neglect. The evaluation of sexual abuse in children. Pediatrics. 2005;116(2):506–12.
23. Committee on Early Childhood, Adoption, and Dependent Care. Health Care of Young Children in Foster Care. Pediatrics. 2002;109(3):536–41.
24. Committee on Practice Ambulatory Medicine, Bright Futures Steering Committee. Recommendations for preventive pediatric health care. Pediatrics. 2007;120(6):1376.
25. Fleiss JL. Design and analysis of clinical experiments, vol. 73. New York, NY: Wiley.com; 1999.
26. Landis JR, Koch GG. The measurement of observer agreement for categorical data. Biometrics. 1977;33(1):159–74.
27. Harris PA, Taylor R, Thielke R, Payne J, Gonzalez N, Conde JG. Research electronic data capture (REDCap)–a metadata-driven methodology and workflow process for providing translational research informatics support. J Biomed Inform. 2009;42(2):377–81.
28. National Resource Center for Child Welfare Data and Technology, Children's Bureau. About Statewide Automated Child Welfare Information Systems (SACWIS). 2013. https://www.acf.hhs.gov/cb/research-data-technology/state-tribal-info-systems/managers. Accessed 21 Jan 2013.
29. National Committee for Quality Assurance. HEDIS 2013 volume 2: technical specifications for health plans, vol. 2012. Washington, DC: NCQA. p. 279–81.
30. Agency for Healthcare Research and Quality. Children's Electronic Health Record Format. United States Health Information Knowledgebase 2013; https://ushik.ahrq.gov/mdr/portals/cehrf?system=cehrf&enableAsynchronousLoading=true. Accessed 13 Jan 2014.
31. Hayrinen K, Saranto K, Nykanen P. Definition, structure, content, use and impacts of electronic health records: a review of the research literature. Int J Med Inform. 2008;77(5):291–304.
32. Centers for Disease Control and Prevention. Immunization Schedules. 2013; http://www.cdc.gov/vaccines/schedules/index.html?s_cid=ostltsdyk_govd_406. Accessed 12 Feb 2013.
33. Ohio Department of Medicaid. Guidelines for Medicaid Lead Testing. Lead Poisoning Prevention and Testing Information for Providers http://medicaid.ohio.gov/FOROHIOANS/Programs/Lead/ProviderLead.aspx. Accessed 15 Jan 2014.

7

A pragmatic controlled trial to prevent childhood obesity within a risk group at maternity and child health-care clinics: results up to six years of age (the VACOPP study)

Taina Mustila[1*], Jani Raitanen[2,3], Päivi Keskinen[4,5] and Riitta Luoto[3]

Abstract

Background: Obesity in childhood appears often during the toddler years. The prenatal environment influences obesity risk. Maternal gestational diabetes, the child's diet, and physical activity in the first few years have an important role in subsequent weight gain. A study was conducted to evaluate effectiveness of a primary health-care lifestyle counselling intervention in prevention of childhood obesity up to 6 years of age.

Methods: The study was a controlled pragmatic trial to prevent childhood obesity and was implemented at maternity and child health-care clinics. The participants ($n = 185$) were mothers at risk of gestational diabetes mellitus with their offspring born between 2008 and 2010. The prenatal intervention, started at the end of the first trimester of pregnancy, consisted of counselling on diet and physical activity by municipal health-care staff. The intervention continued at yearly appointments with a public health-nurse at child health-care clinics. The paper reports the offspring weight gain results for 2–6 years of age. Weight gain up to 6 years of age was assessed as BMI standard deviation scores (SDS) via a mixed-effect linear regression model. The proportion of children at 6 years with overweight/obesity was assessed as weight-for-height percentage and ISO-BMI. Priority was not given to power calculations, because of the study's pragmatic nature.

Results: One hundred forty seven children's (control $n = 76/85\%$ and intervention $n = 71/56\%$) weight and height scores were available for analysis at 6 years of age. There was no significant difference in weight gain or overweight/obesity proportions between the groups at 6 years of age, but the proportion of children with obesity in both groups was high (assessed as ISO-BMI 9.9% and 11.8%) relative to prevalence in this age group in Finland.

Conclusion: As the authors previously reported, the intervention-group mothers had lower prevalence of gestational diabetes mellitus, but a decrease in obesity incidence before school age among their offspring was not found. The authors believe that an effective intervention should start before conception, continuing during pregnancy and the postpartum period through the developmentally unique child's first years.

Keywords: Childhood obesity, Prevention, Diet, Physical activity, Intervention, Gestational diabetes mellitus, Pragmatic

* Correspondence: taina.mustila@fimnet.fi
[1]Seinäjoki Central Hospital, Hanneksenrinne 7, 60220 Seinäjoki, Finland
Full list of author information is available at the end of the article

Background

The prevalence of obesity even among pre-school-age children has increased in recent decades, and this is a global trend [1]. Overweight and obesity prevalence is significant already in the pre-school years: 16.1% and 3.9% of five-year-old girls and 7.5%/3.0% of boys of the same age in Finland are reported to have overweight and obesity, respectively [2]. Early adiposity rebound (AR) has been found to be a marker of higher risk for obesity in children and youth; AR is the point of minimal body mass index (BMI) before the second rise in the BMI curve in childhood, normally between five and 7 years of age (AR is considered to be early if it occurs before the age of 5 years) [3, 4]. Pre-schoolers with obesity tend to become schoolchildren and teenagers with obesity, which leads to increased risk of cardiovascular disease in adulthood and to an intergenerational cycle of these health problems [5, 6]. Results of obesity treatment are not encouraging, and prevention of excess weight gain is considered the most effective way to reduce obesity prevalence both during childhood and in adulthood. Early-childhood obesity has a multifactor origin [7, 8]. Prenatal modifiable factors suspected to promote obesity are mother's obesity before pregnancy, gestational diabetes mellitus (GDM), and smoking during pregnancy, with another being excessive weight gain during pregnancy [7, 9–14], and GDM appears to increase the risk of obesity in offspring even in cases of normal birth weight [15–17]. Large-for-gestational-age newborns have been shown to have a higher risk of obesity; also, infant feeding, sleep duration, and rapid weight gain in the first few months have been shown to influence the risk of children gaining excess weight [18–27].

In light of these potential risk factors, obesity prevention should start early in life. The widespread problem of obesity calls for preventive means that can be integrated into existing health-care settings and also for changes in society that contribute to healthy weight gain in the population [7, 8]. Pragmatic trials are aimed at finding effective preventive programmes that could be incorporated into the usual health-care system [28]. Pregnant mothers and families with small children visit child-welfare clinics regularly in primary health care. They are also interested in the wellbeing of their offspring and hence are receptive to lifestyle counselling. Dietary and physical-activity habits are modifiable during the pre-school years [29, 30]. With lifestyle counselling, a significant effect can be achieved when the target group are known to be at risk of gaining excessive weight. Mothers at risk of developing GDM and their offspring are one such risk group [7]. This group includes pregnant mothers with overweight or obesity, mothers with a history of GDM, a macrosomic newborn or close relatives with type 2 diabetes [31]. These mothers may also have a hereditary predisposition to obesity and type 2 diabetes, with a high risk of passing these risks to their offspring.

To the best of our knowledge, no previous results have been published from intervention studies that have aimed primarily at the prevention of obesity among the offspring and that have started during or before the first trimester of pregnancy. This is at odds with the growing evidence that the time before conception, the prenatal and perinatal periods, and early childhood are the critical windows for effective prevention. Some obesity-prevention studies targeted at infancy have been reported on, with most involving short intervention and follow-up periods [32, 33]. The effect on children's adiposity or weight development, if any, has been found to be slightly positive [34–36]. Some randomised studies are still in progress [37–39]. There are a few studies, originally examining pregnancy outcomes such as excess weight gain during pregnancy, prevention of GDM, or postpartum weight retention, in which, additionally, the offspring's weight development was evaluated for 1–7 years of age [40–44]. Intensified counselling on diet and physical activity (PA) directed at mothers during the infant's first year resulted in offspring's slower weight gain by the age of 4 years in a cluster-randomised pilot study [45]. This intervention when applied during pregnancy did not have the same effect on offspring weight [41]. In a study by Gillman et al., treatment of mild GDM had no effect on the offspring's weight gain by age 4–5 years [40], and likewise no effect on pre-school weight gain was found for the gestational lifestyle intervention of the NELLI Study, the Lifestyle in Pregnancy and Offspring (LiPO) study, or the study by Vesco et al. of a weight-management intervention for limiting gestational weight gain (GWG) a in a group of women with obesity [42–44]. Evidence from the obesity-prevention programmes reported upon has shown that multifaceted intervention could be more effective than targeting a single behaviour [7, 32].

The main results of the controlled lifestyle intervention designed to prevent obesity before school age (the VACOPP, or Vaasa Childhood Obesity Primary Prevention, study) are reported here [46]. The setting of the study was maternity and child health-care clinics in the city of Vaasa, in Western Finland. The intervention started at the end of the first trimester for pregnant mothers and continued with their families until the child was 5 years old. The outcomes presented here cover the offspring's weight gain along with overweight and obesity incidence in the trial groups until the age of 6 years.

Methods

Design and participants

Our study was a non-randomised pragmatic controlled clinical trial. All maternity and child health-care clinics in the city of Vaasa, in Western Finland, participated in the recruitment and intervention. The subjects were recruited from among all eligible GDM risk-group mothers in this city during the chosen recruitment period. Each municipal maternity and child health-care clinic in the city participated in the recruitment. A study nurse recruited GDM risk-group mothers and their offspring born in 2008 to the control group before the offspring reached 1 year of age. The intervention-group mothers were recruited from among the GDM risk-group mothers who were pregnant between February 2009 and April 2010 by public-health nurses. Their offspring comprise the intervention-group children. These criteria were applied for GDM risk: body mass index (BMI) ≥ 25 kg/m^2, macrosomic newborn (birth weight ≥ 4500 g), GDM in any previous pregnancy or an immediate family history of diabetes, and/or age ≥ 40 years. The exclusion criteria were having a multiple pregnancy, being unable to speak Finnish, engaging in substance abuse, and displaying severe psychiatric problems.

Our study was a pragmatic trial, which is why we decided not to give priority to power calculations. In the city chosen, relatively limited number of mothers were expected to participate in the study, so statistical significance in a rigorous sense could not be demanded. The estimate of the mean BMI *z*-score for the control-group offspring is a rough one and yields only an inaccurate power calculation [47]. The design and participants were described in more detail in the protocol article [46].

Intervention

The two group counselling sessions were held in the first and the second trimester of pregnancy. A physiotherapist and a dietician in public health care were the teachers. The recommended consumption of fibre, energy content, quality of carbohydrates, and fat in the diet were emphasised [48]. Mothers were advised to exercise for at least 2.5 h/week (until at least slightly out of breath) and to engage in muscle training twice a week, taking into account what is suitable exercise for pregnant women [49]. The mothers were told also that a healthful diet, exercise, and appropriate weight gain during pregnancy help to prevent GDM, act against perinatal problems for the newborn, and favour the child's healthy weight gain. During the 13 routine visits to the maternity health-care clinics, starting with the tenth week of pregnancy, the public-health nurse (PHN) briefly repeated the counselling to the mother. Breastfeeding until the child is 6 months old was recommended. Intervention-group children had a 30–60-min longer appointment with a PHN at the child health-care clinic at the routine yearly control visits for 1–5 years of age. Counselling on diet, age-appropriate physical exercise, sleep, and screen time was given. The counselling employed a motivating interview method endorsed by the Finnish Heart Association, called 'Smart Family' [46]. The intervention has been described in more detail in the protocol article [46].

Outcome measures

The primary outcomes were BMI-SDS development until age 6 years and the proportion of children at the age of 6 years with overweight or obesity as measured via weight-for-height percentage and ISO-BMI. Weight-for-height curves with percentage deviation of the mean for evaluating overweight/obesity in children are preferred in Finnish health care in addition to ISO-BMI, which is the BMI level equivalent for overweight and obesity in adulthood (≥ 25 kg/m^2 and ≥30 kg/m^2, respectively) were the child's BMI to stay the same until adulthood. The new Finnish growth reference was used [50]. Pregnancy, newborn, and infant outcomes have already been reported [51]. The parents' education levels are defined thus: 'low' corresponds to education as far as vocational school; 'medium' indicates a polytechnic degree and 'high' a university degree (Table 1). The secondary outcomes have been described in the protocol article and in a previous report on this study [46].

Data collection

Child's weight was measured to the nearest 0.1 kg with the child in light clothing on a standard electronic scale by child health-care clinic PHNs at yearly appointments near the child's birthday. Height too was measured during these visits, to the nearest 0.1 cm with a standard stadiometer. The study questionnaires were completed by the parents at these appointments or shortly thereafter. The PHNs submitted the completed questionnaires, along with the child's weight, height, blood pressure, and waist circumference measures. These measurements were recorded also in the health-care centre's electronic database, from which the researcher could check them if needed. Long-term illnesses affecting growth (e.g., severe food allergies) were recorded via this questionnaire. The content of the questionnaire form in full and a description of all data items collected were reported upon in the study protocol article [46].

Statistical methods

The characteristics of the study participants are described in terms of means or frequencies and 95% confidence intervals (Tables 1, 2 and 3). The 95% confidence intervals (CIs) were calculated for continuous variables via the formula mean ± (1.96 * standard error of the mean) and for categorical variables via the Wilson score method without continuity correction, in accordance with Newcombe's work [52]. Group differences were evaluated via Student's *t*-test or Mann–Whitney U-test for normally or non-normally distributed continuous

Table 1 Baseline characteristics of the trial groups participating in the study at offspring age of six years (mean or frequency and 95% confidence interval*)

	Intervention	Control	*p*-value	Missing
N	71	76		
Age of mother before pregnancy (years)	31.8 (30.4 to 33.1)	30.2 (29.0 to 31.5)	0.09[a]	–
Mother's education			0.90[c]	–
Low	29.6% (20.2% to 41.0%)	27.6% (18.8% to 38.6%)		
Medium	42.2% (31.5% to 53.8%)	46.1% (35.3% to 57.2%)		
High	28.2% (19.0% to 39.5%)	26.3% (17.7% to 37.2%)		
Father's education			0.30[c]	–
Low	31.0% (21.4% to 42.5%)	35.5% (25.7% to 46.7%)		
Medium	35.2% (25.1% to 46.8%)	42.1% (31.6% to 53.3%)		
High	33.8% (23.9% to 45.4%)	22.4% (14.5% to 32.9%)		
Mother's pre-pregnancy BMI (kg/m^2)	27.4 (26.3 to 28.5)	26.6 (25.6 to 27.5)	0.25[a]	–
Proportion of mothers with obesity (BMI ≥ 30 kg/m^2)	23.9% (15.5% to 35.0%)	18.4% (11.3% to 28.6%)	0.41[c]	–
Father's BMI (kg/m^2)	26.9 (26.0 to 27.7)	27.1 (26.1 to 28.1)	0.69[b]	2, 3
Proportion of fathers with obesity (BMI ≥ 30 kg/m^2)	17.4% (10.2% to 28.0%)	16.4% (9.7% to 26.6%)	0.88[c]	2, 3
Mother, type 2 diabetes	0.0% (0% to 5.2%)	1.3% (0.2% to 7.1%)	1.00[d]	1, 0
Father, type 2 diabetes	1.4% (0.3% to 7.8%)	1.4% (0.2% to 7.3%)	1.00[d]	2, 2
Proportion of grandparent with obesity (BMI ≥ 30 kg/m^2)	52.3% (40.4% to 64.0%)	56.3% (44.8% to 67.3%)	0.38[c]	6, 5
Parity			0.28[c]	–
Primiparous	59.2% (47.5% to 69.8%)	46.0% (35.3% to 57.2%)		
Second pregnancy	23.9% (15.5% to 35.0%)	32.9% (23.4% to 44.1%)		
At least third pregnancy	16.9% (9.9% to 27.3%)	21.1% (13.4% to 31.5%)		
History of newborn > 4500 g	2.9% (0.8% to 9.8%)	3.9% (1.4% to 11.0%)	0.72[c]	1, 0
Mother smoking during pregnancy	1.4% (0.2% to 7.6%)	9.2% (4.5% to 17.8%)	0.04[c]	–
Mother's physical activity (hours/week) during first trimester of pregnancy (before intervention)	4.5 (3.7 to 5.2)	4.5 (3.6 to 5.3)	0.38[b]	2, 3
OGTT (weeks 26–28 of gestation)				
Pathological OGTT result (0 h ≥ 5.3 or 1 h ≥ 10.0 or 2 h ≥ 8.6 mmol/l)	23.9% (15.5% to 35.0%)	46.1% (35.3% to 57.2%)	0.01[c]	–
Gestational weight gain until 37 weeks (kg)	11.3 (10.2 to 12.4)	12.9 (11.6 to 14.3)	0.08[a]	2, 0
Neonatal outcomes				
Gestational age at birth	39.5 (39.1 to 39.9)	39.4 (39.1 to 39.7)	0.53[b]	–
Sex of newborn (boy)	53.5% (42.0% to 64.6%)	52.6% (41.6% to 63.5%)	0.91[c]	–
Birth weight (grams)	3455 (3333 to 3576)	3509 (3407 to 3611)	0.49[a]	–
Large for gestational age	5.6% (2.2% to 13.6%)	6.6% (2.8% to 14.5%)	0.81[c]	–
Exclusive breastfeeding (months)	3.2 (2.7 to 3.7)	2.7 (2.2 to 3.2)	0.16[b]	1, 0

[a]Independent-samples *t*-test. [b]Mann–Whitney U-test. [c]Chi-squared test. [d]Fisher's exact test
*Wilson score method for interval without continuity correction
BMI body mass index, *OGTT* oral glucose tolerance test (2-h)

variables. Normality was assessed through examination of the skewness and kurtosis of the distributions. Categorical variables were tested via chi-squared test or Fisher's exact test.

The difference in the development of child weight gain between the groups (intervention vs. control) was analysed as BMI-SDS by means of a multilevel mixed-effect linear regression model so as to take into account the within-child correlation between repeated measures. This model included a variable (group) to indicate the difference between groups at baseline and another (age of child) to indicate the changes in BMI-SDS over time. The difference in the change in BMI-SDS from two to 6 years of age between the two groups was tested with a

Table 2 Estimates and 95% confidence intervals for BMI-SDS from two to six years – results from a multilevel mixed-effects linear regression model including group ($n = 171$), age and sex of the child; pre-pregnancy BMI of the mother, and interaction between group and age of the child

	Coefficient (95% CI)	*p*-value
Group (ref. = control)	−0.02 (− 0.70 to 0.65)	0.94
Age of the child	−0.23 (− 0.44 to 0.02)	0.03
Age of the child^2	0.03 (0.00 to 0.05)	0.04
Group * Age of the child	0.02 (−0.28 to 0.32)	0.89
Group * Age of the child^2	−0.00 (− 0.04 to 0.03)	0.81
Maternal pre-pregnancy BMI	0.01 (0.00 to 0.03)	0.02
Sex of the child	−0.02 (− 0.32 to 0.28)	0.88
Constant	−0.41 (−1.38 to 0.55)	0.40

BMI body mass index, *SDS* standard deviation score

term for interaction between group and age of child. To allow for a non-linear individual-specific trajectory across time, a quadratic term for age was included. In addition, we added potential confounding variables to the model: mother's pre-pregnancy BMI and gender of the child. Since BMI-SDS can be calculated from 2 years of age [50], this analysis included 171 children. Overweight or obesity was assessed in terms of weight and height converted to weight-for-height percentages and also ISO-BMI (again, the BMI level equivalent for adulthood overweight and obesity (≥ 25 kg/m^2 and ≥30 kg/m^2, respectively) if the child's BMI level were to stay the same until adulthood) in accordance with the Finnish growth reference [50]. In this study, AR was considered to be early if the child's BMI was lowest at two, three, or 4 years of age and normal if it was lowest at age five or 6 years in this group of 2–6-year-old children. All analyses were performed by means of Stata software (version 13.1 for Windows), from StataCorp LP, Texas, USA.

Results

The study flow is described in Fig. 1. Roughly 700 women per year give birth in the city of Vaasa. In the intervention group, the offspring of 71 of the 127 mothers who started the intervention in pregnancy (56%) were still taking part in the study when the child was 6 years old (i.e., at the planned end of the study), with the corresponding figure for the control group being 76 out of 89 children (85%). Most of the dropouts were cases of moving to another city and hence being unable to remain in the study. We analysed baseline characteristics that might interfere with offspring weight development with regard to those children whose anthropometrics were available when they were 6 years old ($n = 147$) and found no statistically significant differences between the groups (Table 1). The baseline characteristics of children whose anthropometrics were available at age 1 year ($n = 185$) have already been reported [51].

According to the linear mixed-effects model, the BMI-SDS slopes did not differ significantly between the intervention and the control group (the *p*-values for linear and quadratic interactions were 0.89 and 0.81) (Table 2, Fig. 2). Adding gender and mother's pre-pregnancy BMI to the model did not fundamentally affect the results. The proportions (expressed as percentage value deviation from the mean weight-for-height value in line with the Finnish definition of pre-school-age overweight and obesity) of children at the age of 6 years with at least overweight (≥ + 10% weight for height) or with obesity (≥ + 20% weight for height) were not significantly different between the groups. The result was the same when at least overweight and obesity were assessed as ISO-BMI (≥ 25 kg/m^2 and ≥30 kg/m^2, respectively) (Table 3). The difference in equivalent proportions

Table 3 Proportions of children in the study groups at 6 years of age with overweight or obesity (proportion and 95% confidence interval) assessed as ISO-BMI or weight-for-height percentage, where adiposity rebound is presented in two classes

	Intervention	Control	*p*-value	Missing
N	71	76		
Overweight at six years of age				
ISO-BMI ≥ 25	18.3% (11.0% to 28.8%)	19.7% (12.3% to 30.0%)	0.83[a]	
Weight for height ≥ + 10%	20.0% (12.3% to 30.8%)	22.4% (14.5% to 32.9%)	0.73[a]	
Obesity at six years of age				
ISO-BMI ≥ 30	9.9% (4.9% to 19.0%)	11.8% (6.4% to 21.0%)	0.70[a]	
Weight for height > + 20%	12.9% (6.9% to 22.7%)	13.2% (7.3% to 22.6%)	0.96[a]	
Adiposity rebound			0.69[a]	2, 1
Early (< 5 years)	29 (42.0%)	34 (45.3%)		
Normal (≥ 5 years)	40 (58.0%)	41 (54.7%)		

[a]Chi-squared test

ISO-BMI, BMI level equivalent for overweight and obesity in adulthood

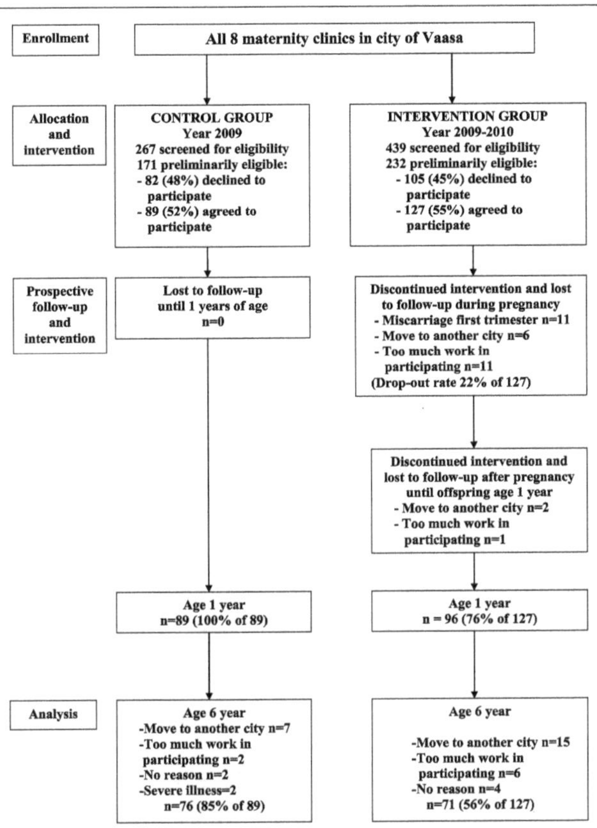

Fig. 1 Flowchart

of early adiposity rebound (< 5 years) between the two groups was not significant either (controls 34/45.3% vs. intervention 29/42.0%, $p = 0.69$) (Table 3).

Discussion

The main result found for our pragmatic lifestyle intervention was a lower occurrence of GDM in the intervention group than in the control group, which result was reported earlier [51], [Table 1]. However, whether the intervention was effective in decreasing excessive weight gain among offspring remains an open question. The non-significant finding might be due also to the low power of the study causing failure to reveal differences between the groups. It has been shown that lower gestational glucose levels may be correlated with a child's lower obesity and type 2 diabetes risk [11, 12, 17]. Rapid weight gain during the first year of life has been demonstrated to predict risk for later obesity [22]. In our study, the offspring's weight gain up to 12 months of age did not differ significantly between groups, but there were slightly more children with overweight in the control group by 1 year of age [51]. Likewise, rapid weight gain in subsequent pre-school years seems to predict obesity in the school years [23]. In addition, early adiposity rebound has been shown to precede obesity in childhood and adulthood and to be a marker of cardiometabolic risk [3, 53]. In our study, no significant difference in the groups' proportions of early vs. normal AR was found, but the proportion of children with early AR in both groups was high, predicting the offspring having the same metabolic risk as their mothers. The proportion of children at the age of 6 years with obesity in both group was high as well (defined as weight for height 12.9% and 13.2%) [2]. These results confirm that our target group for such an intervention may be appropriately chosen.

The offspring's BMI was analysed and adjusted in accordance with the Finnish growth reference, for obtaining the SDS [50]. Weight gain was assessed with a linear mixed-effects model, which allows for a difference between the groups at baseline, intervention effects, and changes over time. No significant differences between the intervention and control group's offspring weight gain during the first year or up to 6 years of age were found. Given that improvements in foetal conditions – such as the mother having a better glucose balance during pregnancy – have been shown to correlate with a good effect on offspring weight gain that emerges in the toddler years. Based on this our intervention had potential to diminish children's overweight/obesity prevalence by age six [11, 12, 17]. However, as we have noted, the insufficient power of the study may have affected the results in this respect.

The overall dropout rate for the intervention group up to 6 years of age was 44% (Fig. 1). The most common reasons for dropping out were moving to a city out of reach of this intervention and the parents experiencing the study intervention or completing the questionnaires as too taxing. Furthermore, the recommendation to participate in blood tests every 2 years was felt to be too taxing for the child in many families, creating reluctance to take part in the study even despite the option of skipping the tests. The dropout rate in our study is acceptable in view of its longer-term intervention and follow-up. There were also dropouts in the control group (15% by age 6 years). It is possible that those families with the healthiest lifestyle and lowest risk of offspring's excess weight gain were more likely to remain in the study, thereby diminishing the difference in proportions of children with overweight and obesity between groups. However, the baseline characteristics were comparable between groups at both 1 year and 6 years of age.

Our target group was mothers at risk of developing GDM and their offspring with a higher risk of unhealthy weight gain. The intervention extended across foetal, infant, and pre-school life, known times of risk for development of obesity. Almost 98% of the mothers in Finland visit municipal maternity health-care facilities, and the high participation percentage holds for child health-care clinic visits. If the intensified counselling is

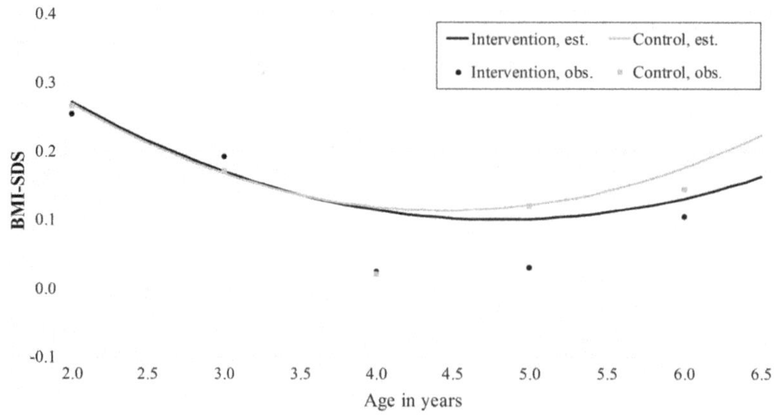

Fig. 2 BMI-SDS in whole group ($N = 171$) from two years to six years of age. Non-linear model including age of child, mother's pre-pregnancy weight, and group × age interaction. Obs., observed; Est., estimated

offered during these routine visits, the at-risk families are conveniently reached. However, those routine visits to child health-care clinics take place only once a year, which may entail too light an intervention for this risk group. Also, evidence is growing that intervention for this purpose should start even before pregnancy, to improve the mother's metabolic health and hence a better prenatal environment in regard of the child receiving a healthier epigenetic heritage [54]. One marked problem is how to reach the risk group with childbearing potential for intensive counselling before pregnancy. Child health-care clinics may be a useful environment for targeting mothers with small children before pregnancy, but this is not true for first-time mothers. In addition, since obesity tends to begin in the early years, focusing more intensive lifestyle counselling also on offspring age 0–2 years within risk-showing families could be effective.

Our study had several limitations. It was not randomised, and the power may not have been sufficient to reveal statistically significant results. We believe also that, as the difference in study-group BMIs proved to be so small, precise primary power calculations would not have shown the number of participants to be sufficient for statistical significance in this intervention trial. An additional factor is that we wanted to perform the trial in this specific relatively large city in Finland, where the protocol is the same across all maternity health care, thereby primarily comparable in that regard. For this pragmatic trial, a randomised controlled design was not considered feasible, because the randomisation process would have been very likely to further reduce the rate of participation in the trial. A case-control study design is the choice in intervention studies when randomisation is not feasible and the study groups are matched as in our study (Table 1). The study design was discussed also in the protocol article [46]. The control group was prospective only from offspring age of 1 year, which may have caused some bias in the results; however, our choice may also have eliminated a possible Hawthorne effect on the control group during the intervention during pregnancy. As is the case with any pragmatic trial, the effectiveness of the counselling situation as a whole might have varied greatly. For example, the motivation of PHNs may vary, and the need for PHN deputies occasionally has an influence on counselling. The recruitment of the intervention group and the paperwork for the study were considered burdensome by some PHNs, mainly for reason of their busy work schedule. Allocating enough time for PHNs to manage the risk-group intervention appointments is crucial also.

One element of our study in its defence is its implementation in real-life practice, which demonstrates the counselling's ability to be a sustainable part of municipal health care. Also, the maternity and child health-care clinics have a good opportunity to identify those at risk for childhood obesity at a stage in life when favourable lifestyle changes promote the offspring's health most. Targeting the at-risk population in a setting that all families in this life situation visit eliminates the risk of stigmatisation. The costs of this study were quite moderate, and the results are generalisable to normal health care, because the study was realised as a part of usual practice at maternity and child health-care clinics.

Conclusions

Obesity with its expensive health effects and economic disadvantages challenges us to initiate solid preventive actions. Primary health-care, maternity, and child health-care clinics reach the beginning of the next generation. Preventive pragmatic trials in real-life settings are needed if we are to target obesity risk groups extensively and economically. In our study, the previously reported improved glucose tolerance during pregnancy demonstrated potential to have a good effect also on offspring weight gain. However, this effect could not be seen in the study. The offspring in both groups showed a high occurrence of early adiposity rebound and high prevalence of obesity, confirming their risk-group status. The knowledge now available suggests that preventive lifestyle interventions should start even before conception, to be able to influence the foetal environment effectively, and also focus on the child's first 2 years, to cover this time with its special risk for obesity development. In addition to applying the right timing, there may be a need for putting more effort and time into the intervention if it is to result in obesity prevention in children in pragmatic settings in health care.

Abbreviations

AR: Adiposity rebound; BMI: Body mass index; CI: Confidence interval; GDM: Gestational diabetes mellitus; GWG: Gestational weight gain; PHN: Public-health nurse; SDS: Standard deviation score

Acknowledgements

We thank the participating families, the public-health nurses at the maternity health-care clinics, and dieticians Diana Markus and Terhi Markkula and physiotherapists Minna Backman and Tuire Rahko-Kinnari at the Vaasa health centre. We also thank research nurses Tiia Krooks and Jenni Siirilä, who participated in the recruitment and training of PHNs for the intervention counselling. In addition, we are grateful to the administrative department for Vaasa municipal health care, especially Dr. Leena Kettunen, for the positive attitude to our study and for being a great help in realising it. Their contribution made this research possible. Thanks also to Marja-Terttu Saha, MD, PhD, who aided in the design of the study.

Funding

This project was funded by the Foundation of Paediatric Research (Finland), The Medical Research.
Fund of the Hospital District of Southern Ostrobothnia (project VTR18), and the Paediatric Research Centre (Tampere, Finland).

Authors' contributions

TM and PK contributed to the design and conception of the study. TM coded the data. TM, RL, PK and JR participated in drafting and revising the manuscript. JR and TM performed the statistical analysis. TM, JR, PK and RL participated in the interpretation of the data. All authors had full access to all of the data (including statistical reports and tables) in the study and can take responsibility for the integrity of the data and the accuracy of the data analysis. All authors read and approved the final version of the manuscript.

Competing interests

The authors declare that they have no competing interests.

Author details

[1]Seinäjoki Central Hospital, Hanneksenrinne 7, 60220 Seinäjoki, Finland. [2]UKK Institute for Health Promotion, Tampere, Finland. [3]Faculty of Social Sciences, University of Tampere, Tampere, Finland. [4]Pediatric Research Centre, 33014 University of Tampere, Tampere, Finland. [5]Tampere University Hospital, 33521 Tampere, Finland.

References

1. Ng M, Fleming T, Robinson M, Thomson B, Graetz N, Margono C, et al. Global, regional, and national prevalence of overweight and obesity in children and adults during 1980–2013: a systematic analysis for the global burden of disease study 2013. Lancet. 2014;384:766–81.
2. Vuorela N, Saha MT, Salo MK. Change in prevalence of overweight and obesity in Finnish children – comparison between 1974 and 2001. Acta Paediatr. 2011;100:109–15.
3. Ip EH, Marshall SA, Saldana S, Skelton JA, Suerken CK, Arcury TA, Quandt SA. Determinants of adiposity rebound timing in children. J Pediatr. 2017;24(17): 30161–0.
4. Hughes AR, Sherriff A, Ness AR, Reilly JJ. Timing of adiposity rebound and adiposity in adolescence. Pediatrics. 2014;134:e1354–61.
5. Gardner DS, Hosking J, Metcalf BS, Jeffery AN, Voss LD, Wilkin TJ. Contribution of early weight gain to childhood overweight and metabolic health: a longitudinal study (EarlyBird 36). Pediatrics. 2009;123:e67–73.
6. Juhola J, Magnussen CG, Viikari JS, Kähönen M, Hutri-Kähönen N, Jula A, et al. Tracking of serum lipid levels, blood pressure, and body mass index from childhood to adulthood: the cardiovascular risk in young Finns study. J Pediatr. 2011;159:584–90.
7. Katzmarzyk PT, Barlow S, Bouchard C, Catalano PM, Hsia DS, Inge TH, et al. An evolving scientific basis for the prevention and treatment of pediatric obesity. Int J Obes. 2014;38:887–905.
8. Blake-Lamb T, Locks LM, Perkins ME, Woo Baidal JA, Cheng ER, Taveras EM. Interventions for childhood obesity in the first 1,000 days. A systematic review. Am J Prev Med. 2016;50:780–9.
9. Oken E, Taveras EM, Kleinman KP, Rich-Edwards JW, Gillman MW. Gestational weight gain and child adiposity at age 3 years. Am J Obstet Gynecol. 2007;196:322.e 1–8.
10. The HAPO Study Cooperative Research Group. Hyperglycaemias and adverse pregnancy outcomes. N Engl J Med. 2008;358:1991–2002.
11. Hillier TA, Pedula KL, Schmidt MM, Mullen JA, Charles MA, Pettitt DJ. Childhood obesity and metabolic imprinting: the ongoing effects of maternal hyperglycaemia. Diabetes Care. 2007;30:2287–92.
12. Chandler-Laney PC, Bush NC, Rouse DJ, Mancuso MS, Gower BA. Maternal glucose concentration during pregnancy predicts fat and lean mass of prepubertal offspring. Diabetes Care. 2011;34:741–5.
13. Wen X, Shenassa ED, Paradis AD. Maternal smoking, breastfeeding, and risk of childhood overweight: findings from a national cohort. Matern Child Health J. 2013;17:746–55.
14. Bammann K, Peplies J, De Henauw S, Hunsberger M, Molnar D, Moreno LA, et al. Early life course risk factors for childhood obesity: the IDEFICS case-control study. PLoS One. 2014;13:e86914.
15. Baptiste-Roberts K, Nicholson WK, Wang NY, Brancati FL. Gestational diabetes and subsequent growth patterns of offspring: the National Collaborative Perinatal Project. Matern Child Health J. 2012;16:125–32. Erratum in: Matern Child Health J. 2012;16:266
16. Zhu Y, Olsen SF, Mendola P, Yeung EH, Vaag A, Bowers K, et al. Growth and obesity through the first 7 y of life in association with levels of maternal glycemia during pregnancy: a prospective cohort study. Am J Clin Nutr. 2016;103:794–800.
17. Gillman MW, Rifas-Shiman S, Berkey S, Field AE, Colditz GA. Maternal gestational diabetes, birth weight, and adolescent obesity. Pediatrics. 2003; 111:221–6.
18. Zhang J, Himes JH, Guo Y, Jiang J, Yang L, Lu Q, et al. Birth weight, growth and feeding pattern in early infancy predict overweight/obesity status at two years of age: a birth cohort study of Chinese infants. PLoS One. 2013;8:e64542.
19. Rogers IS, Ness AR, Steer CD, Wells JC, Emmett PM, Reilly JR, et al. Associations of size at birth and dual-energy X-ray absorptiometry measures of lean and fat mass at 9 to 10 y of age. Am J Clin Nutr. 2006;84:739–47.
20. Griffiths LJ, Smeeth L, Hawkins SS, Cole TJ, Dezateux C. Effects of infant feeding practice on weight gain from birth to 3 years. Arch Dis Child. 2009; 94:577–82.
21. Moorcroft KE, Marshall JL, McCormick FM. Association between timing of introducing solid foods and obesity in infancy and childhood: a systematic review. Matern Child Nutr. 2011;7:3–26.
22. Ong KK, Loos RJ. Rapid infancy weight gain and subsequent obesity: systematic reviews and hopeful suggestions. Acta Paediatr. 2006;95(8):904.
23. Willers SM, Brunekreef B, Smit HA, van der Beek EM, Gehring U, de Jongste C, et al. BMI development of normal weight and overweight children in the PIAMA study. PLoS One. 2012;7:e39517.

24. Glavin K, Roelants M, Strand BH, Júlíusson PB, Lie KK, Helseth S, Hovengen R. Important periods of weight development in childhood: a population-based longitudinal study. BMC Public Health. 2014;14:160.
25. Druet C, Stettler N, Sharp S, Simmons RK, Cooper C, Smith GD, et al. Prediction of childhood obesity by infancy weight gain: an individual-level meta-analysis. Paediatr Perinat Epidemiol. 2012;26:19–26.
26. Buyken AE, Karaolis-Danckert N, Remer T, Bolzenius K, Landsberg B, Kroke A. Effects of breastfeeding on trajectories of body fat and BMI throughout childhood. Obesity (Silver Spring). 2008;16:389–95.
27. Taveras EM, Rifas-Shiman SL, Oken E, Gunderson EP, Gillman MW. Short sleep duration in infancy and risk of childhood overweight. Arch Pediatr Adolesc Med. 2008;162:305–11.
28. Godwin M, Ruhland L, Casson I, MacDonald S, Delva D, Birtwhistle R, Lam M, Seguin R. Pragmatic controlled clinical trials in primary care: the struggle between external and internal validity. BMC Med Res Methodol. 2003;3:28.
29. Timmons BW, Leblanc AG, Carson V, Connor Gorber S, Dillman C, Janssen I, et al. Systematic review of physical activity and health in the early years (aged 0–4 years). Appl Physiol Nutr Metab. 2012;37:773–92.
30. Patrick H, Nicklas TA. A review of family and social determinants of children's eating patterns and diet quality. J Am Coll Nutr. 2005;24:83–92.
31. Farrar D, Duley L, Lawlor DA. Different strategies for diagnosing gestational diabetes to improve maternal and infant health. Cochrane Database Syst Rev. 2011;5:CD007122.
32. Waters E, De Silva-Sanigorski A, Hall BJ, Brown T, Campbell KJ, Gao Y, et al. Interventions for preventing obesity in children. Cochrane Database Syst Rev. 2011;7:CD001871.
33. Wang Y, Cai L, Wu Y, Wilson RF, Weston C, Fawole O, et al. What childhood obesity prevention programmes work? A systematic review and meta-analysis. Obes Rev. 2015;16:547–65.
34. Wen LM, Baur LA, Simpson JM, Rissel C, Wardle K, Flood VM. Effectiveness of home based early intervention on children's BMI at age 2: randomised controlled trial. BMJ. 2012;344:e3732.
35. Daniels LA, Mallan KM, Nicholson JM, Thorpe K, Nambiar S, Mauch CE, et al. An early feeding practices intervention for obesity prevention. Pediatrics. 2015;136:e40–9.
36. Hakanen M, Lagström H, Kaitosaari T, Niinikoski H, Näntö-Salonen K, Jokinen E, et al. Development of overweight in an atherosclerosis prevention trial starting in early childhood: the STRIP study. Int J Obes. 2006;30:618–26.
37. Wen LM, Rissel C, Baur LA, Hayes AJ, Xu H, Whelan A, et al. A 3-arm randomised controlled trial of communicating healthy beginnings advice by telephone (CHAT) to mothers with infants to prevent childhood obesity. BMC Public Health. 2017;17:79.
38. Campbell KJ, Hesketh KD, McNaughton SA, Ball K, McCallum Z, Lynch J, Crawford DA. The extended infant feeding, activity and nutrition trial (InFANT extend) program: a cluster-randomized controlled trial of an early intervention to prevent childhood obesity. BMC Public Health. 2016;16:166.
39. T S, Svensson V, Ek A, Ekstedt M, Karlsson H, Johansson E, et al. A randomised controlled trial for overweight and obese parents to prevent childhood obesityEarly STOPP (STockholm obesity prevention program). BMC Public Health. 2011;11:336.
40. Gillman MW, Oakey H, Baghurst PA, Volkmer RE, Robinson JS, Crowther CA. Effect of treatment of gestational diabetes mellitus on obesity in the next generation. Diabetes Care. 2010;33:964–8.
41. Mustila T, Raitanen J, Keskinen P, Saari A, Luoto R. Lifestyle counselling during pregnancy and offspring weight development until four years of age: follow-up study of a controlled trial. J Negat Results Biomed. 2012;11:11.
42. Kolu P, Raitanen J, Puhkala J, Tuominen P, Husu P, Luoto R. Effectiveness and cost-effectiveness of a cluster-randomized prenatal lifestyle counseling trial: a seven-year follow-up. PLoS One. 2016;11:e0167759.
43. Tanvig M, Vinter CA, Jørgensen JS, Wehberg S, Ovesen PG, Beck-Nielsen H, et al. Effects of lifestyle intervention in pregnancy and anthropometrics at birth on offspring metabolic profile at 2.8 years: results from the lifestyle in pregnancy and offspring (LiPO) study. J Clin Endocrinol Metab. 2015;100:175–83.
44. Vesco KK, Leo MC, Karanja N, Gillman MW, McEvoy CT, King JC, et al. One-year postpartum outcomes following a weight management intervention in pregnant women with obesity. Obesity (Silver Spring). 2016;24:2042–9.
45. Mustila T, Raitanen J, Keskinen P, Saari A, Luoto R. Lifestyle counselling targeting infant's mother during the child's first year and offspring weight development until 4 years of age: a follow-up study of a cluster RCT. BMJ Open. 2012;2:e000624.
46. Mustila T, Keskinen P, Luoto R. Behavioural counselling to prevent childhood obesity – study protocol of a pragmatic trial in maternity and child health care. BMC Pediatr. 2012;12:93.
47. Schulz KF, Grimes DA. Sample size calculations in randomised trials: mandatory and mystical. Lancet. 2005;365:1348–53.
48. Hasunen K, Kalavainen M, Keinonen H, Lagström H, Lyytikäinen A, Nurttila A, et al. The child, family and food: nutrition recommendations for infants and young children as well as pregnant and breastfeeding mothers. Helsinki: Publications of the Ministry of Social Affairs and Health; 2004.
49. Aittasalo M, Pasanen M, Fogelholm M, Kinnunen TI, Ojala K, Luoto R. Physical activity counselling in maternity and child health care – a controlled trial. BMC Womens Health. 2008;8:14.
50. Saari A, Sankilampi U, Hannila ML, Kiviniemi V, Kesseli K, Dunkel L. Finnish growth references for children and adolescents aged 0 to 20 years: length/height-for-age, weight-for-length/height, and body mass index-for-age. Ann Med. 2011;43:235–48.
51. Mustila T, Raitanen J, Keskinen P, Saari A, Luoto R. Pragmatic controlled trial to prevent childhood obesity in maternity and child health care clinics: pregnancy and infant weight outcomes (the VACOPP study). BMC Pediatr. 2013;13:80.
52. Newcombe RG. Two-sided confidence intervals for the single proportion: comparison of seven methods. Stat Med. 1998;17:857–72.
53. González L, Corvalán C, Pereira A, Kain J, Garmendia ML, Uauy R. Early adiposity rebound is associated with metabolic risk in 7-year-old children. Int J Obes. 2014;38:1299–304.
54. Leibowitz KL, Moore RH, Ahima RS, Stunkard AJ, Stallings VA, Berkowitz RI, et al. Maternal obesity associated with inflammation in their children. World J Pediatr. 2012;8:76–9.

8

Extragonadal germ cell tumor of the posterior mediastinum in a child complicated with spinal cord compression

Dong Keon Yon[1], Tae Keun Ahn[2], Dong Eun Shin[2], Gwang Il Kim[3] and Moon Kyu Kim[4*]

Abstract

Background: Germ cell tumors (GCTs) in children are rare neoplasms with diverse pathological findings according to the site and age of presentation. The most common symptoms in children with mediastinal GCTs, which are nonspecific, are dyspnea, chest pain, cough, hemoptysis, vena cava occlusion syndrome, and fatigue/weakness. Because of these nonspecific symptoms, it is difficult to suspect a mediastinal mass. A posterior mediastinal tumor causing spinal cord compression is an important example of an oncologic emergency arising from a neurogenic tumor.

Case presentation: Children with posterior mediastinum GCTs can be easily mistaken as having a neurogenic tumor because of site of tumor origin. We treated our 7-year-old patient with emergency decompression surgery and high-dose steroid pulse therapy to prevent secondary injury to the spinal cord. Primary injury was a result of spinal cord compression due to the initial manifestation of GCT in the posterior mediastinum. Cisplatin-based chemotherapy was also administered. The patient was followed up regularly for 3 years and is undergoing rehabilitation without any signs of recurrence.

Conclusions: We present an extremely rare case of a child with paraparesis caused by extradural spinal cord compression as the initial manifestation of GCT in the posterior mediastinum. The child was treated with emergency decompression surgery and high-dose pulse steroid therapy to prevent secondary injury to the spinal cord.

Keywords: Germinoma, Spinal cord compression, Mediastinal neoplasms, Case report

Background

Germ cell tumors (GCTs) in children are rare neoplasms with diverse pathological findings according to the site and age of presentation. Pediatric GCTs predominantly occur in the midline of the trunk: in the intracranium, mediastinum, gonads, and sacrococcygeum. Histologic subtypes of mediastinal GCTs in children include mature teratoma, 60%; mixed GCTs, 20%; and embryonal carcinoma, 20% (including seminoma/germinoma, immature teratoma, yolk sac tumor, and choriocarcinoma). About 5% of all extragonadal germ cell tumors originate from the mediastinum in children younger than 15 years [1, 2].

The most common symptoms of mediastinal GCTs in children are dyspnea, chest pain, cough, hemoptysis, vena cava occlusion syndrome, and fatigue/weakness [3, 4]. Although survival rates of pediatric GCTs have improved significantly to 80% among patients who receive platinum-based chemotherapy, detection of mediastinal GCTs is challenging because of these nonspecific symptoms. In this article, we report an extremely rare pediatric case of paraparesis caused by extradural spinal cord compression as the initial manifestation of GCT in the posterior mediastinum. This case illustrates the importance of promptness and treatment method, and the prognosis of spinal cord compression caused by GCTs.

* Correspondence: mkkim929@gmail.com
[4]Department of Pediatrics, Severance Hospital, Yonsei University College of Medicine, Seoul, Republic of Korea

Case presentation

We report the case of a 7-year-old boy, who was healthy until the age of 6 years when he presented to a local hospital with progressive intermittent back pain (grade 4 on the Numeric Rating Scale), leg weakness, and poor appetite. Within a month, he was admitted to our pediatric emergency department because he could no longer stand without assistance. At that time, he had no bladder and bowel dysfunction and no history of trauma. On neurological examination, he had significant lower extremity weakness, with a grade 3 in both legs on the Medical Research Council (MRC) scale and with preservation of sensory function. Moreover, he had positive Babinski reflexes in his lower extremities and the presence of ankle clonus. We planned an emergency imaging examination, suspecting spinal cord compression syndrome.

Magnetic resonance imaging (MRI) of the thoracic spine and computed tomography (CT) of the chest revealed a large mass sized 6.1 × 7.4 × 9.5 cm in the right posterior mediastinum from T5 to T11, involving T8 and the T9 vertebral body with extension into the spinal canal and compressing the spinal cord (Fig. 1a, b). Moreover, the tumor showed septal contrast enhancement on coronal T2 view of the thoracic spine MRI and internal dystrophic calcification on the chest CT (Fig. 1c, d). No metastasis was observed on examination with bone scintigraphy, positron emission tomography–CT, and testicular sonography.

Emergency total laminectomy for T6-T10 was performed and histopathological examination of the specimen confirmed a seminoma in the posterior mediastinum. Immunohistochemical staining result was negative for β-human chorionic gonadotropin (HCG), but positive for placental alkaline phosphatase (PALP) and c-KIT (CD117) in the tumor cells (Fig. 2).

Complete blood cell count and an admission panel test revealed no abnormal findings, including levels of lactate dehydrogenase 547 U/L, α-fetoprotein (AFP) < 1.3 ng/mL, and alkaline phosphatase (ALP) 172 U/L (PALP portion was not found). However, β-HCG level was high (30.84 mIU/mL, reference range 0–10 mIU/mL). The patient was treated with methylprednisolone pulse therapy (30 mg/kg/day) postoperatively for 30 h, subsequently followed by maintenance therapy with oral prednisolone for 2 weeks, as well as rehabilitation. Nine cycles of chemotherapy were administered postoperatively, followed by 5 cycles of ICE (Ifosfamide 1500 mg/m^2/day IV on days 1-5, Carboplatin 150 mg/m^2/day IV on days 1-2, Etoposide 100 mg/m^2/day IV on days 1-5) and 4 cycles of BEP

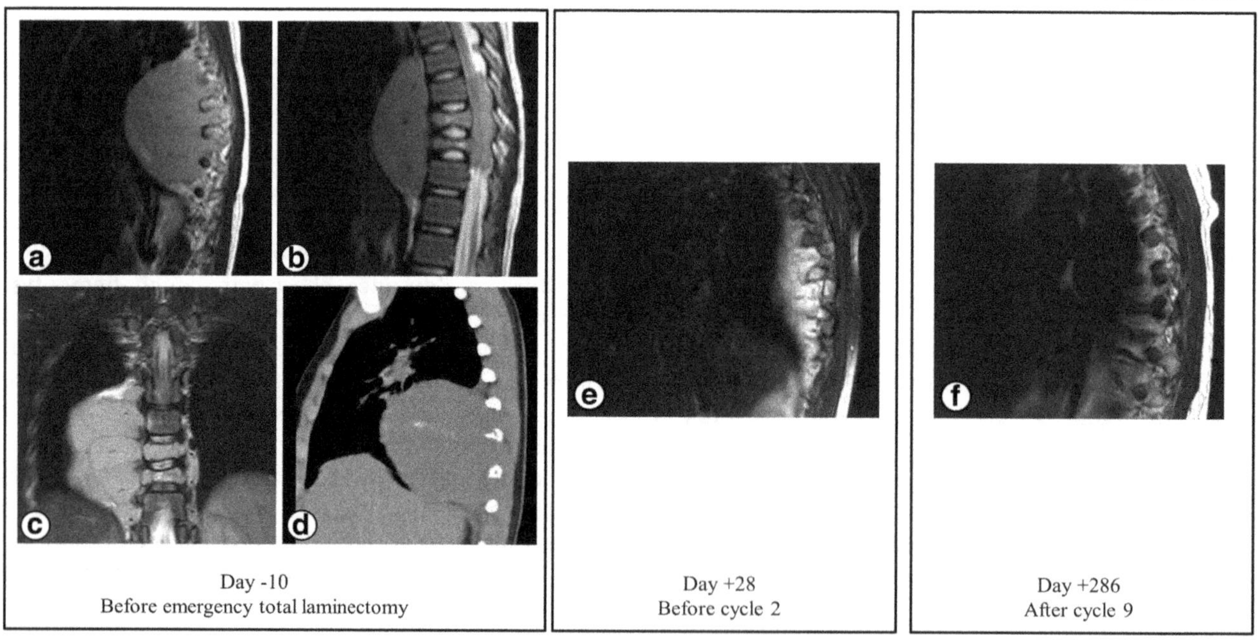

Fig. 1 **a** Sagittal T1 and **b** T2-weighted MRI scans of the thoracic spine reveal a large mass sized 6.1 × 7.4 × 9.5 cm in the right posterior mediastinum from T5-T11, involving the T8 and T9 vertebral body with extension into the spinal canal and compressing the spinal cord. The tumor had a vertebra plana appearance and shows mixed osteolytic and sclerotic bone destruction. **c** The tumor shows septal contrast enhancement on the coronal T2 view and **d** internal dystrophic calcification on CT of the chest. **e** On day + 28 (before the 2nd cycle of chemotherapy), a thoracic spine MRI shows a much-decreased soft tissue tumor in the right posterior mediastinum at T5-T11 level with a residual lesion after removal in the spinal canal from the lower T5 -T9 level with total laminectomy from T6-T10 vertebra. **f** On day + 286 (after the 9th cycle of chemotherapy), a sagittal T2-weighted MRI on follow-up shows that the soft tissue tumor had almost disappeared from the right posterior mediastinal and intercostal space compared with the previous MRIs

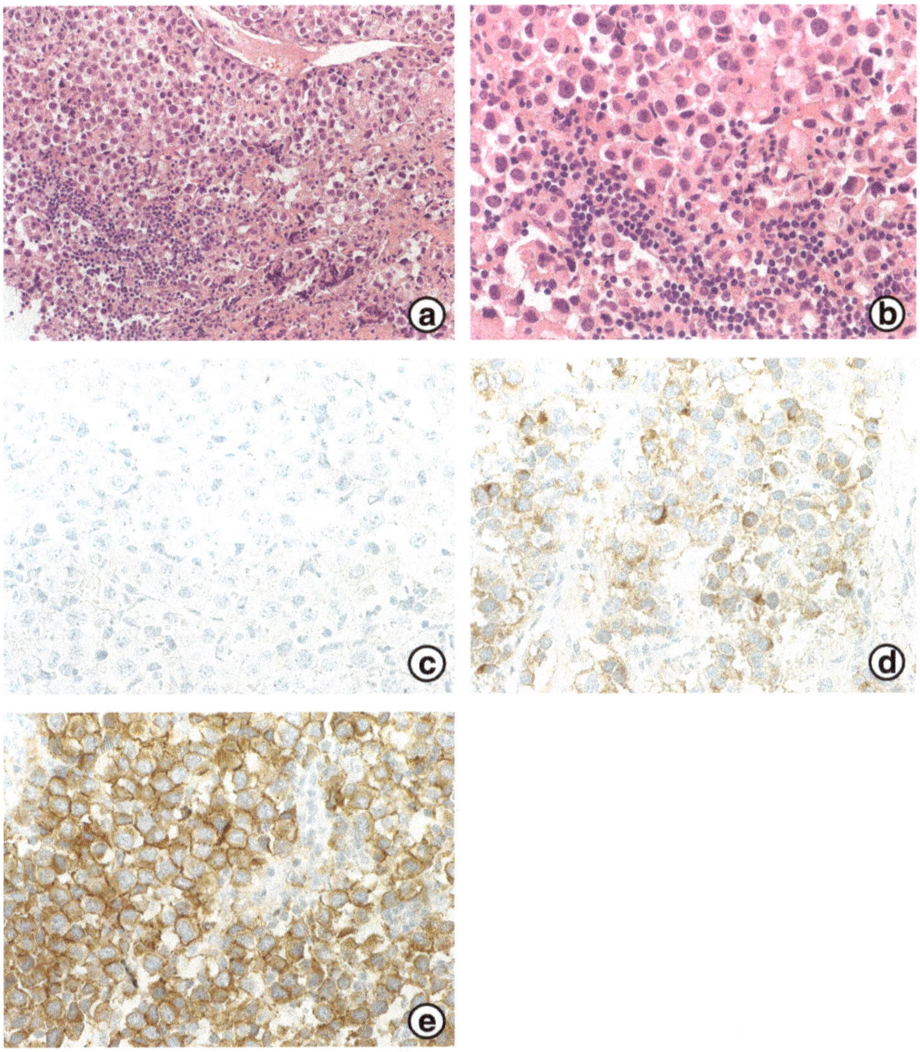

Fig. 2 a Photomicrograph of the surgical specimen showing that the tumor consisted of uniform cells divided into clusters by fine fibrous trabeculae associated with a lymphocytic infiltrate (H&E, 200X). **b** Round or polygonal seminoma cells with a distinct membrane (H&E, 400X). **c** Immunohistochemical staining with β-HCG. The tumor cells were negative for β-HCG (β-HCG, 400X). **d** Seminoma stained with PALP (PALP, 400X). **e** c-KIT showed diffuse positivity in the malignant cells. (c-KIT, 400X)

(Bleomycin 15 mg/m^2/day IV on day 1, Etoposide 100 mg/m^2/day IV on days 1-5, Cisplatin 20 mg/m^2/day IV on days 1-5) alternatively (Fig. 3).

On day 28 (+ 28) after starting chemotherapy, before the 2nd cycle of chemotherapy, β-HCG was undetectable in the blood. Moreover, a thoracic spine MRI showed a much decreased soft tissue tumor in the right posterior mediastinum at T5-T11 level with a residual lesion after removal in the spinal canal from lower T5-T9 level, with the total laminectomy from the T6-T10 vertebra (Fig. 1e).

He underwent video-assisted thoracoscopic exploration and biopsy on day + 91 (after the 3rd cycle of chemotherapy). A grossly visible tumor was not detected and the tissue specimen was free of tumor microscopically.

After the last (ninth) cycle of chemotherapy (on day + 286), a spine MRI revealed an improved state of compressive myelopathy at the T7-T9 region and that the soft tissue tumor had almost disappeared from the posterior mediastinal and intercostal space compared with the initial MRI (Fig. 1f).

The patient has been undergoing regular physical therapy and regular follow ups for 3 years since the chemotherapy ended. On day + 1129, there was no abnormality except for a mild kyphotic curvature on the spine MRI. Moreover, the patient slowly recovered from the neurologic symptoms, improving to grade 4 in lower extremity strength on the MRC scale, and could walk without assistance. He has been wearing a thoracolumbosacral orthosis brace

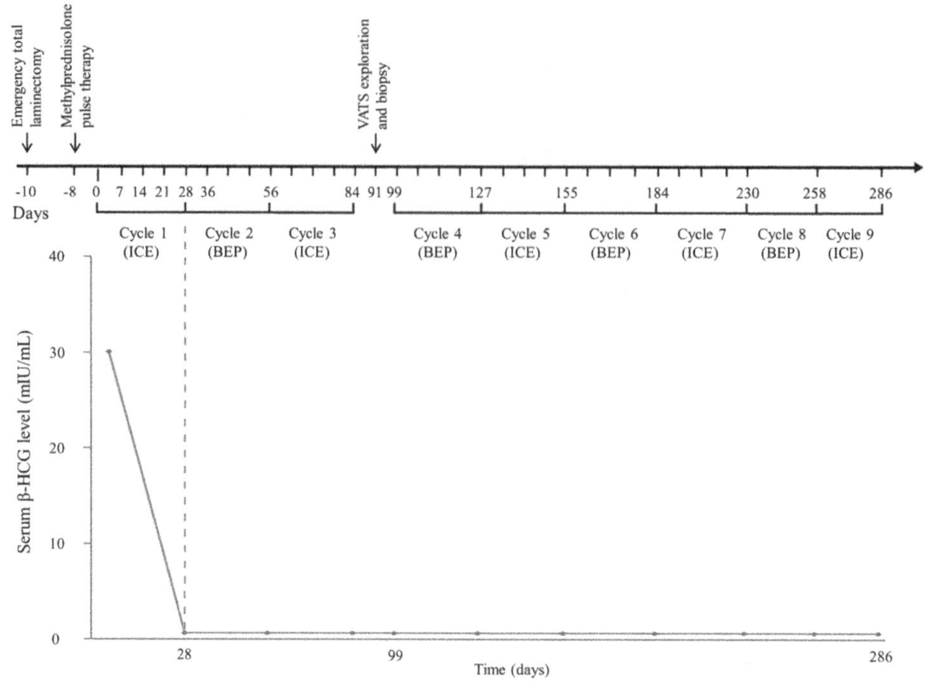

Fig. 3 The timeline of treatment including chemotherapy, surgery, and serum β-HCG concentration. We administered methylprednisolone pulse therapy on day − 8 and alternative ICE and BEP chemotherapy. Moreover, video-assisted thoracoscopic exploration and biopsy were performed on day + 91. In the serum, β-HCG level was 30.84 mIU/mL before cycle 1. β-HCG level was evaluated in every chemotherapy cycle and was undetectable in the blood after cycle 2, as expected

for kyphotic curvature prevention and is undergoing multidisciplinary rehabilitation.

Discussion and conclusion

Spinal cord compression requires accurate diagnosis and rapid treatment to prevent progression to irreversible nerve injury. The most common etiologies of spinal cord compression are lumbar disc herniation, spinal stenosis, and masses including primary and metastatic tumor. The warning signs of back pain identified as spinal cord compression show profound unexplained neurological deficits such as motor or sensory weakness in the lower extremity, recent bowel or bladder dysfunction, and suggest non-musculoskeletal disorders [5]. Additionally, it may be helpful to examine the Babinski sign, presence of clonus, and increased deep tendon reflexes to make a diagnosis.

If the spine is in an unstable condition due to direct compression, which may result in edema, venous congestion, and demyelination, immediate decompression surgery is required for remyelination and recovery of neurologic function [6]. After prolonged compression of the spine and occurrence of spinal cord infarction, it is not possible to achieve a meaningful recovery. However, the optimal treatment for spinal cord compression caused by a primary tumor in children is unclear in a non-emergency condition. The risk of spinal deformity after multi-modality treatment must be considered carefully, especially in younger children [7]. Particularly, radiation therapy for spinal cord compression in younger children was carefully considered because of the potentially irreversible complications of radiation therapy such as spinal deformity, neurological sequelae, and secondary malignant diseases like radiation-induced lymphoma.

Steroid administration after direct decompression surgery aims to prevent secondary injury caused by posttraumatic spinal ischemia, and to improve neurologic function and spinal cord blood flow [8]. The key mechanism in the theory of secondary injury is posttraumatic ischemia in the spinal cord with resultant infarction followed by alterations in microvascular perfusion, inflammation, lipid peroxidation, free radical generation, apoptotic/necrotic cell death, and dysregulation of ionic homeostasis [9]. Based on this theory of secondary injury after direct decompression surgery, the patient received steroid pulse therapy and maintenance therapy at a physiologic dose. In a previous report, preoperative spinal angiography in pediatric inferior posterior mediastinal tumors was used to prevent secondary spinal cord ischemia due to guiding surgical resection [10].

The most common primary malignancies in the posterior mediastinum in children are neurogenic tumors, accounting for 89% of cases, as reported previously, with neuroblastoma being the most common of these [11, 12].

The child with posterior mediastinum seminoma can be easily mistaken as having a neurogenic tumor because of the symptoms and location of tumor origin. Radiographically, these seminomas appear as large, heterogeneous, lobulated soft-tissue masses with areas of hemorrhage and necrosis, and coarse, mottled, ring-shaped calcifications described in approximately 50% of thoracic neuroblastoma [13]. Mediastinal seminomas in children are typically large, homogeneous, lobulated, and well-marginated masses in the anterior mediastinum, but calcification is distinctly uncommon. However, malignant non-seminomatous GCTs differ from those with irregular margins including yolk sac tumor, choriocarcinoma, embryonal carcinoma, and immature teratoma [14, 15].

In this patient, the serum β-HCG level was increased but immunohistochemical staining after total laminectomy was negative for β-HCG. This discrepancy might have been caused by the limited tissue specimen obtained from the emergency surgery for the spinal cord compression, which was not obtained from the main mass. After the surgery, further specimens were unavailable because of the favorable response to chemotherapy.

Survival rates of pediatric GCTs have dramatically improved to more than 80% after the introduction of platinum-based chemotherapy [16]. Current platinum-based chemotherapy protocols are selected based on age, site of origin, histology of tumor, stage, completeness of surgical resection, and treatment response monitored by tumor markers such as AFP and β-HCG, and via imaging studies [17]. The measurement of tumor markers such as AFP and β-HCG helps to ascertain treatment response and determine diagnostic and therapeutic strategies.

An age exceeding 12 years is the most important factor indicative of poor prognosis of event-free survival for extragonadal malignant GCTs in children treated with cisplatin-based therapy. Elevated AFP and advanced tumor stage are also factors indicative of poor prognosis [18, 19]. In this case of a GCT, as the child was 7 years old with a normal serum AFP level and no evidence of metastasis, a good outcome is expected.

Spinal cord compression due to a posterior mediastinal tumor is considered an oncologic emergency and is mostly caused by neurogenic tumors. However, we report an extremely rare case of GCTs not arising from a neurogenic tumor, such as neuroblastoma. We treated the patient with emergency decompression surgery and high-dose steroid pulse therapy to prevent secondary injury to the spinal cord. An ICE/BEP alternative chemotherapy based on cisplatin was administered. He has been followed up regularly for 3 years and is undergoing rehabilitation without any signs recurrence.

Abbreviations

AFP: α-fetoprotein; ALP: Alkaline phosphatase; BEP: Bleomycin, Etoposide, and Cisplatin; CT: Computed tomography; GCTs: Germ cell tumors; HCG: Human chorionic gonadotropin; ICE: Ifosfamide, Carboplatin, and Etoposide; MRC: Medical Research Council; MRI: Magnetic resonance imaging; PALP: Placental alkaline phosphatase; VATS: Video-assisted thoracoscopic surgery

Acknowledgements

The authors would like to thank Dr. Kee Hyun Cho, Dr. Jae woo An, Dr. Joo Young Song, Dr. Yoo Mi Lee in the Pediatrics Department of CHA Bundang Medical Center for excellent care of the patient.

Funding

No financial support was received.

Authors' contributions

DKY was involved in the patient care, and drafted the manuscript. TKA, DES, and GIK were involved in the patient care and helped to draft the manuscript and acquired histological images for illustration. MKK was involved in the patient care and critical revision for content. All authors read and approved the final manuscript.

Consent for publication

Written informed consent was obtained from the parents of the affected child patient for publication of clinical case report and any accompanying images.

Competing interests

The authors declare that they have no competing interests.

Author details

[1]Department of Pediatrics, CHA Bundang Medical Center, CHA University School of Medicine, Seongnam, Republic of Korea. [2]Department of Orthopedic Surgery, CHA Bundang Medical Center, CHA University School of Medicine, Seongnam, Republic of Korea. [3]Department of Pathology, CHA Bundang Medical Center, CHA University School of Medicine, Seongnam, Republic of Korea. [4]Department of Pediatrics, Severance Hospital, Yonsei University College of Medicine, Seoul, Republic of Korea.

References

1. Mosbech CH, Rechnitzer C, Brok JS, Rajpert-De Meyts E, Hoei-Hansen CE. Recent advances in understanding the etiology and pathogenesis of pediatric germ cell tumors. J Pediatr Hematol Oncol. 2014;36(4):263–70.
2. Pinkerton CR. Malignant germ cell tumours in childhood. Eur J Cancer. 1997; 33(6):895–901. discussion 901-892
3. Bokemeyer C, Nichols CR, Droz J-P, Schmoll H-J, Horwich A, Gerl A, Fossa SD, Beyer J, Pont J, Kanz L. Extragonadal germ cell tumors of the mediastinum and retroperitoneum: results from an international analysis. J Clin Oncol. 2002;20(7):1864–73.
4. Si T, Miyoshi S, Ohta M, Minami M, Masaoka A, Matsuda H. Primary germ cell tumors in the mediastinum. Cancer. 2003;97(2):367–76.
5. Sizer PS, Brismée JM, Cook C. Medical screening for red flags in the diagnosis and management of musculoskeletal spine pain. Pain Practice. 2007;7(1):53–71.
6. Patchell RA, Tibbs PA, Regine WF, Payne R, Saris S, Kryscio RJ, Mohiuddin M, Young B. Direct decompressive surgical resection in the treatment of spinal cord compression caused by metastatic cancer: a randomised trial. Lancet. 2005;366(9486):643–8.
7. Sandberg DI, Bilsky MH, Kushner BH, Souweidane MM, Kramer K, Laquaglia

MP, Panageas KS, Cheung N-K. Treatment of spinal involvement in neuroblastoma patients. Pediatr Neurosurg. 2004;39(6):291–8.
8. Tator CH, Fehlings MG. Review of the secondary injury theory of acute spinal cord trauma with emphasis on vascular mechanisms. J Neurosurg. 1991;75(1):15–26.
9. Lu J, Ashwell KW, Waite P. Advances in secondary spinal cord injury: role of apoptosis. Spine. 2000;25(14):1859–66.
10. Nordin AB, Fallon SC, Jea A, Kim ES. The use of spinal angiography in the management of posterior mediastinal tumors: case series and review of the literature. J Pediatr Surg. 2013;48(9):1871–7.
11. Tansel T, Onursal E, Dayıoğlu E, Başaran M, Sungur Z, Çamcı E, Yılmazbayhan D, Eker R, Ertuğrul T. Childhood mediastinal masses in infants and children. Turk J Pediatr. 2006;48:8–12.
12. Saenz NC, Schnitzer JJ, Eraklis AE, Hendren WH, Grier HE, Macklis RM, Shamberger RC. Posterior mediastinal masses. J Pediatr Surg. 1993;28(2):172–6.
13. Hiorns M, Owens C. Radiology of neuroblastoma in children. Eur Radiol. 2001;11(10):2071–81.
14. Drevelegas A, Palladas P, Scordalaki A. Mediastinal germ cell tumors: a radiologic–pathologic review. Eur Radiol. 2001;11(10):1925–32.
15. Carter BW, Okumura M, Detterbeck FC, Marom EM. Approaching the patient with an anterior mediastinal mass: a guide for radiologists. J Thorac Oncol. 2014;9(9):S110–8.
16. Olson TA, Murray MJ, Rodriguez-Galindo C, Nicholson JC, Billmire DF, Krailo MD, Dang HM, Amatruda JF, Thornton CM, Arul GS, et al. Pediatric and adolescent extracranial germ cell tumors: the road to collaboration. J Clin Oncol. 2015;33(27):3018–28.
17. Mann J, Raafat F, Robinson K, Imeson J, Gornall P, Sokal M, Gray E, McKeever P, Hale J, Bailey S. The United Kingdom Children's cancer study Group's second germ cell tumor study: carboplatin, etoposide, and bleomycin are effective treatment for children with malignant extracranial germ cell tumors, with acceptable toxicity. J Clin Oncol. 2000;18(22):3809–18.
18. Marina N, London WB, Frazier AL, Lauer S, Rescorla F, Cushing B, Malogolowkin MH, Castleberry RP, Womer RB, Olson T. Prognostic factors in children with extragonadal malignant germ cell tumors: a pediatric intergroup study. J Clin Oncol. 2006;24(16):2544–8.
19. Baranzelli M, Kramar A, Bouffet E, Quintana E, Rubie H, Edan C, Patte C. Prognostic factors in children with localized malignant nonseminomatous germ cell tumors. J Clin Oncol. 1999;17(4):1212.

9

Health-related quality of life of children and adolescents with osteogenesis imperfecta: a cross-sectional study using PedsQL™

Ana Paula Vanz[1], Juliana van de Sande Lee[2,3], Bruna Pinheiro[1], Marina Zambrano[1], Evelise Brizola[1], Neusa Sicca da Rocha[4], Ida Vanessa D. Schwartz[5,6,7,8], Maria Marlene de Souza Pires[2,3] and Têmis Maria Félix[1,8*]

Abstract

Background: Osteogenesis imperfecta (OI) is a disorder of bone formation leading to low mineral density and fractures. Children and adolescents with OI require periodic medical follow up, corrective surgery, drug therapy and physical therapy, as well as specific daily care practices. In addition, they have an increased incidence of fractures, which require immobilization and cause severe discomfort and short-term disability. This study evaluated the health-related quality of life of children and adolescents with OI in two reference centers for OI treatment in southern Brazil.

Methods: In this prospective cross-sectional study, the Pediatric Quality of Life Inventory (PedsQL™) was applied in two university-affiliated reference centers for OI treatment in southern Brazil. Children and adolescents aged ≥ 5 years with clinical diagnoses of OI were included. Clinical data and socioeconomic status was evaluated.

Results: The sample consisted of 52 children and adolescents with OI (aged 5-17 years); 26 (50%) participants with type I OI, 13 (25%) type IV, 12 (23.1 %) type III, and 1 (1.9%) type V OI. Physical and social functioning domains differed significantly according to clinical presentation of OI with lowest scores in the severe type (OI type III). Pain seems to be the variable that is most associated with impact on the PedsQL domains.

Conclusions: Overall, this study revealed differences in physical functioning and social functioning in relation to OI clinical presentation. These results reinforcing the importance of the clinical management of these patients with the aim of functional improvement and importance of pain control.

Keywords: Osteogenesis imperfecta, Quality of life, Sickness impact profile, Child, Adolescent

Background

Osteogenesis imperfecta (OI) is a disorder of bone formation leading to low mineral density and fractures [1, 2]. The incidence of OI is approximately 1/10,000-20,000 births [1]. It is usually caused by pathogenic mutations in the genes involved in the production of type I collagen, the main building block of bone, leading to reduced collagen production or structural failure. Approximately 80-90% of mutations occur in the *COLIA1* and *COLIA2* genes, which encode the α1 and α2 subunits of type I collagen, respectively [3]. Recently, several molecular studies identified additional genes involved in the biosynthesis of collagen as causing OI. However, the classification of OI that remains in widespread use is based on clinical and radiological features and defines five distinct types (I-V) [4, 5].

Many individuals with genetic disorders struggle with a variety of conditions that accompany chronic disease. Individuals with OI require periodic medical follow up, corrective surgery, drug therapy and physiotherapy, as well as specific daily care practices. In addition, they have an increased incidence of fractures, seen more frequently in children and adolescents, which require immobilization and cause severe discomfort and short-term disability [6]. Thus, OI is assumed to have a major

* Correspondence: tfelix@hcpa.edu.br
[1]Child and Adolescent Health, Universidade Federal do Rio Grande do Sul, Porto Alegre, Brazil
[8]Medical Genetics Service, Hospital de Clinicas de Porto Alegre, Porto Alegre, Brazil

impact on patients' quality of life (QoL). Measurement and analysis of health-related quality of life (HRQoL) in individuals with genetic disorders, particularly OI, are essential for the evaluation not only of treatment outcomes, but also of patients' well-being. This intervention may facilitate the work of professionals by modifying factors that go beyond health outcomes, including environmental, psychosocial, and school-related aspects, which may affect patients' QoL. This study aimed to assess and characterize the HRQoL of children and adolescents with different types of OI.

Methods

Participants in this prospective cross-sectional study were recruited by convenience sampling between December 2013 and January 2015 at two university-affiliated reference centers for OI treatment in two southern Brazilian states: the Clinical Hospital of Porto Alegre in Porto Alegre and Joana Gusmão Hospital in Florianópolis. The study was approved by the research ethics committees of both institutions and was conducted in accordance with the provisions of the Declaration of Helsinki. All parents or guardians provided written informed consent prior to patients' inclusion in the study.

Children and adolescents were invited to participate after routine outpatient visits. No patient presenting for a first visit to the hospital was included in the study. The sample included children and adolescents aged ≥ 5 years with clinical diagnoses of OI type I, III, IV, or V. The OI classification adopted in this study was based on the clinical criteria established by Van Dijk and Sillence [5]. Patients diagnosed with and/or treated for anxiety and depression were excluded from the study.

Participants' socioeconomic status was assessed using a validated Brazilian questionnaire based on the Brazilian Association of Research Companies Economic Classification Criterion [7]. This questionnaire yields a score that can be used to stratify the population into socioeconomic status ranges (A1, A2, B1, B2, C1, C2, D, and E), with "A" corresponding to the highest score and "E" to the lowest score [7].

Bleck's criteria [8], modified by Land et al [9], were used to evaluate mobility: (0) not walking, (1) therapeutic walking, (2) household walking with or without assistance, (3) neighborhood or community walking with or without assistance, and (4) independently walking. For statistical calculations, classifications of 0, 1, and 2 were grouped and compared with classifications of 3 and 4. Two researchers (JVL and APV) collected clinical data.

Given the wide range of patient age at the time of evaluation, we calculated the rate of fracture according to the number of fractures/year. Patients were also asked whether they remembered having felt pain in the last month. Bisphosphonate treatment was investigated in patients receiving intravenous pamidronate (which is usually indicated for the more severe forms of OI with bone quality compromise), alendronate, or no medication.

HRQoL was evaluated using the Pediatric Quality of Life Inventory (PedsQL™ 4.0 Generic Core), a generic assessment instrument that has been validated in Brazilian Portuguese [10]. This self-report instrument consists of 23 items in four domains: physical functioning (8 items), emotional functioning (5 items), social functioning (5 items), and school functioning (5 items). Responses are used to calculate total, psychosocial health, and physical summary scores. Scores were summarized according to a statistical model established by the authors of PedsQL™ 4.0 [11–16]. They were expressed as transformed scores on a 0-100 scale, with higher scores indicating better QoL. Children and adolescents filled out this self-report questionnaire. For children aged 5 to 7 years all questions were read by the researchers and answers were given according to a visual analogic scale as suggested by PedsQL™.

Continuous data were described by mean and standard deviation. Categorical data were presented as counts and percentages. Asymmetrical distribution variables were described by median, interquartile range, and range. Since the PedsQL score followed a nearly symmetrical distribution, mean groups of OI clinical presentation were compared using analysis of variance (ANOVA) with robust standard errors approach when required. Accordingly, the Tukey's and Dunnet's T3 (robust) tests were used for post hoc comparisons. Correlations between continuous symmetrical variables were computed using Pearson's product moment correlation coefficient or Spearman's rank correlation coefficient (rho) for situations where ordinal or not asymmetrical distributed variables we involved. A multiple linear regression model was used to simultaneously evaluate the impact of mobility, medical treatment, annual fracture rate, and pain score on the total PedsQL score and all the other component domains. The selection of these variables was more based on the underlying conceptual framework found in the specialized literature rather than on pure statistical significance. Asymmetrically distributed variables were log transformed before inclusion in the model. The standardized beta coefficient was used to asses and compare the magnitude of association of these factors with the different PedsQL domains in the multiple linear regression model. Statistical significance was set at $p<0.05$. Data were processed and analyzed using R version 3.3.0 and SPSS version 22.0.

Results

The sample was composed of 52 children and adolescents with OI: 12 (23.1%) from the Florianopolis center and 40 (76.9%) from the Porto Alegre center. Patient characteristics are summarized in Table 1. Twenty-six (50%) participants had type I OI, 12 (23.1%) had type III, 13 (25%) had type IV, and one (1.9%) participant had type V OI. Twenty-five (48.1%) patients used pamidronate and one (1.9%) used alendronate; 19 (36.5%) patients were in physiotherapy. Thirteen (25%) patients used a wheelchair and 38 (73.01%) walked with support or independently. One patient was not included in the sample because he had a diagnosis of hyperactivity.

Table 1 Characteristics of study participants

Variable *n*= 52	Frequency no. (%)
Male	29 (55.7)
Age (years)	
5-7	13 (25.0)
8-12	24 (46.2)
13-18	15 (28.8)
Mean (SD)	11.2 ± 4.2
OI type	
I	26 (50.0)
III	12 (23.1)
IV	13 (25.0)
V	1 (1.9)
Treatment	
Sodium pamidronate	25 (48.1)
Sodium alendronate	01 (01.9)
Physiotherapy	19 (36.5)
Mobility[a]	
Wheelchair	13 (25.0)
Walk or walk with support	38 (73.0)
Pain in the last month (n=44)	
Yes	19 (43.2)
No	25 (56.8)
Annual fracture rate[b]	
Median (IQR)	0.91 (0.47 to 1.67)
Minimum to Maximum	0.06 to 6.33
Social assistance (n=42)	
Yes	20 (47.6)
No	22 (52.4)
Socioeconomic status (n=47)	
A	1 (2.1)
B1	3 (6.4)
B2	13 (27.7)
C1	13 (27.7)
C2	9(19.1)
D-E	8 (17.0)

[a]Bleck's criteria [8], modified by Land et al [9], were used to evaluate mobility walking. For statistical calculations, classifications of 0, 1, and 2 were grouped and compared with classifications of 3 and 4. [b]Number of fractures/year.

Thirty-seven (71.2%) children and 15 (28.8%) adolescents completed the PedsQL^{TM}. In the total sample, mean physical functioning scores were lowest and mean social functioning scores were highest. In the analysis of mean domain scores according to clinical presentation, the physical functioning and social functioning scores differed significantly between participants with mild, moderate and severe forms of OI (Table 2).

Clinical presentation was moderately correlated with physical functioning domain (rho = -0.38, p = 0.006) and socioeconomic status was inversely correlated with school functioning domain (rho = -0.31, p = 0.036). Age presented a weak correlation with the social functioning domain score, although significant (r = 0.29, p = 0.037). The annual fracture rate showed no significant correlation with any domain score.

Multiple linear regression analysis showed that pain score was statistically associated with all PedsQL domains except schooling. The pain score presented higher magnitudes of association with the total score, followed by psychosocial health, emotional, social, and physical functioning (Table 3).

Discussion

This study examined self-reported HRQoL of children and adolescents with OI using measures applicable to the age range investigated. Curiously, QoL is not frequently assessed in individuals with genetic disorders. A systematic review published in 2010 [17] identified 58 studies in which QoL was assessed using validated questionnaires in patients with genetic conditions. Only one of these studies examined patients with OI; QoL was assessed in an adult cohort using the SF-36, a validated health self-assessment questionnaire [18]. In a recently published scoping review that addressed the impacts of three genetic musculoskeletal diseases, 15 papers addressing OI were identified, but none focused on children and adolescents or assessed HRQoL with an available and validated inventory [19]. All articles used the term QoL, but the studies evaluated only physical factors such as functionality, and none used a tool designed to measure the QoL construct in children and adolescents.

Parents were formerly believed to be the appropriate informants about their children's HRQoL. The current perspective is that children are able to speak for themselves, enabling researchers to avoid relying solely on parents' opinions, which are influenced by their own experience and backgrounds [20–22]. Children and adolescents with chronic diseases requiring regular healthcare

Table 2 PedsQL™ scores according to OI Clinical Presentation

PedsQL™ score	Total sample	Clinical presentation*			
		Mild	Moderate	Severe	
	n = 52	*n* = 26	*n* = 14	*n=12*	*p***
Total	69.7 ± 13.1	71.3 ± 12.4	71.0 ± 13.2	64.8 ± 14.8	0.349
Physical functioning	61.9 ± 21.1	69.2 ± 17.2[a]	58.5 ± 23.7[a]	50.0 ± 14.8[b]	0.023
Psychosocial health	72.3 ± 12.7	71.9 ± 12.0	75.1 ± 11.7	69.7± 15.7	0.558
Emotional Functioning	66.3 ± 18.1	65.9 ± 16.3	67.0 ± 18.4	66.2 ± 22.9	0.984
Social functioning	77.7 ± 16.3	76.1 ± 19.3[a,b]	85.7 ± 8.0[a]	71.6 ±13.3[b]	0.007
School functioning	73.2 ± 15.2	74.5 ± 10.9	72.6 ± 17.8	71.2 ± 20.2	0.829

Data are presented as means ± standard deviations. *Clinical presentation- Mild (OI type I); Moderate (OI type IV and V); Severe (OI type III). **ANOVA, different index letters represent staticsally significant difference at the post hoc test

acquire knowledge about their health and are able to express their needs related to the disease. Often, their opinions about their health status are much more accurate than those of their parents or caregivers [23]. In this study, for example, two children using wheelchairs responded "never" to the item "It is hard for me to walk more than one block"; that is, their perception of "walking" was appropriate.

As reported by Fano et al [24], we found that patients with moderate and severe OI had lower physical functioning domain than did those with mild OI. This finding shows that the physical health component of QoL is compromised in severely affected patients, making them somewhat "uncomfortable." In a qualitative study of children and adolescents with OI, physical health status was associated with the following themes: being safe and careful, reduced function, pain, fear, isolation, and independence [22]. In another study in which QoL related to olpadronate use was evaluated using the Self-Perception Profile for Children, the athletic performance score was lowest [25]. In the assessment of HRQoL using PedsQL™ in patients with Duchenne muscular dystrophy, the most common inherited pediatric neuromuscular disorder and a cause of significant physical limitation, the physical domain score was lowest in children and adolescents [26].

Multiple linear regression analysis showed that pain affected total, physical functioning, emotional functioning, and psychosocial health scores. In OI, bone fragility results in recurrent fractures, leading to bone pain. Bone deformity also contributes to physical discomfort. A previous analysis of emergency department records demonstrated the need for additional effort and resources to address the under treatment of pain in children and adults with fractures in the emergency setting [27]. The authors stated that special attention should be given to analgesia for the very old and very young. They concluded that the education of providers on nonverbal options for measuring pain, especially in young children, may improve the measurement and documentation of pain status and facilitate recognition and treatment of pain in these vulnerable populations [27].

Socioeconomic status was correlated negatively with school functioning in the present sample, in which 26/52 (50%) patients' family status was classified as B2 or C1. The 2012 Brazilian Institute of Statistics and Public Opinion survey showed that 29% of the Brazilian population belongs to class C1, followed by classes C2 (24%) and B2 (21%). Since 2005, improvement in the population's economic status has been observed [28, 29]. In contrast to the findings of the present study, economic level was not correlated with QoL scores in our previous study of caregivers of individuals with OI [30]. In another study conducted in southern Brazil, socioeconomic level was correlated positively with environmental and social domain scores [31]. The differences can be explained by a small sample size and asymmetric distribution of the socioeconomic status in our study.

Age was positively correlated with the social functioning domain score in the present study. Although the literature does not contain reports of the impact of fractures on the QoL of children and adolescents, fracture is an important modifier of physical condition. It was one the six main themes identified in a qualitative interview-based study involving children and adolescents with OI, as well as their parents [22].

Seikaly et al [32], evaluated the impact of alendronate therapy on QoL in children with OI; however, no specific instrument was used to measure QoL. Their study focused on assessing individuals' self-care and functional ability through application of a visual analog scale for pain and assessment of the number of days without pain. They found significant improvement in subjective well-being, pain, and analgesia use scores in subjects treated with alendronate. In the assessment of HRQoL using PedsQL™, Fano et al [24] also identified pharmacological treatment as a modifying factor in a linear

Table 3 The impacts of selected patient characteristics on PedsQL™ scores, as determined by multiple linear regression

PedsQL™ domain/characteristic	Standardized beta coefficient	*p*
Total		
Mobility	0.22	0.19
Medical treatment	0,28	0.19
Annual fracture rate	-0.28	0.12
Pain score	-0.37	0.009
Physical functioning		
Mobility	0.35	0.03
Medical treatment	0,08	0.67
Annual fracture rate	-0.27	0.34
Pain score	-0.27	0.05
Psychosocial health		
Mobility	0.11	0.52
Medical treatment	0.33	0.12
Annual fracture rate	-0.23	0.20
Pain score	-0.36	0.012
Emotional functioning		
Mobility	0.10	0.56
Medical treatment	0.26	0.23
Annual fracture rate	-0.06	0.72
Pain score	-0.35	0.015
Social functioning		
Mobility	0.62	0.72
Medical treatment	0.20	0.35
Annual fracture rate	-0.20	0.28
Pain score	-0.28	0.015
School functioning		
Mobility	0.09	0.60
Medical treatment	0.27	0.23
Annual fracture rate	-0.27	0.17
Pain score	-0.20	0.18

Ninety-five percent confidence intervals were calculated and the level of significance was set at $p < 0.05$.

regression analysis. The design of the present study did not enable the comparison of treatment regimens; randomized studies are needed to characterize the main effects of drug therapy on OI patients' QoL.

This study has limitations. QoL is a construct with multiple definitions and it is based on qualitative variables, therefore, assessment using generic instruments that produce only quantitative variable values may have limited the analysis in this study. We believe that QoL can be assessed more accurately when quantitative and qualitative tools are used in combination. Moreover, the use of specific questionnaires is ideal for measurement of the impact of chronic disease on QoL with greater accuracy and sensitivity. To date, no specific questionnaire has been validated for patients with OI. Furthermore, the small sample size and convenience sampling limited the power this study. It should be noted that this is a usual finding when studying rare diseases and efforts were made to increase the sample size, recruiting subjects from different centers.

Conclusions

Most chronic illnesses should be seen as stressors that may ultimately affect child development and can restrict children's school and social performance, even in the family context. Estimation of the impact of chronic disease on the lives of children and adolescents is of fundamental importance for the development of interventions that can compensate for these deficits.

The measurement of QoL is gaining momentum and its consideration is having positive effects in health practice, as it allows the development and implementation of comprehensive interventions, rather than focusing only on the health/disease process. Overall, this study revealed differences in physical functioning in relation to OI severity and mobility, reinforcing the importance of the clinical management of these patients with the aim of functional improvement. Further studies in the same population with specific instruments for the measurement of QoL are required to support these results and provide more representative data.

Abbreviations

CAAE: Certificado de Apresentação para Apreciação Ética; HRQoL: Health-related quality of life; OI: Osteogenesis imperfecta; PedsQL™: Pediatric Quality of Life Inventory; QoL: Quality of life

Acknowledgments

We thank the children and adolescents and their parents who participated in this study and the Group for Research and Postgraduate Studies (Grupo de Pesquisa e Pós-Graduação) for their assistance with the statistical analysis, Fundação de Amparo à Pesquisa do Estado do Rio Grande do Sul (FAPERGS) and Hospital de Clínicas de Porto Alegre (FIPE/HCPA). APV received a scholarship from Coordenação de Aperfeiçoamento de Pessoal do Nível Superior (CAPES). TMF is supported by CNPq #306245/2016-7.

Funding

Fundação de Amparo à Pesquisa do Estado do Rio Grande do Sul (FAPERGS) and Hospital de Clínicas de Porto Alegre (FIPE/HCPA).

Author's contributions

APV- planned the approach to the present paper, data collection, performed the statistical analysis and drafted the manuscript. JVSL- planned the approach to the present paper, data collection, analysis and interpretation of results. BP, MZ, EB, NSR and MMSP- participated in analysis and interpretation of results. TMF- participated in the design, data collection and coordination of the study. All authors read and approved the final manuscript.

Ethics approval and consent to participate
All procedures performed in studies involving human participants were in accordance with the ethical standards of the institutional and/or national research committee and with the 1964 Helsinki declaration and its later amendments or comparable ethical standards. The study was approved by the research ethics committees of both institutions and was conducted in accordance with the provisions of the Declaration of Helsinki (Research Ethics Committee at Hospital de Clínicas de Porto Alegre, CAAE: 19041613.7.0000.5327 and Research Ethics Committee at Joana Gusmão Hospital, CAAE: 19041613.7.3001.536). All parents or guardians provided written informed consent prior to patients' inclusion in the study.

Competing interests
Not applicable.

Author details
[1]Child and Adolescent Health, Universidade Federal do Rio Grande do Sul, Porto Alegre, Brazil. [2]Division of Pediatric Endocrinology, Hospital Infantil Joana de Gusmão, Florianópolis, Brazil. [3]Medical Sciences, Universidade Federal de Santa Catarina, Florianópolis, Brazil. [4]Medical Sciences: Psychiatry, Universidade Federal do Rio Grande do Sul, Porto Alegre, Brazil. [5]Medical Sciences, Universidade Federal do Rio Grande do Sul, Porto Alegre, Brazil. [6]Department of Genetics, Universidade Federal do Rio Grande do Sul, Porto Alegre, Brazil. [7]Health Technology Assessment in Clinical Genetics Research Group, Hospital de Clínicas de Porto Alegre, Porto Alegre, Brazil. [8]Medical Genetics Service, Hospital de Clinicas de Porto Alegre, Porto Alegre, Brazil.

References
1. Cole WG. Advances in Osteogenesis Imperfecta. Clin Orthop Relat Res. 2002; 401:6–16.
2. Rauch F, Glorieux FH. Osteogenesis Imperfecta. Lancet. 2004;363:1377–85.
3. Byers PH, Wallis GA, Willing MC. Osteogenesis imperfecta: translation of mutation to phenotype. J Med Genet. 1991;28(7):433–42.
4. Osteogenesis Imperfecta Foundation. Facts about Osteogenesis Imperfecta. [update 2015 Jun 16 cited 2015 Jun 16] Available from http://www.oif.org.
5. Van Dijk FS, Sillence DO. Osteogenesis imperfecta: clinical diagnosis, nomenclature and severity assessment. Am J Med Genet A. 2014;164A(6): 1470–1.
6. Engelbert RH, Uiterwaal CS, Gulmans VA, Pruijs H, Helders PJ. Osteogenesis imperfecta in childhood: prognosis for walking. J Pediatr. 2000;137:397–402.
7. Brasil (2012). ABEP-Associação Brasileira de Empresas de Pesquisa. Critérios de Classificação Econômica Brasil, 2012. [update 2014 Dec 10 cited 2015 Jun 16]. Available from www.abep.org.
8. Bleck EE. Nonoperative treatment of osteogenesis imperfecta: orthotic and mobility management. Clin Orthop Relat Res. 1981;(159):111–22.
9. Land C, Rauch F, Montpetit K, Ruck-Gibis J, Glorieux FH. Effect of intravenous pamidronate therapy on functional abilities and level of ambulation in children with osteogenesis imperfecta. J Pediatr. 2006;148: 456–60.
10. Klatchoian DA, Len CA, Terreri MTRA, Silva M, Itamoto C, Ciconelli RM, et al. Quality of life of children and adolescents from São Paulo: reliability and validity of the Brazilian version of the Pediatric Quality of Life Inventory™ version 4.0 Generic Core Scales. J Pediatr (Rio J). 2008; Aug;84(4):308–15.
11. Varni JW, Seid M, Kurtin PS. The PedsQL™ 4.0: Reliability and validity of the Pediatric Quality of Life Inventory™ Version 4.0 Generic Core Scales in healthy and patient populations. Med Care. 2001; 39(8): 800-812.
12. Varni JW, Seid M, Knight TS, Uzark K, Szer IS. The PedsQL™ 4.0 Generic Core Scales: Sensitivity, responsiveness, and impact on clinical decision-making. J Behav Med . 2002; 25, 175-193.
13. Varni JW, Burwinkle TM, Seid M, Skarr D. The PedsQL™ 4.0 as a pediatric population health measure: Feasibility, reliability, and validity. Ambul Pediatr. 2003; 3, 329-341.
14. Chan KS, Mangione-Smith R, Burwinkle TM, Rosen M, Varni JW. The PedsQL™: Reliability and validity of the Short-Form Generic Core Scales and Asthma Module. Med Care 2005; 43, 256-265.
15. Varni JW, Limbers CA. The PedsQL™ 4.0 Generic Core Scales Young Adult Version: Feasibility, reliability and validity in a university student population. J Health Psychol. 2009; 14, 611-622.
16. Varni JW, Seid M, Rode CA. The PedsQL™: Measurement Model for the Pediatric Quality of Life Inventory. Med Care. 1999; 37(2):126-139.
17. Cohen JS, Biesecker B. Quality of life in rare genetic conditions: A systematic review of the literature. Am J Med Genet Part A. 2010;152A(5):1136–56.
18. Widmann RF, Laplaza FJ, Bitan FD, Brooks CE, Root L. Quality of life in osteogenesis imperfecta. Int Orthop. 2002;26:3–6.
19. Dogba MJ, Rauch F, Douglas E, Bedos C. Impact of three genetic musculoskeletal diseases: a comparative synthesis of achondroplasia, Duchenne muscular dystrophy and osteogenesis imperfecta. Health Qual Life Outcomes. 2014;12(1)
20. Prout A. Representing children: reflections on the children 5–15 programme. Child Soc. 2001;
21. Bryman A. Social Research Methods. 2nd ed. Oxford: Oxford University Press; 2004.
22. Hill CL, Baird WO, Walters SJ. Quality of life in children and adolescents with Osteogenesis Imperfecta: a qualitative interview based study. Health Qual Life Outcomes. 2014;12:54.
23. Mello DB, Moreira MC. The hospitalization and the process of becoming ill through the children's and adolescents' perspective with cystic fibrosis and osteogenesis imperfecta. Cien Saude Colet. 2010;15(2):453–61.
24. Fano V, del Pino M, Rodríguez CM, Buceta S, Obregón MG. Osteogenesis imperfecta: quality of life in children. Arch Argent Pediatr. 2013;111(4):328–31.
25. Kok DHJ, Sakkers RJB, Janse AJ, Pruijs HEH, Verbout A, Castelein RM, Engelbert RHH. Quality of life in children with osteogenesis imperfecta treated with oral bisphosphonates (Olpadronate): a 2-year randomized placebo-controlled trial. European Journal of Pediatrics. 2007;166(11):11–01.
26. Uzark K, King E, Cripe L, Spicer R, Sage J, Kinnett K, Wong B, Pratt J, Varni JW. Health-related quality of life in children and adolescents with Duchenne muscular dystrophy. Pediatrics. 2012; Dec;130(6):e1559–66.
27. Brown JC, Klein EJ, Lewis CW, Johnston PC, Brian D. Emergency Department Analgesia for Fracture Pain. Ann Emerg Med. 2003;42:197–205.
28. Brasil. ABEP-Associação Brasileira de Empresas de Pesquisa. Dados com base no Levantamento Sócio Econômico, 2005. [update 2014 Dec 10 cited 2015 Jun 16] Available from http://www.abep.org/Servicos/Download.aspx?id=07
29. Brasil. ABEP-Associação Brasileira de Empresas de Pesquisa. Critérios de Classificação Econômica Brasil, 2014. [update 2014 Dec 10 cited 2015 Jun 16] Available from http://www.abep.org/criterio-brasil
30. Vanz AP, Félix TM, da Rocha NS, Schwartz IV. Quality of life in caregivers of children and adolescents with Osteogenesis Imperfecta. Health Qual Life Outcomes. 2015;13:41.
31. Rocha NS, Fleck MP. Evaluation of quality of life in adults with chronic health conditions: the role of depressive symptoms. Rev Bras Psiquiatr. 2010; 32(2):119–24.
32. SeikalyMG, Kopanati S, Salhab N, et al. Impact of alendronate on quality of life in children with osteogenesis imperfecta. J Pediatr Orthopaed. 2005;25:786–91.

10

Hospital readmissions with acute infectious diseases in New Zealand children < 2 years of age

Silvia Seibt[1], Catherine A. Gilchrist[2], Peter W. Reed[3], Emma J. Best[2,4], Anthony Harnden[5], Carlos A. Camargo Jr[6] and Cameron C. Grant[2,7*]

Abstract

Background: Infectious diseases are the leading cause of hospital admissions in young children. Hospitalisation with an infectious disease is a recurrent event for some children. Our objective was to describe risk factors for infectious disease readmission following hospital admission with an infectious disease in the first two years of life.

Methods: We performed a national cohort study of New Zealand children, born 2005–2009, with an infectious disease admission before age 24 months. Children readmitted with an infectious disease within 12 months of the first infectious disease admission were identified. Every infectious disease admission was categorised as a respiratory, enteric, skin and soft tissue, urinary or other infection. Independent associations of demographic and child health factors with infectious disease readmission were determined using multiple variable logistic regression.

Results: From 2005 to 2011, there were 69,902 infectious disease admissions for 46,657 children less than two years old. Of these 46,657 children, 10,205 (22%) had at least one infectious disease readmission within 12 months of their first admission. The first infectious disease admission was respiratory (54%), enteric (15%), skin or soft tissue (7%), urinary (4%) or other (20%). Risk of infectious disease readmission was increased if the first infectious disease admission was respiratory (OR = 1.87, 95% CI 1.78–1.95) but not if it was in any other infectious disease category. Risk factors for respiratory infectious disease readmission were male gender, Pacific or Māori ethnicity, greater household deprivation, presence of a complex chronic condition, or a first respiratory infectious disease admission during autumn or of ≥3 days duration. Fewer factors (younger age, male gender, presence of a complex chronic condition) were associated with enteric infection readmission. The presence of a complex chronic condition was the only factor associated with urinary tract infection readmission and none of the factors were associated with skin or soft tissue infection readmission.

Conclusions: In children less than two years old, infectious disease readmission risk is increased if the first infectious disease admission is a respiratory infectious disease but not if it is another infectious disease category. Risk factors for respiratory infectious disease readmission are different from those for other infectious disease readmissions.

Keywords: Infant, Child preschool, Cohort studies, Diarrhea, Hospitalization, Patient readmission, Respiratory tract infections, Skin and soft tissue infections, Urinary tract infections

* Correspondence: cc.grant@auckland.ac.nz
[2]Department of Paediatrics: Child and Youth Health, Faculty of Medical and Health Sciences, University of Auckland, Private Bag 92019, Wellesley Street, Auckland 1142, New Zealand
[7]General Paediatrics, Starship Children's Hospital, Auckland District Health Board, Auckland, New Zealand
Full list of author information is available at the end of the article

Background

Globally, infectious diseases are a leading cause of morbidity and mortality in young children [1]. From 2004 to 2008 in New Zealand (NZ), infectious diseases accounted for 60% of hospitalisations of children < 5 years old [2]. Most infectious disease related hospitalisations were due to lower respiratory tract, enteric, and skin and soft tissue infections [2].

Hospitalisation rates for infectious diseases are higher in NZ than in other developed countries. Children < 2 years old are more than twice as likely to be hospitalised with bronchiolitis in NZ (2006–2010: 45/1000) than in England (2007–2010: 20/1000), or the United States (US) (2000–2009: 16/1000) [3–5]. Hospitalisation rates for pneumonia in children < 2 years old in NZ (2006–2010: 14/1000) are twice those in the US (2007–2009: 7/1000) [3, 6], and children < 1 year old have eight times the US rate of skin infection hospitalisation (NZ 2006–2010: 21/1000, US 2005 2.4/1000) [3, 7]. In recent decades the rate of infectious disease hospital admissions in NZ has increased [2]. This represents a true increase in disease incidence, attributed to ethnic and social inequalities, and to disparities in social determinants of health including household income, housing conditions, and access to healthcare [2].

Hospitalisation with an infectious disease (ID) is a recurrent event for some children. In a US study, the 3% of children with four-or-more recurrent admissions, including but not limited to ID, accounted for 19% of all paediatric hospital admissions [8]. Identifying strategies to prevent readmission is therefore an important component of quality of care improvement [9].

Early identification of children at risk of ID readmission and prevention of repeated illness episodes may prevent subsequent chronic disease. For example, globally almost two-thirds of children with ID-associated bronchiectasis have a history of recurrent acute lower respiratory infections (ALRIs) [10–12]. Bronchiectasis is particularly prevalent in indigenous children from NZ, Australia, Alaska, and Canada and a history of early infant pneumonia and/or recurrent ALRIs is associated with bronchiectasis in over 90% of cases [11, 13, 14].

Our aim was to describe recurrent hospitalisations for infectious diseases in young NZ children, including factors associated with ID readmission. The ability to identify children at risk of recurrent disease when they first present to hospital allows the development and evaluation of interventions targeted to this at-risk group.

Methods

Study design and setting

We created a national cohort study of NZ children born over a five-year period (2005–2009) and described their ID hospitalisations. We identified the children hospitalised with an ID during their first 24 months of life, and the subset of children subsequently readmitted with an ID within 12 months of their initial ID hospitalisation were enrolled in the study. The study protocol was reviewed by the NZ Health and Disabilities Ethics Committee, with the ethics committee determining that ethical approval was not required. The NZ Ministry of Health granted data access, providing data with encrypted NHI numbers to maintain patient anonymity. The Ministry of Health did not grant permission for data sharing.

Study population and sample

Children were eligible if born between 1st January 2005 and 31st December 2009 and a NZ resident at the time of their first ID hospitalisation. Hospitalisation data were collected over six years, from 1st January 2005 to 31st December 2011. Children were excluded if they had an ID admission in their first 24 months of life but died within 12 months of this first admission ($n = 117$). Permission to access data on cause of death was not obtained.

A hospital admission was defined as an overnight stay in a hospital inpatient ward. We excluded episodes where a child was admitted and discharged on the same day. In NZ all acute ID hospital admissions during childhood are to public hospitals.

Hospitalisation data were obtained from the NZ national dataset of hospital admissions, the National Minimum Dataset (NMDS) [15]. We used the national health index (NHI) number, a unique identifier assigned to every person on contact with health services in NZ, to identify all hospitalisations for each child. To maintain anonymity, data provided from the NMDS contained an encrypted unique identifier for each child. Thus, written informed consent was not required.

Identification of infectious disease hospital admissions

Using the approach developed by the US Centers for Disease Control and Prevention [16, 17], and previously used in NZ [2], we defined an ID hospitalisation as one for which the principal International Classification of Disease (ICD-10) code was for an ID (Additional file 1).

Within the NMDS, each hospital admission may include more than one inpatient event. For example, a child admitted to intensive care and then transferred to the inpatient ward is described as two separate events. To ensure each admission was counted only once, consecutive events with the same discharge and admission dates were counted as a single hospitalisation.

Study sample demographics and illness history

Demographic information was obtained from the NMDS. Ethnicity (European, Māori, Pacific, Asian and

Other) was defined as that stated by parents at the first admission. Socioeconomic status was defined using a small area unit level descriptor of household deprivation created from national census data (NZDep2006) grouped as quintiles [18]. As defined by Berry et al. (2011), children with complex chronic conditions (CCC) known to be associated with recurrent hospital admission were identified from the ICD-10 codes listed for the first ID admission [8].

Statistical analyses

ID hospitalisations were grouped into five diagnostic categories: acute respiratory infection (ARI), enteric infection, skin or soft tissue infection (SSTI), urinary tract infection (UTI) and other ID (Additional file 1). Other ID included septicaemia, meningococcal disease, meningitis, osteomyelitis, and septic arthritis. An ID readmission was defined as a second or subsequent hospital admission with an ID principal discharge code, > 1 day after the discharge from the first admission and < 12 months from the original ID admission.

Data were analysed using JMP V10.0 (SAS Inc.). We used multivariable logistic regression to identify independent associations between demographic variables and the risk of hospital readmission with an ID. We determined whether the risk of readmission with an ID varied by type of ID causing the first admission (ARI, enteric, SSTI, UTI or other ID), and, within the ARI group, by type of acute lower respiratory infection (pneumonia, bronchiolitis, influenza and other ARI) (Additional file 2). Within the ARI, enteric, SSTI, UTI or other ID diagnostic groups, we then described the risk factors associated with readmission with a second ID episode within the same ID diagnostic group. Associations were reported using adjusted odds ratios (OR) and 95% confidence intervals (CI).

Results

Study population and sample

There were 659,495 hospital discharge events (from 1st January 2005 and 31st December 2011) for children born between 1st January 2005 and 31st December 2009 (Fig. 1). These events, which included formal transfers and other patient movements, converted to 587,336 hospital admissions, of which 177,545 (30%) included an ID discharge code. We excluded 34,691 admissions (non-acute, to a private hospital or not a NZ resident); and 40,932 admissions lasting < 24 h. Of the 101,922 acute overnight public hospital ID admissions, for 20,186 the ID discharge code was not the principal code, and for 11,834 the first ID admission occurred at age ≥ 2 years.

There were 69,902 ID hospital admissions for 46,657 children < 2 years old, of whom 10,205 (22%) had at least one subsequent ID readmission within the 12 months following their first admission. Therefore, 15% of the national birth cohort from 2005 to 2009 had an ID hospital admission before age two years, with 3% having at least one further ID admission within the next 12 months.

Characteristics of children hospitalised with an infectious disease (Table 1)

The median (interquartile range (IQR)) age at first ID admission was 7.2 (2.4–13.2) months. Compared with the ethnicity of live births in New Zealand in 2010 (27% Māori, 11% Pacific, 11% Asian, and 51% European/other), there were higher percentages of Māori (34%, $p < 0.001$) and Pacific (17%, $P < 0.001$) children among those hospitalised with an ID. By contrast, there were lower percentages of Asian (5%, $P < 0.001$) and European/other (43%, $P < 0.001$) children hospitalised with an ID [19].

Of the 46,540 children hospitalised with an ID, 18,575 (40%) lived in the most deprived households and 894 (2%) had an underlying CCC. The most frequent season of first ID admission was winter (17,285/46,540 37%) and the majority of first admissions were for an ARI (25,256/46,540 54%).

Infectious disease group and readmission risk (Table 2)

Readmission occurred at a median (IQR) of 77 (26–177) days after the first ID admission. Median (IQR) days to ID readmission was 67 (25–157) if the first admission was ARI, 96 (23–198) if it was enteric infection, 100 (34–195) if it was an SSTI and 115 (45–202) if it was a UTI.

Overall, 6735/10,205 (66%) of the ID readmissions were with an ARI. In comparison with all other infections, children whose first ID admission was an ARI were at increased risk (OR = 1.87, 95% CI 1.78–1.95) of readmission, whereas those whose first ID admission was an enteric infection (OR = 0.63, 0.59–0.67), SSTI (OR = 0.62, 95% CI 0.56–0.68), UTI (OR = 0.83, 95% CI 0.74–0.94) or other infection (OR = 0.65, 95% CI 0.62–0.69) were at decreased risk.

Acute respiratory infection group and readmission risk (Tables 3 and 4)

Among children whose first admission was an ARI, the risk of readmission with an ARI was increased if this first admission was with bronchiolitis (OR = 2.21, 95% CI 2.08–2.36) and decreased if the first admission was with pneumonia (OR = 0.66, 95% CI 0.61–0.73), or an ARI that was not bronchiolitis, pneumonia, or influenza (OR = 0.49, 95% CI 0.46–0.53) (Table 3). Among children whose first admission was an ARI, the principal discharge diagnosis of the readmission was lower ARI in 82%. In comparison with those whose first ID admission was an upper ARI, children whose first ID admission

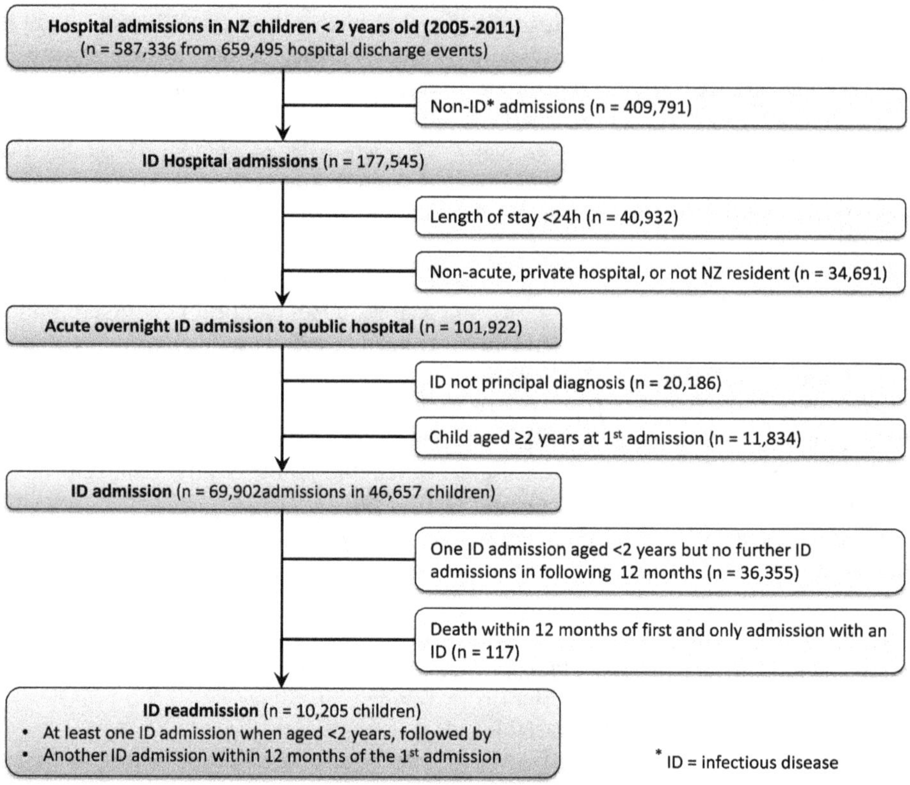

Fig. 1 Flow diagram describing study design

was a lower ARI were at increased risk of readmission with any ID (29% vs. 19%, OR = 1.75, 95% CI 1.63–1.87).

Among children whose first admission was with an ARI, the risk of readmission with any ID was increased if this first admission was with bronchiolitis (OR = 2.27, 95% CI 2.17–2.38) and decreased if the first admission was with pneumonia (OR = 0.91, 95% CI 0.84–0.98), or an ARI that was not bronchiolitis, pneumonia, or influenza (OR = 0.86, 95% CI 0.81–0.92) (Table 4).

Factors associated with readmission with an acute respiratory, enteric, skin or soft tissue, or urinary tract infection

Of the 25,256 children whose first ID admission was ARI, readmission with an ARI occurred in 5521 (22%), with median (IQR) time to readmission of 57 (24–134) days (Additional file 3). Of the 6090 children whose first ID admission was an enteric infection, readmission with an enteric infection occurred in 449 (6%; median time to readmission 39 (5–145) days) (Additional file 4). Of the 3210 children admitted with an SSTI, readmission with an SSTI occurred in 205 (9%; median time to readmission 54 (16–153) days) (Additional file 5). Of the 1826 children admitted with a UTI, readmission with a UTI occurred in 101 (6%; median time to readmission 115 (45–202) days) (Additional file 6).

Children at increased risk of a second ARI admission were of younger age when first admitted with an ARI (age < 6 months vs. 6 to 23 months old, OR = 1.62, 95% CI 1.52–1.73), male gender (OR = 1.20, 95% CI 1.13–1.28), Pacific (OR = 2.14, 95% CI 1.95–2.36) or Māori (OR = 1.98, 95% CI 1.82–2.14) versus European ethnicity, or living in the most (OR = 1.31, 95% CI 1.14–1.51) or second most (OR = 1.21, 95% CI 1.05–1.40) deprived compared with the least deprived quintile of households. The risk of an ARI readmission increased (OR = 1.14, 95% CI 1.01–1.29) for children whose first ARI hospital admission was in autumn compared with summer. Children with a CCC (OR = 3.25, 95% CI 2.73–3.87) or whose first ARI admission was ≥3 days in duration (OR = 1.53, 95% CI 1.43–1.63) were at increased risk of an ARI readmission (Additional file 3).

In contrast with ARIs, demographic and illness factors were less consistently associated with the risk of re-admission with a second enteric infection, SSTI or UTI (Additional files 4, 5 and 6). Children at increased risk of a second enteric infection admission were those aged < 6 months (OR = 1.53, 95% CI 1.24–1.87) when first admitted with an enteric infection, of male gender (OR = 1.25, 95% CI 1.03–1.52) or with a CCC (OR = 3.58, 95% CI 2.03–6.01) (Additional file 4). Children at increased risk of a second UTI were those with a CCC (OR = 3.49,

Table 1 Demographic and illness characteristics of children aged less than 2 years admitted to hospital with an infectious disease from 1st January 2005 to 31st December 2011

Variable	Children admitted to hospital with an infectious disease before age 2 years $n = 46{,}540$
Demographic characteristics	
Age in months, median (IQR)	7.2 (2.4–13.2)
Age, *n* (%)	
Less than 6-months-old	19,028 (41)
6- to 23-months-old	27,512 (59)
Gender, *n* (%)	
Male	26,038 (56)
Female	20,502 (44)
Ethnicity[a], *n* (%)	
Pacific	7902 (17)
Māori	15,876 (34)
Asian	2499 (5)
Other	740 (2)
European	19,411 (42)
Household deprivation[b], *n* (%)	
Dep 9 & 10 (most deprived)	18,575 (40)
Dep 7 & 8	10,996 (24)
Dep 5 & 6	7226 (16)
Dep 3 & 4	5171 (11)
Dep 1 & 2 (least deprived)	4435 (10)
Season of admission[c], *n* (%)	
Autumn	8586 (18)
Winter	17,285 (37)
Spring	13,162 (28)
Summer	7507 (16)
Illness characteristics	
Length of stay in days, median (25th, 75th centile)	3 (2, 4)
Diagnostic group of first admission, *n* (%)	
Acute respiratory infection (ARI)	25,256 (54)
Enteric infection	6909 (15)
Skin and soft tissue infection (SSTI)	3210 (7)
Urinary tract infection (UTI)	1826 (4)
Other	9339 (20)
Presence of complex chronic conditions, *n* (%)	
All complex chronic conditions	894 (2)
Neuromuscular	45 (0.1)
Cardiovascular	403 (0.9)
Respiratory	116 (0.2)
Renal	43 (0.1)
Gastrointestinal	78 (0.2)
Haematologic and immunologic	38 (0.1)
Metabolic	3 (0.01)
Other congenital or genetic defect	133 (0.3)
Malignancy	35 (0.1)

Table 1 Demographic and illness characteristics of children aged less than 2 years admitted to hospital with an infectious disease from 1st January 2005 to 31st December 2011 *(Continued)*

[a]Ethnicity not stated, $n = 112$
[b]Area-level socio-economic deprivation was measured using the NZ Index of Deprivation (NZDep06), grouped into quintiles [18]. Data were missing for 137 (0.2%) children
[c]Autumn = March to May; Winter = June to August; Spring = September to November; Summer = December to February
CI Confidence interval
IQR Interquartile range

95% CI 1.45–7.51) (Additional file 6). None of these factors was associated with the risk of a second SSTI (Additional file 5).

Discussion

In this national study, 15% of children in the 2005–2009 NZ birth cohort were hospitalised with an ID in the first two years of life, 40% of whom lived in the most deprived 20% of households. Twenty-two percent of these children (3% of the birth cohort) had at least one further ID admission within 12 months of their first admission. Two-thirds of the first ID admissions were for an ARI and over one-quarter of these children had a subsequent ARI admission. In contrast, a first ID admission for an enteric ID, SSTI or UTI was not associated with an increased risk of readmission within the same ID category.

In multivariable models, the risk factors associated with ARI readmission were younger age, male gender, Pacific or Māori ethnicity, living in a more deprived household, a first ARI admission during autumn, the presence of a CCC, or a first ARI admission of ≥3 days duration. Only younger age, male gender and presence of a CCC were associated with an increased risk of enteric ID readmission, and only presence of a CCC with an increased risk of UTI readmission. None of these factors were associated with the risk of SSTI readmission.

A strength of our study was the ability to describe ID hospital admissions for the national birth cohort. In NZ, discharge data for admissions to public hospitals are loaded into the NMDS within 21 days of discharge. We are confident, therefore, that our description of ID admissions is complete. By studying a five-year birth cohort (2005–2009) we minimised the effect of an isolated

Table 2 Risk of any infectious disease readmission within a 12 month period based upon infectious disease discharge diagnosis category at first admission

Infectious disease diagnosed at admission	Any infectious disease readmission within 12 months			
	n (row %)		Unadjusted odds ratio (95% CI)	Forest Plot
	Yes n = 10,205	No n = 36,335		
Respiratory infection	6,735 (27)	18,521 (73)	**1.87 (1.78-1.95)**	
Non-respiratory infections	3,470 (16)	17,814 (84)	1.00	
Enteric infection	1,090 (16)	5,819 (84)	**0.63 (0.59-0.67)**	
Non-enteric infections	9,115 (23)	30,516 (77)	1.00	
Skin and soft tissue infection	487 (15)	2,723 (85)	**0.62 (0.56-0.68)**	
Non-skin and soft tissue infections	9,718 (22)	33,612 (78)	1.00	
Urinary tract infections	348 (19)	1,478 (81)	**0.83 (0.74-0.94)**	
Non-urinary tract infections	9,857 (22)	34,857 (78)	1.00	
Non-respiratory, non-enteric, non-SSTI and non-UTI infection	1,545 (17)	7,794 (83)	**0.65 (0.62-0.69)**	
Respiratory or enteric or SSTI or UTI infection	8,660 (23)	28,541 (77)	1.00	

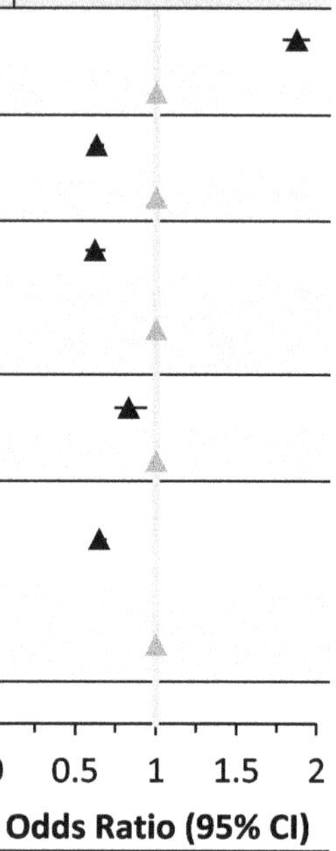

CI Confidence interval, *SSTI* Skin or soft tissue infection, *UTI* Urinary tract infection

Table 3 Risk of respiratory disease readmission within a 12 month period based upon respiratory illness present at the first admission

Respiratory illness diagnosed at admission	Respiratory infection readmission within 12 months			
	n (row %)		Unadjusted odds ratio (95% CI)	Forest Plot
	Yes n = 5,521	No n = 19,735		
Bronchiolitis	3,644 (28)	9,222 (72)	**2.21 (2.08-2.36)**	
Non-bronchiolitis respiratory infection	1,877 (15)	10,513 (85)	1.00	
Pneumonia	655 (16)	3,324 (84)	**0.66 (0.61-0.73)**	
Non-pneumonia respiratory infection	4,866 (23)	16,411 (77)	1.00	
Influenza	68 (20)	267 (80)	0.91 (0.70-1.19)	
Non-influenza respiratory infection	5,453 (22)	19,468 (78)	1.00	
Non-bronchiolitis, non-pneumonia, non-influenza respiratory infection	1,154 (14)	6,922 (86)	**0.49 (0.46-0.53)**	
Bronchiolitis, pneumonia or influenza	4,367 (25)	12,813 (75)	1.00	

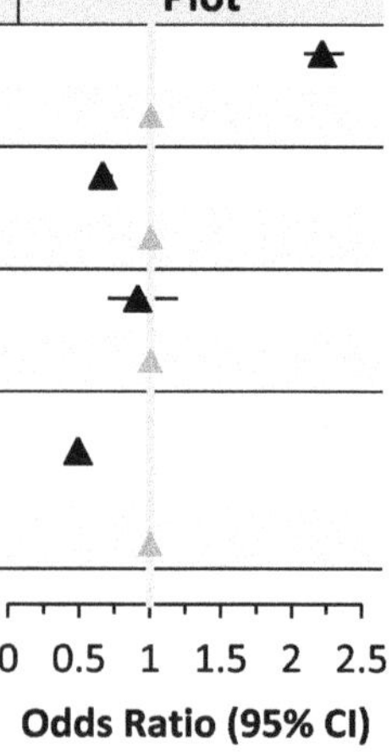

CI Confidence interval

Table 4 Risk of any infectious disease readmission within a 12 month period based upon respiratory illness present at the first admission

Respiratory illness diagnosed at admission	Any infectious disease readmission within 12 months n (row %) Yes n = 10,205	No n = 36,335	Unadjusted odds ratio (95% CI)	Forest Plot
Bronchiolitis	4,229 (33)	8,637 (67)	**2.27 (2.17-2.38)**	
All other infections	5,976 (18)	27,698 (82)	1.00	
Pneumonia	814 (20)	3,165 (80)	**0.91 (0.84-0.98)**	
All other infections	9,391 (22)	33,170 (78)	1.00	
Influenza	86 (26)	248 (74)	1.24 (0.96-1.59)	
All other infections	10,119 (22)	36,087 (78)	1.00	
Non-bronchiolitis, non-pneumonia, non-influenza respiratory infection	1,606 (20)	6,471 (80)	**0.86 (0.81-0.92)**	
All other infections	8,599 (22)	29,864 (78)	1.00	

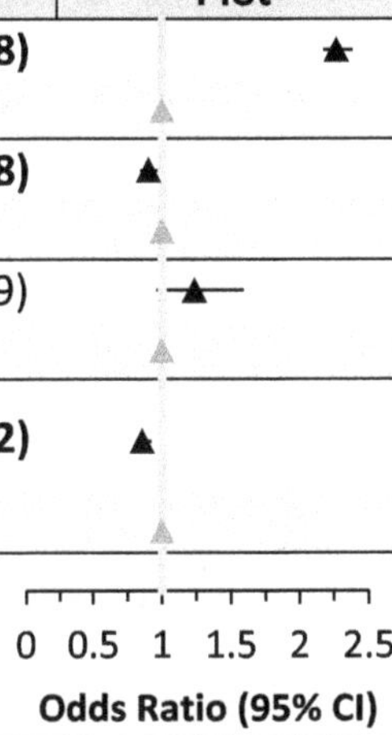

CI Confidence interval

epidemic, for example that caused by the 2009 H1N1 influenza pandemic [20].

By limiting to ID principal discharge codes, our study underestimated the total number of ID admissions. However, limitation to principal codes was necessary to clearly describe the relationship between first and subsequent ID admissions. Our analyses were restricted to NMDS data and therefore the influence of other factors, such as cigarette smoking, or primary care received, was not evaluated, as they are not included in a national data set.

Our case definition was limited to overnight hospital admissions. This excludes very short-term hospital admissions, which may be more likely to occur due to systemic failure in the delivery of acute care in primary care and emergency departments [21].

Children with CCC and children supported with medical technology, for example a tracheostomy or ventriculo-peritoneal shunt, are especially vulnerable to events requiring hospital admission [8]. Whilst children with an underlying CCC were at an increased risk of ID readmission, in our study they accounted for only 2% of all of the children hospitalised with an ID before age 2 years.

Our data suggest that identification of children at risk of recurrent admission and intervention during the first admission may reduce total ID hospitalisation burden. Our study findings imply that such strategies should focus on preventing ARI readmission, given that the risk of ID readmission was increased for ARI but not for enteric infections, SSTIs or UTIs.

Providing specialist health care outside of the hospital is one such potential strategy. In England, the concept of "Hospital-at-Home" with paediatric nurse home care visits accessible 24 h per day was recently evaluated as an alternative to inpatient care for children with breathing difficulties, diarrhoea and vomiting, or fever [22]. Whilst the hospital-at-home care was well accepted by families, it did not result in any reduction in risk of hospital readmission in the subsequent 90 days [22].

Clinical pathways including specific admission and discharge criteria can help to reduce the rate of readmission within two weeks of the first admission, as shown in a recent Australian study of children < 12 months old hospitalised with bronchiolitis [23]. This clinical pathway included improved discharge planning, including specific discharge criteria, a discharge plan developed in consultation with parents, and communication with the primary care physician [23].

Can ARI readmissions over the longer term be prevented, beyond those due to the same respiratory illness that caused the first admission? A recent meta-analysis of 25 randomised controlled trials, which enrolled 11,321 participants aged 0 to 95 years, showed that vitamin D supplementation prevents ARIs [24]. Supplementation is of most benefit to those who are vitamin D deficient, and when daily or weekly vitamin D dosing regimens without bolus doses are used [24]. In Auckland, daily vitamin D_3 supplementation during pregnancy and infancy was shown to reduce the proportion of children making a primary care ARI visit up to age 18 months [25]. Therefore, vitamin D_3 supplementation following ARI hospital admission could potentially prevent ARI readmissions. We are currently conducting a randomised clinical trial to determine if vitamin D supplementation prevents ARI healthcare visits in children under two-years-old (Trial ID: ACTRN12616000659404).

Hospital admission also provides an immunisation update opportunity. Children with more acute illness visits are at increased risk of delayed immunisations [26]. The pneumococcal conjugate vaccine prevents a proportion of ARI hospital admissions, including a spectrum of ARI without radiographic evidence of pneumonia [27]. Our study shows that infants who present in autumn are more likely to represent with ARI. Hence offering seasonal influenza vaccination prior to hospital discharge, provided the child does not have a temperature > 38 °C [28], may reduce the risk of the winter readmission of these children.

Children of Māori and Pacific ethnicity and those living in deprived households continue to be at increased risk of hospital admission and readmission with infectious diseases [2]. Characteristics of the child's home environment, such as overcrowding, dampness and mould, can increase the risk of contracting and being hospitalised with an ARI [29–32]. A recent NZ study found that the risk of ARI hospitalisation before age five years was increased for children living in households where there was gas heating in the bedroom the child slept in during their first year of life [33]. Thus, identification, during the first ARI admission, of the type of heating used in the child's household and replacing gas heating with electric heating, particularly in the room where the child sleeps, could prevent ARI readmissions.

In summary, children hospitalised with an ARI in the first 2 years of life, and in particular a lower ARI, are a group for whom strategies are required to reduce the risk of ARI readmission. Contemporary evidence indicates potential interventions including vitamin D supplementation, ensuring immunisation status is up to date and replacing gas heating in the child's bedroom. Randomised controlled trials of these interventions are necessary to determine which, if any, are sufficiently cost-effective for general implementation.

Conclusions

Hospitalisation rates for infectious diseases continue to be high for NZ children. Of the 15% of children hospitalised with an infectious disease before age two years, one-in-five will have an infectious disease readmission within 12 months of their first admission. The risk of readmission is increased when the first infectious disease is respiratory, but not when it is an enteric, skin or urinary tract infection. Strategies to prevent infectious disease readmission should focus on children hospitalised prior to age two years with lower respiratory infections.

Additional files

Additional file 1: Organ system, infectious disease diagnostic groups and associated ICD-10 codes [2, 34].

Additional file 2: Acute lower respiratory infection syndromes and associated ICD-10 codes [2, 34].

Additional file 3: Associations of demographic and illness characteristics with risk of hospital readmission with a second acute respiratory infection within 12 months of a first hospital admission with an acute respiratory infection.

Additional file 4: Associations of demographic and illness characteristics with risk of hospital readmission with a second enteric infection within 12 months of a first hospital admission with an enteric infection.

Additional file 5: Associations of demographic and illness characteristics with risk of hospital readmission with a second skin and soft tissue infection within 12 months of a first hospital admission with a skin and soft tissue infection.

Additional file 6: Associations of demographic and illness characteristics with risk of hospital readmission with a second UTI within 12 months of a first hospital admission with a UTI.

Abbreviations

ARI: Acute Respiratory Infection; CCC: Complex Chronic Condition; CI: Confidence Interval; ICD-10: International Classification of Disease-10; ID: Infectious Disease; IQR: interquartile range; NHI: National Health Index; NMDS: National Minimum Dataset; NZ: New Zealand; OR: Odds Ratio; SSTI: Skin or Soft Tissue Infection; US: United States; UTI: Urinary Tract Infection

Acknowledgements

We acknowledge the assistance of Ilya Ratine, Senior Information Analyst, Analytical Services, NZ Ministry of Health, for assistance with accessing the National Minimum Dataset.

Funding

None.

Authors' contributions

SS conceived and designed the study, obtained the data, interpreted the data and prepared a first draft of the manuscript. PWR conceived and designed the study, analysed and interpreted the data, and edited the manuscript. CAG, EJB, AH, and CAC interpreted the data and edited the manuscript.CCG conceived and designed the study, communicated with the Ethics Committee, obtained the data, interpreted the data, and completed the final draft of the manuscript. All authors approved the final submitted version of the manuscript and agree to be accountable for all aspects of the work.

Competing interests

The authors have no competing interests to declare.

Author details

[1]Paediatrics, Taranaki Base Hospital, New Plymouth, New Zealand. [2]Department of Paediatrics: Child and Youth Health, Faculty of Medical and Health Sciences, University of Auckland, Private Bag 92019, Wellesley Street, Auckland 1142, New Zealand. [3]Children's Research Centre, Starship Children's Hospital, Auckland, New Zealand. [4]Infectious Diseases, Starship Children's Hospital, Auckland District Health Board, Auckland, New Zealand. [5]Nuffield Department of Primary Care Health Sciences, University of Oxford, Oxford, England. [6]Emergency Medicine, Massachusetts General Hospital, Harvard Medical School, Boston, USA. [7]General Paediatrics, Starship Children's Hospital, Auckland District Health Board, Auckland, New Zealand.

References

1. Kassebaum N, Kyu HH, Zoeckler L, Olsen HE, Thomas K, Pinho C, Bhutta ZA, Dandona L, Ferrari A, Ghiwot TT, et al. Child and adolescent health from 1990 to 2015: findings from the global burden of diseases, injuries, and risk factors 2015 study. JAMA Pediatr. 2017;171(6):573–92.
2. Baker MG, Barnard LT, Kvalsvig A, Verrall A, Zhang J, Keall M, Wilson N, Wall T, Howden-Chapman P. Increasing incidence of serious infectious diseases and inequalities in New Zealand: a national epidemiological study. Lancet. 2012;379(9821):1112–9.
3. Craig E, Adams J, Oben G, Reddington A, Wicken A, Simpson J. Service NCaYE: The Health Status of Children and Young People in New Zealand. In: Department of Women's and Children's Health at the University of Otago's Dunedin School of Medicine: University of Otago; 2013.
4. Hasegawa K, Tsugawa Y, Brown DF, Mansbach JM, Camargo CA, Jr.: Trends in bronchiolitis hospitalizations in the United States, 2000-2009. Pediatrics 2013, 132(1):28–36.
5. Cheung CR, Smith H, Thurland K, Duncan H, Semple MG. Population variation in admission rates and duration of inpatient stay for bronchiolitis in England. Arch Dis Child. 2013;98(1):57–9.
6. Griffin MR, Zhu Y, Moore MR, Whitney CG, Grijalva CG. U.S. hospitalizations for pneumonia after a decade of pneumococcal vaccination. N Engl J Med. 2013;369(2):155–63.
7. Friedman B, Berdahl T, Simpson LA, McCormick MC, Owens PL, Andrews R, Romano PS. Annual report on health care for children and youth in the United States: focus on trends in hospital use and quality. Acad Pediatr. 2011;11:263–79.
8. Berry JG, Hall DE, Kuo DZ, Cohen E, Agrawal R, Feudtner C, Hall M, Kueser J, Kaplan W, Neff J. Hospital utilization and characteristics of patients experiencing recurrent readmissions within children's hospitals. JAMA. 2011;305(7):682–90.
9. Berry JG, Toomey SL, Zaslavsky AM, Jha AK, Nakamura MM, Klein DJ, Feng JY, Shulman S, Chiang VK, Kaplan W, et al. Pediatric readmission prevalence and variability across hospitals. JAMA. 2013;309(4):372–80.
10. Brower KS, Del Vecchio MT, Aronoff SC. The etiologies of non-CF bronchiectasis in childhood: a systematic review of 989 subjects. BMC Pediatr. 2014;14(1):4.
11. Chang AB, Masel JP, Boyce NC, W G, Torzillo PJ. Non-CF Bronchiectasis: clinical and HRCT evaluation. Pediatr Pulmonol. 2003;35(6):477–83.
12. Singleton RJ, Valery PC, Morris P, Byrnes CA, Grimwood K, Redding G, Torzillo PJ, McCallum G, Chikoyak L, Mobberly C, et al. Indigenous children from three countries with non-cystic fibrosis chronic suppurative lung disease/bronchiectasis. Pediatr Pulmonol. 2014;49(2):189–200.
13. Singleton R, Morris A, Redding G, Poll J, Holck P, Martinez P, Kruse D, Bulkow LR, Petersen KM, Lewis C. Bronchiectasis in Alaska native children: causes and clinical courses. Pediatr Pulmonol. 2000;29(3):182–7.
14. Das L, Kovesi TA. Bronchiectasis in children from Qikiqtani (Baffin) region, Nunavut, Canada. Ann Am Thorac Soc. 2015;12(1):96–100.
15. National Health Board Business Unit. National Minimum Dataset (Hospital Events) Data Dictionary. Wellington: Ministry of Health; 2010.
16. Pinner RW, Teutsch SM, Simonsen L, Klug LA, Graber JM, Clarke MJ, Berkelman RL. Trends in infectious diseases mortality in the United States. JAMA. 1996;275(3):189–93.
17. Simonsen L, Conn LA, Pinner RW, Teutsch S. Trends in infectious disease hospitalizations in the United States, 1980-1994. Arch Intern Med. 1998;158(17):1923–8.
18. Salmond C, Crampton P, Atkinson J. NZDep2006 index of deprivation. Wellington: Department of Public Health, University of Otago; 2007.
19. Ministry of Health. Report on Maternity, 2010. Wellington: Ministry of Health; 2012.
20. Falagas ME, Koletsi PK, Baskouta E, Rafailidis PI, Dimopoulos G, Karageorgopoulos DE. Pandemic a(H1N1) 2009 influenza: review of the southern hemisphere experience. Epidemiol Infect. 2011;139(1):27–40.
21. Gill PJ, Goldacre MJ, Mant D, Heneghan C, Thomson A, Seagroatt V, Harnden A. Increase in emergency admissions to hospital for children aged under 15 in England, 1999-2010: national database analysis. Arch Dis Child. 2013;98(5):328–34.
22. Sartain SA, Maxwell MJ, Todd PJ, Jones KH, Bagust A, Haycox A, Bundred P. Randomised controlled trial comparing an acute paediatric hospital at home scheme with conventional hospital care.[see comment]. Arch Dis Child. 2002;87(5):371–5.
23. Cheney J, Barber S, Altamirano L, Medico C, Cheney M, Williams C, Jackson M, Yates P, O'Rourke P, Wainwright C. A clinical pathway for bronchiolitis is effective in reducing readmission rates. J Pediatr. 2005;147(5):622–6.
24. Martineau AR, Jolliffe DA, Hooper RL, Greenberg L, Aloia JF, Bergman P, Dubnov-Raz G, Esposito S, Ganmaa D, Ginde AA, et al. Vitamin D supplementation to prevent acute respiratory tract infections: systematic review and meta-analysis of individual participant data. BMJ. 2017;356:i6583.
25. Grant CC, Kaur S, Waymouth E, Mitchell EA, Scragg R, Ekeroma A, Stewart A, Milne T, Rowden J, Wall CR, et al. Reduced primary care respiratory infection visits following pregnancy and infancy vitamin D supplementation: a randomised-controlled trial. Acta Paediatr. 2014;
26. Turner N, Grant C, Goodyear-Smith F, Petousis-Harris H. Seize the moments: missed opportunities to immunize at the family practice level. Fam Pract. 2009;26(4):275–8.
27. Centers for Disease Control and Prevention. Pneumonia hospitalizations among young children before and after introduction of pneumococcal conjugate vaccine–United States, 1997-2006. MMWR Morb Mortal Wkly Rep. 2009;58(1):1–4.
28. Ministry of Health: Immunisation Handbook. In: 2017; Wellington: Ministry of Health; 2017.
29. Fisk WJ, Lei-Gomez Q, Mendell MJ. Meta-analyses of the associations of respiratory health effects with dampness and mold in homes. Indoor Air. 2007;17(4):284–96.
30. Fisk WJ, Eliseeva EA, Mendell MJ. Association of residential dampness and mold with respiratory tract infections and bronchitis: a meta-analysis. Environ Health. 2010;9:72.
31. Colosia AD, Masaquel A, Hall CB, Barrett AM, Mahadevia PJ, Yogev R. Residential crowding and severe respiratory syncytial virus disease among infants and young children: a systematic literature review. BMC Infect Dis. 2012;12:95.
32. Baker MG, McDonald A, Zhang J, Howden-Chapman P. Infectious diseases attributable to household crowding in New Zealand: A systematic review and burden of disease estimate. Wellington: He Kainga Oranga/ Housing and Health Research Programme, University of Otago, 2013; 2013.
33. Tin Tin S, Woodward A, Saraf R, Berry S, Atatoa Carr P, Morton SM, Grant CC. Internal living environment and respiratory disease in children: findings from the growing up in New Zealand longitudinal child cohort study. Environ Health. 2016;15(1):120.
34. O'Sullivan CE, Baker MG. Proposed epidemiological case definition for serious skin infection in children. J Paediatr Child Health. 2010;46(4):176–83.

Community health education improves child health care in Rural Western China

Weifeng Liang[1†], Yuan Xing[2†], Miaomiao Pang[3], Duolao Wang[4] and Hong Yan[1*]

Abstract

Background: Rural infant growth failure has been highlighted as a priority for action in China's national nutrition and child development policies. The aim of this paper was to evaluate the effect of community-based intervention project on child feeding, child health care and child growth.

Methods: From 2001 to 2005, UNICEF and China's Ministry of Health worked together to develop holistic strategies for child health care. All the interventions were implemented through the three-tier (county-township-village) rural health care network.In this study, 34 counties were included in both surveys in 2001 and 2005. Among these 34 counties, nine were subjected to the intervention and 25 counties were used as controls. In nine intervention counties, leaflets containing information of supplemental feeding of infants and young children were printed and distributed to women during hospital delivery or visit to newborn by village doctors. Two cross-sectional surveys were both conducted from July to early September in 2001 and 2005. We calculated Z-scores of height-for-age (HAZ), weight-for-age (WAZ) and weight-for-height (WHZ), with the new WHO growth standard. HAZ < -2 was defined as stunting, WAZ < -2 was defined as underweight, and WHZ < -2 was defined as wasting.

Results: Following the four-year study period, the parents in the intervention group showed significantly better infant and young child feeding practices and behaviors of child care than did their control group counterparts. In addition, all three anthropometric indicators in 2005 in the intervention group were better than in the control, with stunting 4.9% lower ($p < 0.001$), underweight 2.2% lower ($p < 0.001$), and wasting 1.0% lower ($p < 0.05$).

Conclusions: We concluded that the health care education intervention embed in government had the potential to be successfully promoted in rural western China.

Keywords: Rural western China, Child feeding practices, Breastfeeding, Complementary foods, Stunting

Background

Physical growth is often considered as a good global indicator of children's well-being, because infections and unsatisfactory feeding practices, or more often a combination of the two, are major factors affecting their physical growth and mental development [1]. Many studies have shown an association between increased severity of anthropometric deficits and infant and child mortality, and a substantial contribution to child mortality is made by all degrees of malnutrition [2–4].

Child malnutrition may also have an adverse effect on children's intellectual development [2]. Child growth retardation is associated with adult life dysfunction [3, 4], decreased ability to work, affecting economic productivity [5].

Child development refers to the orderly appearance of the interdependent skills of sensory, cognitive and social emotional functions. This emergence depends on, and is interlinked with, a child's good nutrition and health. As "A World Fit for Children" states, "...children should be physically healthy, mentally alert, emotionally secure, socially competent and ready to learn" [6]. The most important years for a child's survival, growth, and development are prenatally through the transition to school, with the fastest period of growth occurring during the first three to four years of life, when the child's brain is

* Correspondence: xjtu_yh.paper@aliyun.com
Yuan Xing regarded as first joint authors.
†Equal contributors
[1]Department of Epidemiology and Health Statistics, School of Public Health, Xi'an Jiaotong University College of Medicine, P.O. Box 46, No.76 West Yanta Road, Xi'an, Shaanxi 710061, People's Republic of China

rapidly growing and adapting to the environment. During this period, the developing brain is most sensitive to the effects of malnutrition, toxins, stress, and lack of nurturing or brain stimulation [7].

A common model of health promotion to improve nutrition and child development has three major components [8]: (i) enhancing nutritional intake (including exclusive breastfeeding up to six months of life, appropriate provision of weaning foods, and micronutrient supplementation); (ii) improving health and sanitation services; and (iii) enhancing the level of child care, such as early childhood stimulation programmes and monitoring children's growth and development.

Rural infant growth failure was highlighted as a priority for action in China's national nutrition and child development policies [9]. It was considered important to both enhance the nutritional status of rural children and to find effective ways to improve early childhood development. Thus UNICEF and China's Ministry of Health developed a wide ranging programme of strategies for child health care intervention, including the "Rural Primary Health Care project (RPHC)" from January 1, 2002 to December 31, 2005.. This study was designed to evaluate the effect of this project on child feeding, child health care and child growth.

Methods

Population and setting

The RPHC project was implemented in 10 provinces of rural western China, where there is a total land area of 151,548 km^2, a population of 19.1 million, and 52 nationalities [10].

A 1999 Chinese national survey in children under three years of age in rural western areas reported the prevalence of stunting was 23.0%, while underweight and wasting were 22.6% and 7.5%, respectively [11].

Study design

Through a quasi experimental design, changes in anthropometric indices from 2001 to 2005 were evaluated between intervention and control arm. Nine counties were subjected to the intervention and 25 counties were used as controls.

RPHC intervention

The Rural Primary Health Care project (RPHC) was a province-level government-led integrated intervention project, which targeted children aged less than 3 years. The main objectives were: (i) to promote healthy growth and reduce the incidence of malnutrition in infants and young children through the use of recommended feeding and dietary practices [12], (ii) to monitor child growth and development; (iii) to improve the Hepatitis B vaccination rate, (iv) to improve vitamin A supplementation intake rate among children. All the interventions were implemented through the three-tier "county-township-village" rural health care network, which is the standard channel through which all national health policies are implemented.

The county-level staffs were responsible for policy supervision across the whole county. Township-level staffs were responsible for the hepatitis B vaccination initiative for all the township's children. Village-level staffs were responsible for vitamin A supplementation supply for all the village's children, monitoring each child's growth and provision of appropriate nutrition guidance and health education for parents.

Data collection

Two cross-sectional surveys were used for data collection, one at the beginning and one at the end of intervention (2001 and 2005, respectively). The two samples were obtained using a stratified multistage cluster random sampling method, taking into account the hierarchical structure of Chinese administrative districts and the imbalanced population distribution between the different provinces. In each county, five townships were selected with probability proportional to total population (from the countries' demographic data). In each selected township, four villages were selected randomly, also with probability proportional to population size. Finally in each village 16 children less than three years old were randomly selected from all the children aged < 3 years in this village.

All participants were interviewed face-to-face by trained professional interviewers from the Xi'an Jiaotong University College of Medicine. The children's mothers were interviewed and a questionnaire was used to collect information on the child and family socio-demographic characteristics, child health care, mothers' feeding/caring practices, hepatitis B vaccination status, and vitamin A supplementation intake. The age of each child was obtained from their Permanent Residence Registration, where birth dates are recorded (Additional files 1 and 2).

Anthropometric measurements

Lengths were measured in children from birth to 36 completed months using a standard calibrated board (accurate to 1 mm). Weights were measured using portable electronic scales with measurement accuracy to 0.1 kg. All equipment was newly purchased, recommended by UNICEF and calibrated daily.

Data management and statistical analysis

A database was established using Epi Info Version 6.0 (CDC, Atlanta, GA, USA), and data were double-entered to reduce data entry errors.

We hypothesized that the intervention would lead to improved feeding practices, child care, and growth among children in the areas of the intervention. The main outcomes variables were: (1) Feeding practices (including early initiation of breastfeeding, exclusive breastfeeding, and child feeding index); (2) Child care (including give separate cooking for children, attendance rate at a health service for cold symptoms in two weeks, attendance rate at a health service for diarrhea in two weeks, vitamin A supplementation intake rate, and hepatitis B vaccination rate); (3) Anthropometric status (including stunting, underweight, and wasting).

A household wealth index was constructed from an inventory of five levels of household assets or facilities from both the intervention and control groups for 2001 and 2005, using a principal component analysis method, and this index was categorized as tertiles as indicators of the least, middle, and wealthiest households [13].

Early initiation of breastfeeding was used as an indicator to assess breastfeeding practices [14]. Exclusive breastfeeding of infants up to 6 months old was used to assess the feeding practices of children less than 6 months of age. The child feeding index was used to assess the feeding practices of children over 6 months of age (Table 1) [15, 16].

We calculated Z-scores of height-for-age (HAZ), weight-for-age (WAZ) and weight-for-height (WHZ), with the new WHO growth standard [17]. HAZ < − 2 was defined as stunting, WAZ < − 2 was defined as underweight, and WHZ < − 2 was defined as wasting [18]. Before calculating these indicators, length was converted into height if a child whose age was two years or older. Grossly improbable z-scores were excluded before data analysis (HAZ: <− 6 or > 6; WAZ: <− 6 or > 5; WHZ: <− 5 or > 5).

Bivariate analyses were performed using *t* tests for continuous outcome variables and χ^2 tests for categorical variables. A multiple logistic regression model was used to assess the influence of the intervention on each of the child health care outcomes (including: early initiation of breastfeeding, exclusive breastfeeding, child feeding index, cook food separately for children, attendance rate at a health service for cold symptoms in two weeks, attendance rate at a health service for diarrhea in two weeks, vitamin A supplementation intake rate, hepatitis B vaccination rate, stunting, underweight and wasting), after adjusting for economic and sociodemographic factors. In the logistic regression, we defined each outcome 0 = no and 1 = yes. Covariates were defined as follows: group 0 = control and 1 = intervention; place of birth 0

Table 1 Variables and scoring system used to create the child

Variables	Item Score	6–9 month	9–12 month	12–36 month
Breastfeeding	2	No = 0; Yes = 2	No = 0; Yes = 2	No = 0; Yes = 1
Milk and related products				0–2 times/w = 0
				1–4 times/w = 1
				5+ times/w = 2
Cereals	1	0–1 time/d = 0	0–2 times/d = 0	
		1+ time/d = 1	2+ times/d = 1	
Beans and related products	2	0–1 time/m = 0	0–1 time/m = 0	0–1 time/m = 0
		1 time/m-4 times/w = 1	1 time/m-4 times/w = 1	1 time/m-4 times/w = 1
		5+ times/w = 2	5+ times/w = 2	5+ times/w = 2
Egg	2	0–1 time/m = 0	0–1 time/m = 0	0–1 time/m = 0
		1 time/m-4 times/w = 1	1 time/m-4 times/w = 1	1 time/m-4 times/w = 1
		5+ times/w = 2	5+ times/w = 2	5+ times/w = 2
Fish	2	0–1 time/m = 0	0–1 time/m = 0	0–1 time/m = 0
		1 time/m-4 times/w = 1	1 time/m-4 times/w = 1	1 time/m-4 times/w = 1
		5+ times/w = 2	5+ times/w = 2	5+ times/w = 2
Meat	2	0–1 time/m = 0	0–1 time/m = 0	0–1 time/m = 0
		1 time/m-4 times/w = 1	1 time/m-4 times/w = 1	1 time/m-4 times/w = 1
		5+ times/w = 2	5+ times/w = 2	5+ times/w = 2
Dietary diversity	2	0 kind = 0	0 kind = 0	kind = 0
		1–3 types = 1	1–3 types = 1	1–3 types = 1
		4 + types = 2	4+ types = 2	4+ types = 2
Total score		13 points	13 points	13 points

[1]Time/d: times per day; time/w: times per week; time/m: times per month

= not in township or higher level hospital and 1 = in township or higher level hospital; child's age, mother's education, wealth index and size of family were treated as continuous variables.

SPSS Version 13.0 (Statistical Package for Social Science, Inc., Chicago, IL, USA) was used for all analyses. The significance of hypothesis testing was determined as $P < 0.05$ with two-tailed tests.

Human participants and ethical considerations

The project was approved by the Human Research Ethics Committee of the Xi'an Jiaotong University College of Medicine prior to conducting the research. Written consent was received from the parents of the children who voluntarily participated in the study. All the data collected were kept confidential.

Results

Sample characteristics

In the 2001 survey, the information from 2673 (92.8% of the total survey participants) children represented the intervention group and 9031 (97.3%) children for the control. In the 2005 survey, the information from 2693 (93.5%) children represented the intervention group and 8425 (90.8%) children for the control. The following were excluded from the analysis: children or their parents who were unavailable for measurement, children whose birth date was unknown, and children with grossly improbable Z-scores. Table 2 shows the characteristics of the participants before and after the intervention.

Feeding practices

In 2001, early initiation of breastfeeding occurred in 15.4% of the intervention group and 20.0% of the control group ($p < 0.001$). After the intervention, in 2005, the early initiation of breastfeeding had improved to 51.9% in the intervention group, which was higher than in the control group (41.8%, $p < 0.001$). There was no difference between the two groups in the prevalence of exclusive breastfeeding in 2001 (13.8% vs 14.1%, $p > 0.05$). In 2005, this increased to 24.7% in the intervention group, which was significantly higher than in the control group (14.6%, $p < 0.001$) (Table 3).

The median of child feeding index score varied from 3 to 8 in intervention group, and which varied from 4 to 7 in control group. Before the intervention, the mean child feeding score for the intervention group was lower than that for the control group (3.0 vs 4.0, $p < 0.001$), while after the intervention, the mean score was higher for the intervention group (8.0 vs 7. 0, $p < 0.001$) (Fig. 1).

Child care

Table 3 shows that more than half of the mothers were cooking separate meals for their children in 2001. After the intervention, more mothers in the intervention than in the control group were cooking separately for their children (73.1% vs 54.4%, $p < 0.001$). The attendance rate at a health service for colds/diarrhea in a two-week period also improved in the intervention group, but the rates of diarrhea cases showed no significant difference in 2005. Vitamin A supplementation intake rates improved significantly, rising to 79.9% in the intervention and 49.0% in the control. The Hepatitis B vaccination rate showed no significant difference between the intervention and control group in 2005 (96.9% vs 97.1%, $p > 0.05$).

Anthropometric status

There was no difference in stunting or wasting for the two groups in the 2001 (Table 3), although there was a small difference for underweight with the prevalence in the intervention group 1.5% lower than in the control. Following the intervention, all three anthropometric indicators in 2005 in the intervention group were better than in the control, with stunting 4.9% lower ($p < 0.001$), underweight 2.2% lower ($p < 0.001$), and wasting 1.0% lower ($p < 0.05$).

Table 2 Socio-demographic characteristics of participants in 2001 and 2005

Characteristics	2001				2005			
	Intervention (n = 2673)	Control (n = 9031)	T/X^2	*P*-value	Intervention (n = 2693)	Control (n = 8425)	T/X^2	*P*-value
Age of child in months,mean *(SD)*	18.6 (9.2)	18.5 (9.9)	0.466	0.641	15.8 (9.5)	17.9 (9.9)	9.675	0.001
Male sex, *n (%)*	1564 (58.5)	5170 (57.2)	1.141	0.285	1579 (58.6)	4858 (57.7)	0.790	0.374
Place of birth, in hospital, *n (%)*	1057(39.5)	4944 (54.7)	190.7	0.0001	2452 (91.1)	6914 (82.1)	124.1	0.0001
Age of mother in years, mean *(SD)*	27.0 (3.9)	26.6 (4.0)	4.567	0.001	27.1 (4.4)	27.2 (4.9)	0.944	0.345
Mother's education in years, mean *(SD)*	5.8 (3.2)	6.0 (3.2)	2.838	0.004	6.9 (2.9)	6.5 (3.1)	5.919	0.001
Household wealth index, *(SD)*	−0.01 (0.05)	−0.00 (0.06)	7.84	0.001	0.02 (0.03)	0.01 (0.06)	8.322	0.001
Size of family, *n (SD)*	4.3 (1.5)	4.7 (1.6)	11.51	0.001	4.6 (1.6)	4.8 (1.6)	5.646	0.001
Drinking Water Source,, *n (%)*	728 (27.2)	2365 (26.2)	1.164	0.281	1023 (38.0)	3367 (40.0)	3.338	0.068

[1] *P*-values for continuous variables were calculated by Student's 2-sided t test; *P*-values for categorical variables were calculated using Pearson's χ^2 test

Table 3 Intervention effects on feed practices, child care, and anthropometric status of children in 2001 and 2005: Univariate analysis

Outcomes (%)	2001				2005				Change	
	Intervention	Control	X^2	*P*-value[1]	Intervention	Control	X^2	*P*-value[a]	Intervention	Control
Feed practices										
Early initiation of breastfeeding	15.4	20.0	41.02	0.0001	51.9	41.8	84.52	0.0001	36.5	21.8
Exclusive breastfeeding	13.8	14.1	0.145	0.703	24.7	14.6	147.06	0.0001	10.9	0.5
Child feeding index (score ≥ 6)	5.2	10.0	58.56	0.0001	85.2	80.0	36.00	0.001	80.0	70.0
Child care[a]										
Give separate cooking for children, > 6 *mo*	59.6	55.9	11.50	0.001	73.1	54.4	295.41	0.0001	13.5	−1.5
Attendance rate at a health service for cold symptoms in two weeks[b]	91.4	94.0	22.68	0.001	97.6	95.1	30.71	0.001	6.2	1.1
Attendance rate at a health service for diarrhea in two weeks[c]	81.2	82.5	2.465	0.116	93.2	91.7	6.29	0.01	12	9.2
Vitamin A intake rate	9.2	37.4	767.3	0.0001	89.1	86.4	13.05	0.001	79.9	49
Hepatitis B vaccination rate	82.3	66.2	253.9	0.0001	96.9	97.1	0.247	0.619	14.6	30.9
Anthropometric status										
Stunting	25.4	26.9	2.360	0.124	13.1	18.0	34.96	0.001	−12.3	−8.9
Underweight	12.0	10.5	4.876	0.027	5.6	7.8	14.54	0.001	−6.4	−2.7
Wasting	3.7	3.0	3.32	0.068	3.1	4.1	5.65	0.017	−0.6	1.1

[a]P-values were calculated using Pearson's χ^2 test
[b]proportion of attending at a health service for cold symptoms among children who had symptoms of cold in two weeks
[c]proportion of attending at a health service for diarrhea among children who had diarrhea in two weeks

Evaluation of intervention

The difference between two groups in 2005 was modeled in Table 4. It shows that for child health care behaviors, the intervention group made much more progress than did the control. After adjusting for the socio-demographic characteristics, we found that the intervention was associated significantly with early initiation of breastfeeding, exclusive breastfeeding, child feeding index (score ≥ 6), giving separate cooking for children, attendance at a health service for cold symptoms in two weeks, and vitamin A supplementation intake. The prevalence of stunting was reduced by 3.4% more in the intervention group than in the control (Odds ratio: 0.82, 95%CI: 0.72 to 0.94), and wasting was reduced by 1.7% of more in intervention than in control (Odds ratio: 0.75, 95%CI: 0.59 to 0.97). However, for

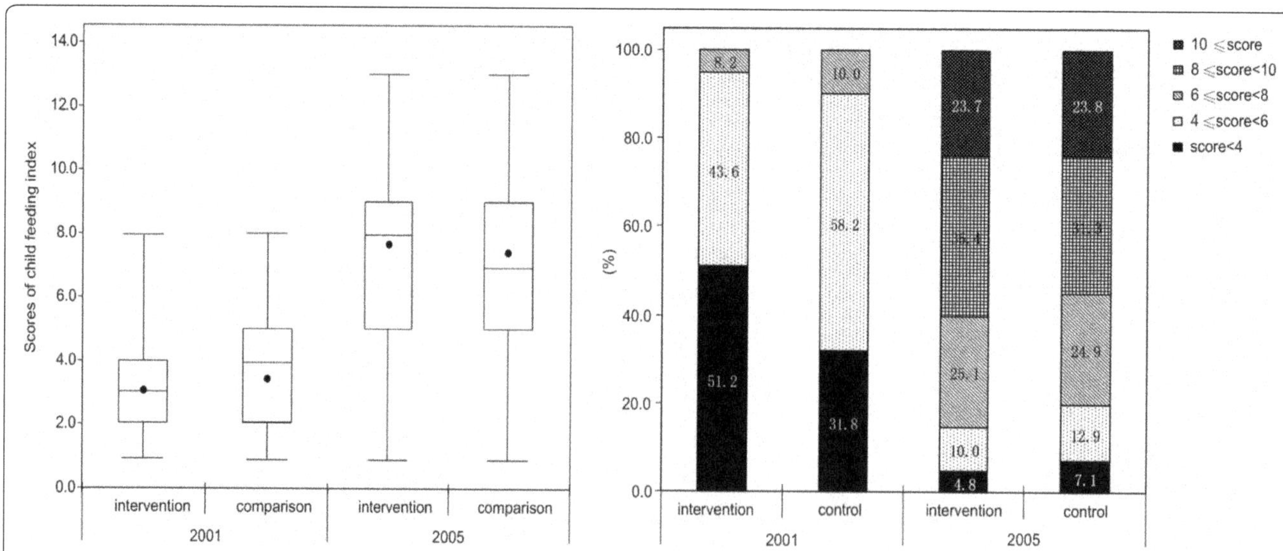

Fig. 1 Distribution of scores of child feeding index in 2001 and 2005

Table 4 Intervention effects on feed practices, child care, andanthropometric status of children in 2005: Multiple logistic

Outcomes	Odds ratio (95% CI)	*P*-value
Feed practices		
Early initiation of breastfeeding	1.30 (1.19,1.42)	< 0.001
Exclusive breastfeeding	2.32 (1.72, 3.13)	< 0.001
Child feeding index (score ≥ 6)	1.12 (1.01, 1.25)	< 0.05
Child care		
Give separate cooking for children	1.79 (1.62, 1.97)	< 0.001
Attendance at a health service for cold symptoms in two weeks	2.16 (1.07, 4.37)	< 0.05
Attendance at a health service for diarrhea in two weeks	1.12 (0.51, 2.48)	NS
Vitamin A supplementation intake	1.16 (1.02, 1.31)	< 0.05
Hepatitis B vaccination	1.20 (0.78, 1.84)	NS
Anthropometric status		
Stunting	0.85 (0.74, 0.97)	< 0.05
Underweight	0.85 (0.71, 1.03)	NS
Wasting	0.75 (0.58, 0.97)	< 0.05

The multiple logistic regression model was used to assess intervention effect of the cross sectional results in 2005 on each outcome after adjusting for child's age, mother's education, wealth index, size of family and child's birth place

the attendance at a health service for diarrhea in two weeks and underweight, no significant intervention effects were observed ($p > 0.05$).

Discussion

This four-year child health care intervention was aimed to promote child growth and reduce the incidence of malnutrition of infants and young children by encouraging recommended feeding and dietary practices, as well as to improve the rate of Hepatitis B vaccination and the vitamin A supplementation intake rate in rural China.

For child growth the intervention seemed successful in reducing the prevalence of stunting. The intervention group saw the risk of stunting lowered by 12.3%. This result could be explained by the following reasons. First, breastfeeding was reported to have a stronger effect on linear growth than on weight gain during late infancy and preschool years [19]; Second, primary disease prevention education was part of the intervention, and may have resulted in improved hygiene and sanitation, which have also been reported to improve linear growth [20]; and third, the increased intake of complementary foods such as milk-based gruels or cereal-pulse mixes may represent improved nutrient quality intake [21]. The effect of intervention on reducing the prevalence of stunting should be interpreted with the fact that rapid economic growth occurred in China from 2001 to 2005 with increase over 8.0% per year.

In the community-based health education program, the messages need to be well disseminated so as to reach the target population. This study demonstrates the value of using the existing primary health care management channels of "county-township-village" for message delivery, wide dissemination of messages related to optimal exclusive breastfeeding, and instruction on complementary feeding practices and other child health care practices. This was a government-led project, so the assessment results of project progress reflected on the work performance of government health officials. As such, strong political support was consistently provided throughout the project. Another feature of this intervention was that the government was responsible for training and supervising those involved in carrying out the project, the village doctors in particular, and for hiring MCH complementary foods specialists at the county level to supervise and support the village educators until the feeding practices had improved more widely [22]. This study not only reached large numbers of the target audience but also reached them frequently enough to stimulate lasting behavioral changes. For an organization with limited funding, it can be very difficult to devote a large amount of manpower and a long period of time to complete such a project as this one without support from different levels of government.

The majority of child feeding practice studies have focused their evaluations on single behaviors, and it may be difficult to summarize a series of interrelated behaviors into one or a few variables that accurately reflect these practices. Based on a study by Ruel [15], we used the child feeding index to assess child feeding behaviors. Using this indicator, we were able to conduct a quantitative evaluation of the intervention effect on child feeding behaviors. Even though a study conducted in rural Senegal reported that a young child feeding index was not associated with either height-for-age or height velocity [23]. Another Chinese study found significant correlations between the feeding index and height-for-age or weight-for-age [16].

In this study, although early initiation of breastfeeding and exclusive breastfeeding among the intervention group showed more improvement than among the control, the results were still not as significant as we had expected. In 2005, the intervention group's prevalence of early initiation of breastfeeding was about 50% but the rate of exclusive breastfeeding was no more than 25%. The same phenomenon was observed in previous studies in rural China [22] but there was a very strong secular trend to having delivery in hospital among both the intervention and control groups. Early initiation of breastfeeding is easier in hospital-based deliveries.

Traditional beliefs regarding child feeding practices may be the main reason for the relatively low rates of breastfeeding. In the study areas, we found that mothers used to be restricted to bed rest for an extended period of time after giving birth, believing that breastfeeding should not begin immediately after delivery. As a result, many women feed newborn infants with only water or sugar water. Furthermore, in rural areas, mothers involvement in farm work limited them to commit to exclusive breastfeeding.

After adjusting for socio-demographic characteristics, we found that the intervention significantly increased the attendance rate at a health service for cold symptoms in two weeks; but for attendance rate at a health service for diarrhea, the intervention results were not satisfactory. There are some possible explanations for this. Through education, parents can more easily recognise the symptoms of a cold, and take a child immediately for treatment. Although most cases of diarrhea in children can be discovered in a timely manner, due to economic factors among rural residents, non-severe diarrhea is often not considered a condition requiring treatment.

This study had some limitations. First, the intervention and control groups were not randomly allocated. As a result, the observed treatment differences may be subject to unobserved confounding factors. Second, during the intervention, although the household wealth index was used, we could not completely rule out the confounding factor of concurrent socioeconomic development that would also improve child health care conduct within the control group. Third, another confounding factor arose from our finding was that the hepatitis B vaccination rate of the control group was higher after the intervention. This is because during the implementation of the intervention, the Chinese government carried out a hepatitis B vaccination program free of charge nationwide. Therefore, it is likely that the health education initiative was not responsible for any significant effect on the vaccination rate. Fourthly, some findings were based on participants' subjective response. They were not as objective as growth outcomes because the intervention emphasizes them. Fortunately, outcomes based on participants' response showed similar pattern as growth outcomes. Two types of outcomes could serve the purpose to evaluate the effect of health education.

Conclusion

Based on the results from this study, we concluded that this health care education intervention embed in government had the potential to be successfully promoted in rural western China. Community-based intervention on child feeding, child health care and child growth can effectively promote the growth and development of children.

Abbreviations

CI: Confidence interval; HAZ: Height-for-age; RPHC: Rural primary health care project; UNICEF: United nations international children's emergency fund; WAZ: Weight-for-age; WHO: World health organization; WHZ: Weight-for-height

Acknowledgements

We are grateful to Dr. Ray Yip and Dr. Bin Liu, UNICEF, Beijng, Dr. Zuguo Mei and Dr. Parvanta Ibrahim, Division of Nutrition and Physical Activity, Centers for Disease Control and Prevention, Dr. Tong Zhang, director of Project Office of MCH. We also thank Quanli Wang, Qiang Li, and Yuan Shen for data arrangement and entry.

Funding

This article was sponsored and funded by the Ministry of Health, People's Republic of China and the United Nations Children's Fund (YH 001).

Authors' contributions

WL and YX conceived the work, conducted the analyses and draft the first version of the manuscript. HY and DW designed the study, supervised data collection and participated in data analysis. MP participated in data analysis and contributed to the first draft of the manuscript. All authors gave final approval of the version to be published.

Competing interests

The authors declare that they have no competing interests.

Author details

[1]Department of Epidemiology and Health Statistics, School of Public Health, Xi'an Jiaotong University College of Medicine, P.O. Box 46, No.76 West Yanta Road, Xi'an, Shaanxi 710061, People's Republic of China. [2]Xi'an Center for Disease Control and Prevention, Xi'an, Shaanxi 710054, People's Republic of China. [3]Shaanxi Provincial Corps Hospital of Chinese People's Armed Police Force, Xi'an, Shaanxi 710054, People's Republic of China. [4]Department of Clinical Sciences, Liverpool School of Tropical Medicine, Liverpool L3 5QA, UK.

References

1. de Onis M, Frongillo EA, Blossner M. Is malnutrition declining? An analysis of changes in levels of child malnutrition since 1980. Bull World Health Organ. 2000;78:1222–33.
2. Pelletier DL, Frongillo EA Jr, Schroeder DG, Habicht JP. The effects of malnutrition on child mortality in developing countries. Bull World Health Organ. 1995;73:443–8.
3. Nguyen, et al. Physical growth during the first year of life. A longitudinal study in rural and rban areas of Hanoi, Vietnam. BMC Pediatr. 2012:12–26.
4. Martorell RRJ, Kaplowitz H, Pollit E. Long-term consequences of growth retardation during early childhood. International Congress Series; Human growth: Basic and clinical aspects. 1992. p. 143–9.
5. Spurr GB, Barac-Nieto M, Maksud MG. Productivity and maximal oxygen consumption in sugar cane cutters. Am J Clin Nutr. 1977;30:316–21.
6. The Lacent. A world fit for children? Lancet. 2007 Dec 15;370:1975.
7. UNICEF. Programming Experiences in early child development. New York: Early Child Development Unit Programme Director's Office; 2006.
8. Harold A. Improving nutrition through community growth promotion: longitudinal study of the nutrition and early child development program in Uganda. World Dev. 2007;35:1376–89.
9. Chen CM. Food and nutrition policies in China–using nutrition surveillance data. 16th International Congress of Nutrition. Canadian Federation Biological Societies Ottawa. Montreal,Canada; 1997.
10. Li DS. China Statistical Yearbook 2004. China Press statistics; 2004.
11. Dang SN, Yan H, Zeng LX, Wang QL, Li Q, Xie H, Xiao SB, Kang YJ. Assessment on nutritional status among children under 3 years using anthropometry in 40 counties of western China. Chinese Journal of Epidemiology. 2005;26:177–81.

12. AFE Development. Recommended feeding and dietary practices to improve infant and maternal nutrition. Washington, DC: Academy for Educational Development 1825 Connecticut Avenue NW; 1999. p. 39.
13. Filmer D, Pritchett LH. Estimating wealth effects without expenditure data–or tears: an application to educational enrollments in states of India. Demography. 2001;38:115–32.
14. WHO. Indicators for assessing infant and young child feeding practices : conclusions of a consensus meeting held 6–8 November 2007 in Washington D.C., USA. In: WHO, editor. Geneva: World Health Organization; 2008.
15. Ruel MT, Menon P. Child feeding practices are associated with child nutritional status in Latin America: innovative uses of the demographic and health surveys. J Nutr. 2002;132:1180–7.
16. Lai JQ, Yin SA, Yang XG, Ma GS. Distribution of feeding index and association between feeding index and growth of infants and young child aged 6 - 24 months. Wei Sheng Yan Jiu. 2005;34:617–9.
17. de Onis M, Onyango AW. WHO child growth standards. Lancet. 2008;371:204.
18. Physical status: the use and interpretation of anthropometry. World Health Organ. 1995;30(6):786–7.
19. Onyango AW. Breastfeeding and growth in rural Kenyan toddlers. Adv Exp Med Biol. 2000;478:151–62.
20. Esrey SA, Habicht JP, Casella G. The complementary effect of latrines and increased water usage on the growth of infants in rural Lesotho. Am J Epidemiol. 1992;135:659–66.
21. Bhandari N, Mazumder S, Bahl R, Martines J, Black RE, Bhan MK. An educational intervention to promote appropriate complementary feeding practices and physical growth in infants and young children in rural Haryana, India. J Nutr. 2004;134:2342–8.
22. Guldan GS, Fan HC, Ma X, Ni ZZ, Xiang X, Tang MZ. Culturally appropriate nutrition education improves infant feeding and growth in rural Sichuan. China J Nutr. 2000;130:1204–11.
23. Ntab B, Simondon KB, Milet J, Cisse B, Sokhna C, Boulanger D, Simondon F. A young child feeding index is not associated with either height-for-age or height velocity in rural Senegalese children. J Nutr. 2005;135:457–64.

12

Implementing paediatric early warning scores systems in the Netherlands

J. F. de Groot[1*], N. Damen[1], E. de Loos[2], L. van de Steeg[1,7], L. Koopmans[1,8], P. Rosias[3,9], M. Bruijn[4,10], J. Goorhuis[5] and C. Wagner[1,6]

Abstract

Background: Paediatric Early Warning Scores (PEWS) are increasingly being used for early identification and management of clinical deterioration in paediatric patients. A PEWS system includes scores, cut-off points and appropriate early intervention. In 2011, The Dutch Ministry of Health advised hospitals to implement a PEWS system in order to improve patient safety in paediatric wards. The objective of this study was to examine the results of implementation of PEWS systems and to gain insight into the attitudes of professionals towards using a PEWS system in Dutch non-university hospitals.

Methods: Quantitative data were gathered at start, midway and at the end of the implementation period through retrospective patient record review ($n = 554$). Semi-structured interviews with professionals ($n = 8$) were used to gain insight in the implementation process and experiences. The interviews were transcribed and analysed using an inductive approach.

Results: Looking at PEWS systems of the five participating hospitals, different parameters and policies were found. While all hospitals included heart rate and respiratory rate, other variables differed among hospitals. At baseline, none of the hospitals used a PEWS system. After 1 year, PEWS were recorded in 69.2% of the patient records and elevated PEWS resulted in appropriate action in 49.1%. Three themes emerged from the interviews: 1) while the importance of using a PEWS system was acknowledged, professionals voiced some doubts about the effectiveness and validity of their PEWS system 2) registering PEWS required little extra effort and was facilitated by PEWS being integrated into the electronic patient record 3) Without a national PEWS system or guidelines, hospitals found it difficult to identify a suitable PEWS system for their setting. Existing systems were not always considered applicable in a non-university setting.

Conclusions: After 1 year, hospitals showed improvements in the use of their PEWS system, although some were decidedly more successful than others. Doubts among staff about validity, effectiveness and communication with other hospitals during transfer to higher level care hospital might hinder sustainable implementation. For these purposes the development of a national PEWS system is recommended, consisting of a "core set" of PEWS, cut-off points and associated early intervention.

Keywords: Paediatric early warning score, PEWS, Implementation, Quality improvement

* Correspondence: j.degroot@nivel.nl
[1]NIVEL Netherlands Institute for Health Services Research, Otterstraat 118-124, 3513 CR Utrecht, the Netherlands
Full list of author information is available at the end of the article

Background

While paediatric resuscitation in hospitalized patients is rare, outcomes are poor [1]. Therefore, Paediatric Early Warning Scores (PEWS) are increasingly being used for early identification of clinical deterioration in paediatric patients. PEWS consist of a predefined set of parameters with age specific cut-off points. The idea behind PEWS is early recognition of clinical deterioration and thereby preventing mortality and/or morbidity related to resuscitation or avoidable deterioration of the child's status. The calculation of PEWS is based on selected routine parameters in paediatric patients, such as heart rate, respiratory rate, respiratory distress, temperature, and oxygen saturation, but can also include information on behaviour and mental status [2–6]. A higher PEWS indicates a worse clinical condition and should ideally be followed up by early intervention by nursing and/or medical staff to prevent further deterioration [6].

Several authors, as well as the NHS Institute for Innovation and Improvement, argue that in order for PEWS to positively influence inpatient paediatric care, it is essential that they are part of a Pediatric Early Warning Scores *System* [7, 8]. This requires, next to monitoring and registering symptoms and scores, clear guidelines for rapid decision-making on appropriate actions following elevated PEWS [6, 9]. Examples of such actions include calling a pediatrician or more frequent monitoring of the patient.

Because of the expected benefits of using a PEWS system and its role in optimizing safety and preventing avoidable damage in pediatric hospital care, the Dutch national patient safety program "Prevent Harm, Work Safely" in 2011 advised that all Dutch hospitals should implement a PEWS system. With this program, implementation of a PEWS system became part of the accreditation of Dutch hospitals (VMS Safety Program, 2011) [10]. At the same time though, the national patient safety program did not provide hospitals with guidelines regarding the content of the PEWS system to be used. E.g. which and how many parameters to use to calculate a score, which cut-off points to use, which patients to include, or a description of the associated actions as a result of elevated PEWS. Clear (inter)national standards for PEWS are lacking, which has resulted in multiple PEWS having been developed worldwide over the past decades. PEWS may differ regarding the included number of physiological and behavioural parameters and/or the cut-off points for intervention [5, 11].

During the same time of the VMS program in the Netherlands, a joint action was started within the European Union Network for Patient Safety and Quality of Care (PaSQ) (www.pasq.eu). This initiative aimed to support European hospitals in implementing several safe clinical practices, including the implementation of a PEWS system. In the Netherlands, five non-university hospitals participated in this PaSQ project from September of 2013 through December 2014 as an incentive to start the implementation of a PEWS system in their hospital.

The objectives of the current study were to evaluate the implementation of a PEWS system in five non-university hospitals within the European Union Network for PaSQ initiative in the Netherlands. For this purpose a mixed-methodology was used to 1) describe and compare the specific PEWS scores and protocols for early intervention (together a PEWS system) in each hospital; 2) evaluate the level of implementation of the PEWS system within each hospital, and 3) gain insight into the attitudes of nurses and paediatricians towards implementation of the PEWS system in their hospital.

Methods

Design and setting

Two of the participating hospitals were located in highly urbanized areas in the western part of the Netherlands, two were located in the south, and one was located in a more rural region in the eastern part of the country. See Table 1 for a description of hospital type and size.

The goal of the five hospitals was to implement a PEWS system in at least one paediatric and/or maternity ward in their hospital. Due to a lack of a validated national PEWS system, hospitals were free to choose their own clinical symptoms to be included, scoring methods, cut-off points, and procedures following elevated PEWS. At the start of the PaSQ project, every participating hospital had developed a PEWS system, including a description of the selected parameters and associated actions for elevated PEWS, but none were actively working with a PEWS system.

The Dutch PaSQ team consisted of the Netherlands Institute for Health Services Research (NIVEL) and the Dutch Institute for Healthcare Improvement (CBO), with CBO providing the hospitals with implementation support throughout the project and NIVEL being responsible for the independent evaluation of the implementation. The PaSQ team organized national meetings for multidisciplinary hospital teams, as well as two webinars. The meetings were aimed at exchanging

Table 1 Description of included hospitals

	Type of Hospital	Number of beds	ICU present	PICU
1	General Hospital	425	Yes	No
2	General Hospital	633	Yes	No
3	General Hospital	290	Yes	No
4	Tertiary Teaching Hospital, non-university	1070	Yes	No
5	Tertiary Teaching Hospital, non-university	724	Yes	No

information on implementation progress, implementation training, and experiences in daily practice. CBO also held frequent individual conference calls with project leaders of the multidisciplinary hospital teams to discuss implementation progress and provide advice on how to carry out further implementation. The hospitals were made aware of the open accessible PaSQ website, the PaSQ implementation toolbox and PaSQ activities, such as webinars and exchange meetings. The online PaSQ toolbox consisted of information on the origin and background of PEWS, evidence on the effectiveness, and implementation advice. Additionally, a selection of specific tools, such as videos, checklists, and guidelines were provided, which could be used and/or adapted by health care organizations implementing a PEWS system. In order to provide participating hospitals with insight into their implementation progress, during the project NIVEL sent performance reports regarding the level of implementation to the hospitals at the start (September–October 2013), at midterm (May–June 2014), and at the end (November–December 2014) of the PaSQ project.

Sample and data collection

In each hospital a paediatrician and paediatric nurse was appointed as contact person assisting the researchers in the organisation of data collection in the hospital. These contact persons also provided the researchers with the PEWS protocol as developed within their hospital, including chosen parameters, cut-off points, and local procedures. The independent evaluation of PEWS implementation consisted of two parts: 1) quantitative patient record review, and 2) qualitative semi-structured interviews.

Patient record review

A random sample of patient records was reviewed at the start, midterm and end of the PaSQ project. The sample consisted of records from discharged patients aged ≤18 years, with a length of hospital stay ≥24 h, admitted in October/November 2013, May/June 2014, or November/December 2014. We aimed to include at least 40 patient records per data collection period for each hospital, from either the paediatric or maternity/neonatal ward.

From these individual patient records, we determined the frequency of PEWS registration in the patient record, the number of elevated scores and the number of times that an elevated score lead to the appropriate action by nursing staff and/or medical staff as described in the hospital's own protocol.

Semi-structured interviews

To gain insight into the implementation process and the attitude towards working with a PEWS system, semi-structured interviews were conducted during the second phase of the project (between January 2015 and March 2015) with the contact persons for the PASQ project. This meant that in each participating hospital one paediatric nurse and one paediatrician involved in the project was interviewed about the implementation process of PEWS scores and system at their paediatric ward. During these interviews, information was gathered on the method of introducing and implementing the PEWS system as well as their experiences with and attitudes towards a PEWS system (see Fig. 1 for topic guide). All interviews were held face-to-face and interviewees were assured that the gathered interview data remained confidential. With the participants' consent, interviews were audiotaped for further analysis.

Data analyses

Data from the patient record review were analysed using STATA 13.1. Descriptive statistics were used to describe hospital and patient characteristics, as well as the level of PEWS implementation per hospital.

Interview data were analysed using a grounded theory approach [12]. In doing so,, the interviews were transcribed verbatim into Microsoft Word. Next, open and thematic coding was used in order to identify generic themes related to the implementation of PEWS scores and the PEWS system. Two researchers (LK and LvdS) independently analysed the interviews, by coding the sections of the transcripts to find submerging themes. When coding disagreements arose, the researchers discussed the responses and selected the most appropriate code for each response. Qualitative data analyses were performed using MAXQDA 11.

Topic guide:

- Why were the PEWS scores and the PEWS system implemented in your hospital?
- How were the PEWS scores and the PEWS system implemented in your hospital?
- What are your experiences with implementing PEWS scores and PEWS system in your hospital?
- How easy to use are PEWS-scores and the PEWS system?
- What are your views regarding PEWS-scores and the PEWS system?
- What is the effectiveness according to you of monitoring PEWS scores and using a PEWS system?

Fig. 1 Topic guide for interviews with pediatric nurses and pediatricians

Results

Description and comparison of PEWS scores and systems per hospital

Hospitals used different parameters and had different protocols for required action following elevated PEWS (see Tables 2 and 3). All hospitals assessed heartrate and breathing rate as part of the PEWS parameters, whereas four included respiratory effort (#1,2,4,5) or capillary refill time (#1,2,3,4) and three the use of supplementary O_2. Other parameters, e.g. O_2 saturation, temperature, systolic blood pressure, color, behavior and nurse's concern were part of PEWS in two of the five hospitals. In existing literature, level of consciousness is often considered part of behavior, so combining these two items, behavior was part of the PEWS scoring system in four hospitals in our sample.

When looking at policies and required actions following elevated PEWS, most differences concerned the general policy for when to use PEWS, ranging from all patients every 8 h (#2 and 4), to all patients twice every 24 h (#5), to monitoring only on admission or patients on monitors and/or considered high risk (#1 and 3). In all hospitals, PEWS had to be calculated at least once for all paediatric inpatients. The cut-off points used by the hospitals all differed, but the actions of nursing staff following elevated PEWS would mostly include increasing the frequency of calculating the PEWS, consulting with a paediatrician and/or attending physician, or interventions aimed at directly improving the condition of the patient, such as administering oxygen or pain medication. With regards to the cut-off points, it is important to realize that PEWS scores are not comparable between hospitals as they are the results of different variables leading to a PEWS score.

Level of implementation in patients' records

A total of 554 paediatric patient records were included in the study. One hospital (hospital # 2) dropped out during the last part of the implementation phase due to internal reorganization. A description of the patient characteristics can be found in Table 4.

Table 5 shows registration of PEWS at the different time points during the implementation. None of the hospitals were recording PEWS at the start of the study, and that at midterm only three hospitals (#2, #3 and #5) had started registering PEWS. One year after implementation, all hospitals had started to record PEWS. The registration of PEWS differed considerably, from 25.0% (#1) to 97.9% (#5), with an average of PEWS being recorded in 69.2% of the paediatric patients admitted (see Table 5).

Next to PEWS being reported, elevated PEWS increasingly led to appropriate action as described in the hospitals' own protocols (see Table 6). After 6 months of implementation, required action was taken in 10.3% of cases (3/29), whereas this number increased to 49.1% (27/55) after 1 year of implementation.

Overall, the patient records showed that after 1 year of implementation there was a positive trend towards improvement in using a PEWS system; PEWS were not only being recorded in more patients, but elevated PEWS led to appropriate action by the nursing and/or medical staff more often.

Interview findings: Implementation process and attitudes of professionals towards using a PEWS system

Eight semi-structured interviews were held with the contact persons for the project, consisting of paediatric nurses ($n = 4$) and paediatricians ($n = 4$) from the four

Table 2 List of items used in PEWS scores of the five participating hospitals

Item	Hospital 1	Hospital 2	Hospital 3	Hospital 4	Hospital 5
Heart rate	x	X	x	x	x
Breathing rate	x	X	x	x	x
Respiratory Effort	x	X		x	x
Capillary Refill Time	x	X	x	x	
Use of O_2 therapy	x		x		x
O_2 saturation	x		x		
Systolic Blood Pressure	x		x		
Temperature	x		x		
Colour		X		x	
Behaviour		X		x	
Consciousness			x		x
Nurse Concern			x		x
Total items	8	6	9	6	6

Table 3 Summary of PEWS systems used within each hospital

	General policy when to use PEWS	Cut-off points and associated actions
Hospital 1	High risk patient every 8 h PEWS ≤2 every 24 h	PEWS 4–5: assess PEWS every 4 h PEWS 6–7: assess PEWS every hour PEWS ≥8: consult pediatrician
Hospital 2	All patients every 8 h	PEWS 2: assess PEWS every 3 h PEWS 3: assess PEWS every hour and consult attending physician PEWS 4–5: call pediatrician and attending physician PEWS 6: consult with pediatrician within 30 min
Hospital 3	Patients on monitors every 8 h Other patients at least once, on admissions	PEWS ≥3: call pediatrician and assess PEWS every 2 h
Hospital 4	All patients every 8 h	PEWS 3: consider consulting pediatrician or attending physician PEWS ≥4: consult with pediatrician within 15 min
Hospital 5	All patients twice in 24 h	PEWS 3–4: re-assess PEWS after 4 h, consider assessment of blood pressure and O_2 saturation PEWS 5–6: call pediatrician and measure blood pressure and O_2 saturation

remaining hospitals in the last phase. The mean age of the interviewees was 44 years (range 27–50 years) and on average they had 15 years of experience in paediatrics (range 6–27 years of experience). They spoke from both personal experience as well as experiences from colleagues within their department. The findings from the interviews will be presented here, grouped into three themes that emerged from the interviews regarding the attitudes of the healthcare professionals towards and experiences regarding the implementation of the PEWS system in their hospital.

Theme 1: Using a PEWS system is important, but...

Most interviewed paediatric nurses and paediatricians were introduced to PEWS because it was part of the national VMS program in the Netherlands. They indicated that they already had a high registration burden, and showed some resistance to having to register yet another score. Nevertheless, they were motivated to use a PEWS system, indicating that they did acknowledge the importance of registering PEWS scores and working with a PEWS protocol for early intervention.

"I think using the PEWS has added value. Just this week we had a boy who looked good clinically. But then we measured his blood pressure, and realised it was really low. He appeared to have hypotension. So yeah... we would not have noticed that otherwise, with only temperature and pulse. [...] We always call each other a lot. Our paediatrician is easily approachable."

Nurse and care coordinator

Table 4 Patient characteristics of the reviewed records

Characteristic (*n* = 554)	
Sex (% male)	52.0
Mean age in years (SD)	4.5 (5.6)
Ward (%)	
Pediatrics	92.8
Maternity/neonatal care	7.2

Despite the fact that they considered working with PEWS important, they also voiced doubts about the effectiveness of using a PEWS system. Interviewees indicated that they considered evaluating the effectiveness of using the PEWS system as the next priority. They wondered how many children had been identified only because of an elevated PEWS, that would otherwise not have been identified.

"I think that when a child is unstable, the doctor is often already alerted. [...] When you are worried or it does not feel right, you warn the doctor. That does not rely on a score. It is not that I only start calling the doctor when I have a PEWS of 3-4-5, because you probably already did so because you are worried about the child. So in that respect, I do not think that we call the doctor faster by using PEWS-scores."

Nurse

"I am not sure whether using PEWS really has an added value. [...] We now want to investigate whether we are really able to identify those children at risk. Are there a lot of false positives? What could be the disadvantages of using PEWS? I do not immediately have a positive feeling about it. I do know that I almost never get called with the request 'the PEWS is elevated, will you come by?'"

Pediatrician

Table 5 Registration of PEWS scores (n) at start, midterm and end of implementation

	Start (month = 0)	Midterm (month = 6)	End (month = 12)	Total records (n)
Hospital 1	0% (42)	0.0% (35)	25.0% (40)	117
Hospital 2	0% (42)	10.0% (40)	(0)	82
Hospital 3	0% (40)	72.4% (29)	61.4% (44)	113
Hospital 4	0% (45)	0.0% (33)	92.5% (40)	118
Hospital 5	0% (38)	92.3% (39)	97.9% (47)	124
Average	0% (207)	34.9% (176)	69.2% (171)	554

Although interviewees indicate that a PEWS can help in early identification of clinical deterioration in paediatric patients, early identification should not depend solely on elevated PEWS. Easily approachable nurses and physicians, as well as good communication, were considered to be vital for timely intervention in cases of clinical deterioration in paediatric patients.

Theme 2: Easy to register and calculate especially when using an integrated system

In general, interviewees found the PEWS were easy to calculate because the underlying measurements were often already part of nurses' daily work routine, and therefore required little behavioral changes in their daily work. Some interviewees found that exclusion of the peripheral blood pressure measurement would made the PEWS easier to use. Some quotes to illustrate these findings:

> *"..... So I think that some people, at least that is what I heard in the beginning, were like 'yet another score'. Of course you look at the child and you pay attention to the child, but you spend so much time behind the computer just to register everything. That creates resistance sometimes. I hear that, and I think: 'yes of course you can see when a child deteriorates, but the registration, and being able to find it back in the computer, is important'."*
>
> Nurse

> *"[...] I am under the impression that measuring PEWS does not require a lot of extra work from the nurses."*
>
> Pediatrician

Once the PEWS scores and the protocol for early intervention were selected, the implementation of the PEWS system showed few difficulties and improved when nurses were aware of the reason why PEWS scores were calculated and realised that it was not a lot of extra work.

Facilitators for the implementation of registration of PEWS included the integration of PEWS scores into the electronic patient records. While this effort was time consuming and difficult, it proofed worthwhile to facilitate implementation.

> *"It took a very long time to embed PEWS in our department. Why? On the one hand I think that we did not clearly formulate the purpose of measuring PEWS to the team. The intention we had concerning PEWS was unclear and everyone thought it made the workload heavier: another extra activity. [...] But now, in hindsight, you realise that you already do perform many of these measurements on a daily basis. But now you put them in a format, which you didn't do before. So, actually it only takes you a very short time, but instantly gives you an idea of the child's situation. [...]"*
>
> Nurse

> *"We also connected the acute medication list to filling out the PEWS. So, when we enter the child's information, it then provides a list that assists the nurses. This way nurses are motivated to first obtain and enter the score and in order to get that list. It provides information and lets you know how much and what you can give. Almost everyone does that. But whether it is really done a couple of times a day, I cannot say."*
>
> Care coordinator

Table 6 Distribution of elevated PEWS and frequency of required action (PEWS system)

Month	Number of records	Registration of PEWS score	Action required[a](n)	Action taken (n)
Start	207	0%	NA	NA
Midterm	176	34.9%	29	10.3% (3)
End	171	69.2%	55	49.1% (27)

[a] = Based on information of the PEWS systems provided by the participating hospitals (see Table 3)

One hospital (#1) had not included PEWS in their electronic patient records yet, but interviewees from this hospital indicated that this was desirable.

Theme 3:National guidelines versus local applicability

The implementation advice and practical tools provided during the first face-to-face meeting were taken to heart by several project leaders and applied in practice. This led to project leaders involving the end users in selecting specific PEWS variables and developing a project plan for their hospital.

Hospitals found it difficult to identify a suitable PEWS system for their setting. The nursing and medical staff felt that the available systems were all developed for use in university hospitals, making them not necessarily applicable in their non-academic setting. This was partly due to the absence of an paediatric intensive care, where for instance intra-arterial measurements and monitoring are often used to calculate PEWS. In addition, nurses and paediatricians indicated that they would have liked to be provided with one national, uniform PEWS system that all hospitals could use. Because such a national system as lacking, all hospitals searched for their own suitable PEWS system. Most hospitals did so on their own, for example by instating a working group, by researching the literature, or by asking information from other hospitals (including regional university medical centres).

> *"At first we decided to await a national development of a PEWS system, so we didn't have to "re-invent the wheel". But that took a very long time and we had to get started with PEWS in our hospital, so we decided to set up our own PEWS. [...] Of course every nurse wants to identify that one child you would otherwise miss. But having to fill in something, again, like with the pain score... All the checks you have to do create resistance."*
>
> Nurse

Discussion

The objectives of the current mixed methods study were to 1) describe and compare the specific PEWS and protocols for early intervention (together a PEWS system) in each hospital; 2) evaluate the level of implementation of a PEWS system within each hospital and 3) gain insight into the attitudes of nurses and paediatricians towards implementation of a PEWS system in their hospital.

While implementation of a PEWS system became part of accreditation of Dutch hospitals, national guidelines regarding which clinical symptoms to be included, which scoring methods, cut-off points, and procedures to use were lacking. Therefore, it came as no surprise that the five hospitals all developed their own criteria, scoring and policies regarding the use of PEWS. A recent study showed that in 68 Dutch hospitals that had implemented a PEWS system, 45 different versions were being used, including 200 different parameters, with not one parameter being used in all hospitals [13]. Using different parameters, elevated scores are not necessarily comparable between hospitals. This situation, of each hospital developing or adapting their own PEWS criteria and policies, is similar to the situation in the United Kingdom and North America [6]. On one hand, different contexts and clinical populations justify different PEWS variables, but at the same time, these differences are barriers to communication between hospitals and the developing evidence for effective and validated systems [8]. This was also reflected in the doubts by the interviewed professionals, while they intuitively thought of PEWS system as a positive value in the daily care of children, they also voiced doubts about the validity and effectiveness of registering PEWS scores. This clearly indicates the need for nationally agreed guidelines when developing a PEWS system.

While PEWS have been validated for more specific settings such as university hospitals [9], questions can be raised regarding the use of the same list of parameters in other settings, such as non-university hospitals. At the same time however, most of our included hospitals did base their parameters on internationally published PEWS, such as the "Brighton PEWS-score" [3, 14], using parameters concerning the cardiovascular and respiratory system and behaviour. While for the point of view of validating and evaluating effectiveness, one standard set of PEWS parameters might be preferred, it is important to keep in mind that non-university settings often include different populations of patients and thus a different a-priori chance of developing acute deterioration based on physiological markers. This was also reflected in the interviews with professionals. While they acknowledged the importance and the purpose of PEWS, they also expressed doubts regarding the effectiveness of the PEWS in their own hospital. They felt the parameters of PEWS were developed in and for university or specialized hospitals with more complex pathology. Because acute clinical deterioration was a rare occurrence in the participating hospitals, the nurses and paediatricians felt that they had not yet the opportunity to observe and experience the usefulness of PEWS in practice.

For example, elevated temperature and heart rate in an otherwise healthy child could carry a very different risk of further escalation than those same symptoms in a child after bone marrow transplantation at a specialized oncology unit. The solution for this tension between on one hand PEWS variables that are appropriate for specific settings and on the other the call for a more standardized PEWS, could be to develop a core set of PEWS that can be used effectively in all settings, while still leaving room for specific populations and different settings. The development of a core set of PEWS and standardized protocols for follow up to be used in all Dutch hospitals would also enable these hospitals to more easily compare results and exchange information on quality improvement efforts. In the Netherlands, the Dutch Society for Paediatricians (NVK) and the Dutch society for Nurses (V&VN) are collaborating in a national working group to further support the development of a core data set for PEWS scores and early intervention for different settings.

Looking at the success of implementation, a couple of things stand out. Findings from the patient records seem to indicate that the registration of PEWS had improved during the PaSQ project, although the extent of implementation differed across hospitals ranged from 25 to 98%. While the staff was motivated to implement a PEWS system, because they believed in the goal of the PEWS system, they had doubts about whether the currently used often non-validated scores and protocols would lead to the desired outcomes. In contrast to studies from the United States reporting that the introduction of PEWS improved nurses' and paediatricians' abilities to recognize early signs of deterioration [15, 16], the interviewed professionals in our study were not convinced of this effect. Nurses and paediatricians indicated that prior to the introduction of PEWS, they already communicated effectively regarding the deterioration of patients, without experiencing hierarchical boundaries. This may point to a cultural difference between countries in how nurses and pediatricians work together.

These doubts and lack of obvious better ability to detect clinical deterioration could be part of the reasons why still more than 50% of the elevated scores did not lead to action as required by the local hospital policy. Therefore these doubts from professionals should be taken seriously in future improvement projects, as attitude and believes are important factors in implementation and sustainability of using a PEWS systems in non-university hospitals [17]. These concerns are supported by the mixed existing evidence regarding the effectiveness of using a PEWS system, with some studies showing positive effectiveness of PEWS in improving patient care, while other studies showing no positive effects [18, 19].

On a positive note, interviewees indicated that the relative ease with which a PEWS system could be incorporated in daily practice, facilitated implementation. Because many of the measurements underlying PEWS scores were already part of daily routine - and thus familiar to nurses - the practical use and registration of PEWS required little extra nursing effort, while the administrative burden of entering them into a system was perceived as high in some hospitals. A good digital system for entering and analysing the PEWS was mentioned during the interviews as a facilitating factor for implementation. This was in line with our findings from the patient record review. The two hospitals showing almost 100% implementation of PEWS (hospitals 4 and 5) were those where PEWS were incorporated in the electronic patient records. At the same time, these two hospitals were the two tertiary teaching hospitals in the sample, often dedicated to more complex care. In the Netherlands, general hospitals provide good quality basic care, where the non-university tertiary teaching hospitals and university hospitals provide more complex and specialized care. While all hospitals in the sample had access to an ICU, only the eight university hospitals have a paediatric ICU. This means that when a patient deteriorates or when PEWS are elevated, the child may have to be transferred to a higher level care hospital. During transition of care, good communication is essential for continuation of care [20]. With hospitals all using their own set of parameters and scoring procedures, important information may be missed during an acute transfer. This is another reason, professionals argue for the development of a core set of PEWS scores for Dutch hospitals.

Recent literature on change management research emphasizes the importance of small changes to existing behaviours in determining the success of implementation of new guidelines and protocols. The smaller the differences between current work processes and the new work processes [21], the easier the implementation process. In our study, successful implementation required very little change from nurses, whereas the less successful hospitals required nurses to use different systems for the administration of PEWS and the administration of regular patient information. The results of this study also shows less complex behaviour, in this case recording the PEWS, was easier to implement than the more complex changes, e.g. implementation of the early intervention protocols following an elevated PEWS score.

What we also learn from this study is that implementation of new policies takes time. At 6 months PEWS were registered in 34.9% and elevated PEWS led to appropriate action in 10.3%, whereas at 6 months this number increased to respectively 69.2% and 49.1%.

This study has several limitations. One of them being the methodology of using patient records. While this method is being used extensively in paediatric patient safety research [18, 22, 23] and has been proven a reliable way to assess patient safety [24], it is limited by the information that is actually being recorded by the healthcare professionals and by the quality of the patient records. Therefore, it is recommended to include different sources of information when evaluating (paediatric) patient safely issues [25]. For that reason we did enhance the patient record data with interviews with representatives of the wards and used the individual hospital protocols in the analysis. Even using a mixed methods approach, it is still difficult to understand the less than 50% rate of follow up after elevated PEWS. Recommendations for future research into the effectiveness of PEWS include a more process oriented evaluation, including experiences by patients and parents, patient safety culture assessment throughout the wards and using cases from where PEWS might have "saved" a child instead of the focus on adverse events which in paediatrics are small in number [18].

Secondly, the outcomes of the study are limited to a small sample of non-university hospitals, limiting generalizability of these results. At the same though, the number of patients included in this study was high ($n = 554$) and the hospitals were selected from different regions and different levels of urbanization and therefore a representative mix of non-university hospitals in the Netherlands.

Conclusion

Hospitals participating in the PaSQ project showed improvements in the use of their PEWS system, although some were decidedly more successful than others. Facilitating factors included the small amount of change in professional behavior that was required, in combination with a system integrated into the EPD for entering and analysing the PEWS. However, doubts among staff about validity and effectiveness might hinder further sustainable implementation. More evidence is needed regarding effectiveness of using a PEWS system. For this purpose the development of a national PEWS system is highly recommended, existing of a "core set" of PEWS and clinical decision making rules for elevated scores in different clinical settings.

Abbreviations

CBO: Dutch Institute for Healthcare Improvement; NIVEL: Netherlands Institute for Health Services Research; NVK: Dutch society for pediatricians; PaSQ: Patient Safety and Quality of Care; PEWS: Paediatric early warning scores; V&VN: Dutch Society for Nurses

Acknowledgements

We gratefully acknowledge the participating hospitals and their staff. We would also like to thank S. van Schoten, J. Hoogervorst-Schilp, M. Broekens, and L. Peppel for contributing to study design and the data collection.

Funding

Dutch participation in PaSQ has been co-funded by the European Commission within the Public Health Programme, and the Dutch Ministry of Health, Welfare and Sports.

Authors' contributions

CW and EdL contributed to the study design. CW conceived the study, and led the application for funding. EdL, LK, PR, MB, JG were responsible for the implementation of PEWS. JG, LvdS and ND were involved in the acquisition of data. LvdS, JdG, LK, LvdS and ND were involved with data analysis. JdG, ND and LvdS drafted the manuscript. All authors contributed to interpretation of the findings. All authors read, revised and approved the final manuscript.

Ethics approval and consent to participate

The study has been granted ethical approval by the medical ethical review board at VU University Medical Centre, in Amsterdam, the Netherlands. All interviews were held face-to-face and interviewees were assured that the gathered interview data remained confidential. With the participants' verbal consent at the start of the interview recorded on tape at the start of the interview. The verbatim interview was checked by all participants for accurateness prior to further analysis. Signed consent to participate in the project and evaluation was provided at hospital level.

Competing interests

The authors declare that they have no competing interests.

Author details

[1]NIVEL Netherlands Institute for Health Services Research, Otterstraat 118-124, 3513 CR Utrecht, the Netherlands. [2]Netherlands Federation of University Medical Centres-Consortium Quality of Care, NIAZ & CBOimpact Dutch Institute for Healthcare Improvement, Utrecht, the Netherlands. [3]Zuyderland Medical Centre Sittard, Sittard, the Netherlands. [4]Noord West Ziekenhuisgroep, Alkmaar, the Netherlands. [5]Medisch Spectrum Twente, P.O Box 50 000, 7500 KA Enschede, the Netherlands. [6]APH Amsterdam Public Health Institute, VU University Medical Centre, Amsterdam, the Netherlands. [7]Ecorys, P.O. Box 4175, 3006 AD Rotterdam, the Netherlands. [8]TNO Healthy Living, Schipholweg 77-89, 2316 ZL Leiden, the Netherlands. [9]Department of Pediatrics, Zuyderland Medical Center, PO Box 5500, 6130 MB Sittard, The Netherlands. [10]Department of Pediatrics, Northwest Clinics, P.O.Box 501, 1800 AM Alkmaar, The Netherlands.

References

1. Girotra S, Spertus JA, Berg RA, Nadkarni VM, Chan PS. Survival trends in pediatric in-hospital cardiac arrests. Circ Cardiovasc Qual Outcomes. 2013;6:42–9.
2. Monaghan A. Detecting and managing deterioration in children. Paediatr Nurs. 2015;17:32–5.
3. Akre M, Finkelstein M, Erickson M, Liu M, Vanderbilt L, Billman G. Sensitivity of the paediatric early warning score to identify patient deterioration. Pediatrics. 2010;125(4):e763–9.
4. Parshuram CS, Duncan HP, Joffe AR, Farrell CA, Lacroix JR, Middaugh KL, Hutchison JS, Wensley D, Blanchard N, Beyene J, Parkin PC. Multicentre validation of the bedside paediatric early warning system score: a severity of illness score to detect evolving critical illness in hospitalised children. Crit Care. 2011;15(4):R184.
5. Robson MA, Cooper CL, Medicus LA, Quintero MJ, Zuniga SA. Comparison of three acute care paediatric early warning scoring tools. J Pediatr Nurs. 2013;28(6):e33–41.
6. Roland D, Oliver AM, Edwards ED, Mason BW, Powell CVE. Use of paediatric early warning systems in great Britain: has there been a change of practice in the last 7 years? Arch Dis Child. 2014;99:26–9.
7. McCAbe A, Duncan H, Heward Y. Paediatric early warning systems: where do we go from here? Paediatr Nurs. 2009;21(1):14–7.
8. Pearson G, Duncan H. Early warning systems for identifying sick children. Paediatr Child Health. 2011;21(5):230–3.
9. Fuijkschot J, Vernhout B, Lemson J, Draaisma JMT, Loeffen JLCM. Validation of a Paediatric early warning score: first results and implications of usage. Eur J Pediatr. 2015;174(1):15–21.

10. VMS Veiligheidsprogramma. Safe care for sick children. 2011. [in Dutch] http://wmszorg.nl.
11. Seiger N, Maconochie I, Oostenbrink R, Moll HA. Validity of different paediatric early warning scores in the emergency department. Paediatrics. 2013;132(4):e841–50.
12. Glaser BG, Strauss AL. The discovery of grounded theory: strategies for qualitative research. New Brunswick and London: Aldine Transaction Sociology Press; 1967.
13. Saambeeck V, et al. De PEWS en veilige(re) zorg in Nederland. Praktische pediatrie. 2016;1:10–4.
14. Solevåg AL, Eggen EH, Schröder J, Nakstad B. Use of a modified paediatric early warning score in a department of paediatric and adolescent medicine. PLoS One. 2013;8(8):e72534.
15. Bonafide CP, Roberts KE, Weirich CM, Paciotti B, Tibbetts KM, Keren R, Barg FK, Holmes JH. Beyond statistical prediction: qualitative evaluation of the mechanisms by which paediatric early warning scores impact patient safety. J Hosp Med. 2013;8(5):248–53.
16. Kaul M, Snethen J, Kelber ST, Zimmanck K, Maletta K, Meyer M. Implementation of the bedside Paediatric early warning system (BedsidePEWS) for nurse identification of deteriorating patients. J Spec Pediatr Nurs. 2014;19(4):339–49.
17. Michie S1, Johnston M, Abraham C, Lawton R, Parker D, Walker A. "Psychological theory" group. Making psychological theory useful for implementing evidence based practice: a consensus approach. Qual Saf Health Care. 2005;14(1):26–33.
18. Panesar R, Polikoff LA, Harris D, Mills B, Messina C, Parker MM. Characteristics and outcomes of paediatric rapid response teams before and after mandatory triggering by an elevated paediatric early warning system (PEWS) score. Hosp Pediatr. 2014;4(3):135–40.
19. Bonafide CP, Localio AR, Roberts KE, Nadkarni VM, Weirich CM, Keren R. Impact of rapid response system implementation on critical deterioration events in children. JAMA Pediatr. 2014;168(1):25–33.
20. Zegers M, de Bruijne MC, Wagner C, Hoonhout LHF, Waaijman R, Smits M, et al. Adverse events and potentially preventable deaths in Dutch hospitals: results of a retrospective patient record review study. Qual Saf Heal Care. 2009;18:297–302.
21. Clay-Williams R, Hounsgaard J, Hollnagel E. Where the rubber meets the road: using FRAM to align work-as-imagined with work-as-done when implementing clinical guidelines. Implement Sci. 2015;10:125.
22. Unbeck M, Lindemalm S, Nydert P, Ygge BM, Nylén U, Berglund C, Härenstam KP. Validation of triggers and development of a paediatric trigger tool to identify adverse events. BMC Health Serv Res. 2014;14:655.
23. Davalos MC, Samuels K, Meyer AN, Thammasitboon S, Sur M, Roy K, Al-Mutairi A, Singh H. Finding Diagnostic Errors in Children Admitted to the PICU. Pediatr Crit Care Med. 2017;18(3):265-71.
24. Hanskamp-Sebregts M, Zegers M, Vincent C, van Gurp PJ, de Vet HC, Wollersheim H. Measurement of patient safety: a systematic review of the reliability and validity of adverse event detection with record review. BMJ Open. 2016;6(8):e011078.
25. Hanskamp-Sebregts M, Zegers M, Boeijen W, Westert GP, van Gurp PJ, Wollersheim H. Effects of auditing patient safety in hospital care: design of a mixed-method evaluation. BMC Health Serv Res. 2013;13:226.

13

Risk factors for carriage of *Streptococcus pneumoniae* in children

Maria G. Koliou[1,2,3*], Kyriaki Andreou[4], Demetris Lamnisos[5], Giagkos Lavranos[5], Paris Iakovides[6], Christos Economou[6] and Elpidoforos S. Soteriades[3,7]

Abstract

Background: During the past decades *Streptococcus pneumoniae* has developed significant resistance to many classes of antimicrobial drugs. Potential risk factors for colonization of the nasopharynx by *Streptococcus pneumoniae* in children and for carriage of drug resistant strains were examined.

Methods: Between 2007 and 2008 nasopharyngeal swabs were collected from 402 children 6 months to 5 years old visiting the public sector immunization centers and outpatient departments as well as offices of paediatricians from private practice in Nicosia district in Cyprus. Information on demographic characteristics and potential risk factors of participating children were collected using a standardized questionnaire distributed to parents.

Results: In multivariable analyses we found that attendance at day care center, having siblings in the family and having both parents originating from Cyprus, statistically increased the risk of pneumococcal colonization. Full immunization with PCV7 appears to be a protective factor against colonization by pneumococcus. Previous administration of antimicrobials during the last month prior to specimen collection appeared to be the most consistent risk factor for carrying a non susceptible strain of *Streptococcus pneumoniae* to either penicillin or erythromycin. Factors such as age, nationality, previous or current breastfeeding, passive exposure to cigarette smoke and attendance in a day care center do not appear as independent risk factors for colonization by non susceptible strains.

Conclusions: Prudent use of antibiotics especially for upper respiratory tract infections in children as well as increased vaccination coverage by the pneumococcal conjugate vaccines could prove effective in reducing levels of colonization by drug resistant pneumococcal strains.

Keywords: *Streptococcus pneumoniae*, Colonization, Risk factors, Drug resistance, Vaccination, Cyprus

Background

Streptococcus pneumoniae is a common cause of meningitis, pneumonia and bacteraemia particularly among children and the elderly. It is also the most frequent pathogen causing acute otitis media in children and the most frequent bacterial cause of disease in children younger than 3 years of age [1]. Colonization of the nasopharynx by *S. pneumoniae* is considered a prerequisite for invasive disease and has a key role in the transmission of the pathogen to other individuals leading to pathogen spread in the community [2, 3]. Therefore strains colonizing the nasopharynx reflect the strains circulating in the community leading to different infections [4].

During the past decades, global development of resistance of *S. pneumoniae* to several antimicrobials appears to pose a significant challenge to the successful treatment of infections [5]. Development of pneumococcal conjugate vaccines has led to a significant decrease of pneumococcal infections in general and also to infections caused by drug resistant strains [6]. Conjugate vaccines act by decreasing infections caused by vaccine serotypes. They also reduce colonization by the same serotypes; a result which appears to account for a significant herd effect noted in older age groups who have not been vaccinated [7].

Vaccine serotypes account for the highest percentage of resistance in most countries. Several factors appear to

* Correspondence: mkoliou@spidernet.com.cy
[1]Department of Paediatrics, Archbishop Makarios III Hospital, Nicosia, Cyprus
[2]School of Medicine, University of Cyprus, Nicosia, Cyprus
Full list of author information is available at the end of the article

influence the type and frequency of pneumococcal isolates colonizing the nasopharynx. Environmental and socioeconomic factors, overcrowding conditions and overconsumption of antimicrobials have been reported in various studies [8–11].

In Cyprus, the PCV7 (Pneumococcus 7-valent conjugate vaccine) was introduced in 2004 only in the private sector and was not subsidized by the state until 2010 when the 10-valent vaccine was introduced in the public sector and was offered free of charge. In 2011 the 13-valent vaccine was also introduced in Cyprus but only by the private sector. Therefore population coverage of children by the PCV7 vaccine in 2007–2008 when the current study was conducted remained relatively low. Data from the tri-annual survey performed in Cyprus by the Ministry of Health among children 17–24 months old in 2009, revealed full coverage by the PCV7 vaccine only in 37.5%, partial coverage in 42% and no vaccine coverage in 20.5% of children [12]. The susceptibility pattern and the circulating serotypes of *S. pneumoniae* isolated in Cypriot children have been reported elsewhere [13]. So far, no previous studies have been reported in Cyprus examining potential risk factors for colonization by pneumococcus in Cypriot children. The objective of our study was to evaluate the potential risk factors among Cypriot children associated with colonization of nasopharynx by *S. pneumoniae* and those risk factors that may be associated with the carriage of drug resistant strains.

Methods

Design and setting of the study

The study was conducted in Nicosia district (capital); the largest district of Cyprus, between November 2007 and May 2008. The population of Nicosia district at the end of 2007 was 301,103 people representing 38.8% of the total population of the Republic of Cyprus. The target population of the study was children 6 months to 5 years old, who visited the government immunization centers in urban and rural areas, the outpatient department of Archbishop Makarios III Hospital or those who visited the offices of 4 major pediatric units of the private sector. Due to the absence of a National health care system in Cyprus, health services are currently offered independently in the public and private sector. The public sector in Cyprus provides health coverage to about 80% of the population, which is eligible for medical care, including current and former public sector employees and their families, individuals with low income and other EU (European Union) nationals residing in Cyprus with recognized medical coverage in their country of origin. On the other hand, the private health sector in Cyprus currently offers its services to a particular segment of the population, who either pay out of pocket or maintain coverage from private health insurance plans. For each child participating in the study, written informed consent was taken from the parents or legal guardians. The study was approved by the National Bioethics Committee of the Republic of Cyprus.

Epidemiological and demographic data were collected through standardized questionnaires which were addressed to the parents at the time of specimen collection. Information was gathered on age, gender, parent nationality, exposure to passive smoking, previous or current breastfeeding, number of siblings, attendance to day care centers, immunization with PCV7 vaccine, current illness, whether the sample was taken from a public sector center or from a private paediatrician's office (specimen origin) and on recent use of antibiotics. Children suffering from a bacterial infection or being on antibiotics at the day of specimen collection were excluded from the study. Specimens were taken from only one child from each family.

Sampling procedure

Nasopharyngeal specimens were collected using sterile Rayon swabs on flexible wire (Medical Wire and Equipment Co. Ltd.,Corsham, Wilts., England) and were plated within two hours on Blood agar plates supplemented with 5% defibrinated horse blood and chocolate agar plates and incubated in 5% CO_2 for 24 h at 35 °C. *S. pneumoniae* strains were identified by optochin sensitivity and bile solubility as described before [14].

Susceptibility testing

Susceptibility testing was performed on Mueller-Hinton agar supplemented with 5% defibrinated horse blood as follows: All strains were tested by the disk diffusion methods for susceptibility to oxacillin, cefotaxime, erythromycin, clindamycin, trimethoprim – sulfamethoxazole, tetracycline, vancomycin, linezolid and levofloxacin and by assessing the MIC (Minimum Inhibitory Concentration) of all strains to penicillin. MIC was determined by the Etest method (AB Biodisk, Solna, Sweden) [15]. MIC was also determined for all antibiotics to which *S. pneumoniae* appeared non susceptible by the disk method.

Subsequently, the results of susceptibility to penicillin were interpreted based on the new definitions issued by the CLSI (Clinical and Laboratory Standards Institute) at the beginning of 2008 as applied for a non-meningitis infection if antibacterial is administered orally [16]. A strain is considered sensitive to penicillin if MIC is < 0.06 μg/ml, intermediate resistant if MIC is between 0.12–1 and resistant if MIC is $> = 2$ μg/ml.

Statistical analysis

The following factors were examined as possible risk factors for colonization and carriage of drug resistant strains for *S. pneumoniae* in the children population: gender, age, parent nationality, exposure to passive smoking, previous or current breastfeeding, number of siblings, attendance to day care centers, immunization with PCV7 vaccine, whether the sample was taken from a public sector center or from a private paediatrician's office (specimen origin) and on recent use of antibiotics. These factors were first analyzed by a series of univariable analyses. Then, to control simultaneously for the possible confounding effects of the different variables, the risk of colonization and carriage of drug resistant strains of *S. pneumoniae* was estimated by multiple logistic regression analyses that simultaneously included all factors as predictor variables in the model. In both analyses, the association was expressed in OR (odds ratios) and 95% CI (confidence intervals). Statistical analyses were performed using the statistical package SPSS 20. Statistical significance was set at $p < 0.05$.

Results

Demographics

One nasopharyngeal specimen was taken from each of 402 children who represented 2.4% of the total population of the children of same age in the district of Nicosia. In Table 1 we present the socioeconomic and demographic characteristics of the children enrolled in the study. A total of 143 children attended a variety of 19 different day care centers while 33 children were cared for during the morning hours by an adult who also provided care for a small number of other children. The majority of children (226) stayed at their home supervised by an adult family member. A total of 60.3% of the specimens were obtained from children visiting a public sector center and 39.8% from the offices of private paediatricians. We found that 35.3% of the children in the sample were colonized by *S. pneumoniae.*

Table 1 Sociodemographic characteristics

Characteristics/variables	Categories	Frequency (%)
Gender	Boy	207 (51.5)
	Girl	195 (48.5)
Age	< 1 year	130 (32.3)
	1–2	123 (30.6)
	> 2 years	149 (37.1)
Nationality	Both parents Cypriots	273 (67.9)
	Others	128 (31.9)
	Missing	1(0.2)
Breastfeeding	Yes	300 (74.6)
	No	97 (24.1)
	Missing	5 (1.2)
Exposure to smoking	Yes	142 (35.3)
	No	255 (63.4)
	Missing	5 (1.2)
Day care attendance[a]	Yes	170 (42.3)
	No	226 (56.2)
	Missing	6 (1.5)
Siblings	No	168 (42.5)
	1	140 (35.4)
	> = 2	87 (22.0)
Vaccinated	Full	91 (22.6)
	Incomplete	53 (13.2)
	No	226 (56.2)
	Missing	32 (16)
Origin of specimen	From a public center	241 (60.3)
	From the private sector	159 (39.8)
Colonized	Yes	142 (35.3)
	No	260 (64.7)

[a]Includes children who were supervised during the morning hours by an adult who also cared for at least 3 other children

Risk factors for carriage

In Table 2 we delineate the association of different risk factors with the colonization of nasopharynx of children by *S. pneumoniae.* In multivariable analyses, we did not find any association between age or gender and the risk of colonization with *S. pneumoniae.* Furthermore, we did not find any statistically significant association between history of breastfeeding, exposure to passive smoking and specimen origin (obtained from a child attending the public sector versus the private sector) and the risk of colonization. Day care attendance or having siblings (one or more) appeared to increase the risk by nearly 3 fold. If both parents were Cypriot nationals in comparison with any other nationality also appeared to increase the risk of colonization by more than two times. On the other hand, full immunization status by PCV7 was associated with a protective effect (two-fold lower risk).

Risk factors for drug resistant strains

The risk factors associated with colonization of children by a drug resistant strain to penicillin (full and intermediate resistance) are presented in Table 3. The only factor that was associated with an increased risk of colonization by drug resistant strains to penicillin was the use of antibiotics within the previous month before specimen collection [3-fold increased risk, OR: 2.83 (95% CI 1.09, 7.74)]. Two factors that appeared to be protective against colonization by resistant strains were female gender, [2.5 times lower risk, OR: 0.39 (95% CI 0.16, 0.90)], and the origin of the specimen from the office of a private paediatrician [3 times

Table 2 Association between potential risk factors and colonization by pneumococcal isolate

Variable/risk factor	Category	Percentage of colonized children (%)	Unadjusted OR (95% CI)	Adjusted OR[d] (95% CI)	*p*-value[¶]
Gender	Boy	37.7%	Ref [a]	Ref [a]	
	Girl	32.8%	0.81 (0.54, 1.22)	0.91 (0.57, 1.47)	0.71
Age	< 1 year	26.2%	Ref	Ref	
	1–2	30.9%	1.26 (073, 2.19)	0.93 (0.50, 1.74)	0.83
	> 2 years	47.0%	**2.50 (1.52, 4.18)**[c]	1.31 (0.63, 2.72)	0.47
Nationality	Both parents Cypriots	41.0%	**2.27 (1.43, 3.70)**[c]	**2.31 (1.29, 4.21)**[c]	**< 0.01**[c]
	Other	23.4%	Ref	Ref	
Breastfeeding	Yes	36.0%	1.09 (0.68, 1.78)	1.28 (0.73, 2.27)	0.40
	No	34.0%	Ref	Ref	
Exposure to smoking	Yes	37.3%	1.13 (0.74, 1.73)	1.43 (0.86, 2.40)	0.17
	No	34.5%	Ref	Ref	
Day care attendance[b]	Yes	51.2%	**3.34 (2.18, 5.15)**[c]	**2.88 (1.62, 5.20)**[c]	**< 0.01**[c]
	No	23.9%	Ref	Ref	
Siblings	No	25.6%	Ref	Ref	
	1	41.4%	**2.06 (1.27, 3.35)**[c]	**2.72 (1.55, 4.86)**[c]	**< 0.01**[c]
	> = 2	46.0%	**2.47 (1.44, 4.29)**[c]	**2.78 (1.47, 5.34)**[c]	**< 0.01**[c]
Vaccination	Full	29.7%	0.85 (0.50, 1.43)	**0.48 (0.25, 0.92)**[c]	**0.03**[c]
	Incomplete	47.2%	1.80 (0.98, 3.30)	1.64 (0.79, 3.38)	0.18
	No	33.2%	Ref	Ref	
Origin of specimen	From a public center	34.0%	Ref	Ref	
	From a private center	37.7%	1.17 (0.77, 1.78)	1.05 (0.62, 1.77)	0.85

[a]Ref means reference group
[b]Includes children who were supervised during the morning hours by an adult who also cared for at least 3 other children
[c]Statistically significant associations are marked in bold
[d]Adjusted for gender, age, nationality, breastfeeding, exposure to smoking, day care attendance, siblings, vaccination and origin of specimen
[¶] *p*-values for multiple logistic regression model

lower risk, OR: 0.32 (95% CI 0.12, 0.82)]. Percentages of resistance to penicillin are also presented in Table 3.

In Table 4 we present identified risk factors associated with drug resistant isolates (full and intermediate resistance) to erythromycin. Univariable as well as multi-variable analyses showed that the administration of anti-microbials to a child within the previous 30 days or the previous 3 months before specimen collection, both increased the risk of colonization by at least 3-fold (OR: 3.00 95% CI 1.15, 8.17). However, obtaining the specimen from a private paediatrician's office versus the public sector outpatient clinic was associated with a protective effect for colonization [2.8 times lower risk, OR: 0.36 (95% CI 0.13,0.93)].

Discussion

To our knowledge, this is the first study in Cyprus to examine the association of various potential risk factors for carriage of *S. pneumoniae* and also for carriage of drug resistant isolates. Attendance at a day care center was identified as a risk factor for colonization by nearly 3-fold increased risk. Other studies have also reported similar findings and this is maybe due to the increased exposure of children to other children colonized or even suffering from a pneumococcal upper respiratory tract infection [9, 17]. Having siblings in the family has also been identified as a risk factor in the multi-variable analyses. Even one sibling increased the risk by at least 2.5 times. Other studies have also reported similar findings, which may be attributed to additional exposure to carriage or infections from siblings [9, 18].

Children with both parents originating from Cyprus had a significantly increased risk of colonization by *S. pneumoniae* isolates. The risk was increased by more than two times. This finding requires further investigation however, a possible explanation could be that these children may have a higher socioeconomic status compared to children from immigrants or other visitors due to the unique conditions of healthcare access in Cyprus discussed above. Higher socioeconomic status has been found among the risk factors associated with higher carriage of *S. pneumoniae* in one study from Greece [19].

Factors such as age, gender, history of breastfeeding, and passive exposure to smoking do not appear to be statistically significantly associated with the risk of

Table 3 Risk factors associated with colonization by a penicillin non-susceptible strain

Variable/Risk factor	Category	Percentage of resistance[a] (%)	Unadjusted OR (95% CI)	Adjusted OR[d] (95% CI)	p value[¶]
Gender	Boy	48.7%	Ref [b]	Ref [b]	
	Girl	32.8%	0.51 (0.26, 1.01)	**0.39 (0.16, 0.90)**[c]	**0.03**[c]
Age	< 1 year	44.1%	Ref	Ref	
	1–2	47.4%	1.14 (0.45, 2.91)	0.89 (0.23, 2.76)	0.85
	> 2 years	37.1%	0.75 (0.33, 1.73)	0.47 (0.14, 1.55)	0.22
Nationality	Both parents Cypriots	41.1%	0.91 (0.40, 2.09)	0.93 (0.29, 3.03)	0.91
	Others	43.3%	Ref	Ref	
Breastfeeding	Yes	41.7%	1.10 (0.50, 2.48)	1.36 (0.52, 3.76)	0.54
	No	39.4%	Ref	Ref	
Exposure to smoking	Yes	43.4%	1.16 (0.58, 2.32)	1.45 (0.59, 3.57)	0.41
	No	39.8%	Ref	Ref	
Day care attendance	Yes	41.4%	1.03 (0.52, 2.06)	1.45 (0.54, 4.02)	0.47
	No	40.7%	Ref	Ref	
Siblings	No	41.9%	Ref	Ref	
	1	41.4%	0.98 (0.44, 2.19)	0.98 (0.35, 2.76)	0.97
	> = 2	40.0%	0.93 (0.38, 2.23)	0.67 (0.21, 2.06)	0.49
Vaccination	Full	29.6%	0.63 (0.23, 1.59)	0.81 (0.24, 2.63)	0.72
	Incomplete	56.0%	1.91 (0.77, 4.85)	2.55 (0.82, 8.32)	0.11
	No	40.0%	Ref	Ref	
Origin of specimen	From a public center	47.6%	Ref	Ref	
	From a private center	33.3%	0.55 (0.27,1.09)	**0.32 (0.12, 0.82)**[c]	**0.02**[c]
Antibiotics last month	Yes	60.6%	**2.86 (1.29, 6.55)**[c]	**2.83 (1.09, 7.74)**[c]	**0.04**[c]
	No	35.0%	Ref	Ref	
Antibiotics last trimester	Yes	48.5%	1.80 (0.91, 3.63)	2.24 (0.95, 5.48)	0.07
	No	34.3%	Ref	Ref	

[a]Strain with intermediate and full resistance to penicillin are included
[b]Ref: means a reference group
[c]Statistically significant associations are marked in bold
[d]Adjusted for gender, age, nationality, breastfeeding, exposure to smoking, day care attendance, siblings, vaccination, origin of specimen and antibiotic use the last month
[¶] *p*-values for multiple logistic regression model

colonization with *S. pneumoniae.* On the other hand, full immunization with PCV7 in comparison to non vaccinated children appeared to have a protective effect against colonization (two-fold decreased risk). Because of the herd effect, non immunized children can also benefit from the PCV7 vaccine. However the comparison between the groups revealed a protective effect of the vaccine against colonization. This has not been shown in other studies as in most countries the situation before and after the introduction of a conjugate vaccine is usually compared.

As shown in Tables 3 and 4, the most consistent and common factor associated with carriage of drug resistant isolates to either penicillin or erythromycin was the previous use of antibiotics during the month prior to specimen collection, raising the risk by more than 3 times. Use of antimicrobials even at 3 months prior to specimen collection was also a risk factor for colonization by drug resistant strains to both penicillin and erythromycin (2 to 3-fold increased risk). Many studies support our findings and have reported similar associations [10, 20, 21]. The association between high antibiotic use and high levels of antibiotic resistance in an area or a country is well documented [22, 23]. It is well known that the sub-inhibitory concentrations of anti-microbials allow *S. pneumoniae* to exhibit increased mutation frequency. Such increase in mutation frequency may give the bacterium a selective advantage as it helps to cope with the stress induced by the antimicrobials [24]. Selection of non-susceptible strains in colonization is likely to occur also by favoring the Growth and acquisition of non-susceptibility. Furthermore, horizontal gene transfer is considered a major cause of adaptability and spread of resistance genes within pneumococci and other mitis Group streptococci [25].

Table 4 Risk factors associated with carriage by an erythromycin non–susceptible strain

Variable/risk factor	Category	Percentage of resistance[a] (%)	Unadjusted OR (95% CI)	Adjusted OR[d] (95% CI)	*p*-value[¶]
Gender	Boy	43.6%	Ref [b]	Ref [b]	
	Girl	37.5%	0.77 (0.39, 1.52)	0.74 (0.32, 1.70)	0.48
Age	< 1 year	41.2%	Ref	Ref	
	1–2	44.7%	1.16 (0.45, 2.97)	1.39 (0.46, 4.31)	0.56
	> 2 years	35.7%	0.79 (0.34, 1.86)	0.92 (0.28, 3.02)	0.89
Nationality	Both parents Cypriots	41.1%	1.39 (0.61, 3.36)	3.04 (0.94, 10.70)	0.07
	Others	33.3%	Ref	Ref	
Breastfeeding	Yes	41.7%	1.43 (0.64, 3.33)	2.27 (0.84, 6.65)	0.12
	No	33.3%	Ref	Ref	
Exposure to smoking	Yes	41.5%	1.13 (0.56, 2.26)	1.62 (0.66, 4.00)	0.29
	No	38.6%	Ref	Ref	
Attendance at a Day care	Yes	39.1%	0.93 (0.47, 1.88)	1.04 (0.39, 2.80)	0.94
	No	40.7%	Ref	Ref	
Siblings	No	48.8%	Ref	Ref	
	1	39.7%	0.69 (0.31, 1.53)	0.65 (0.24, 1.76)	0.40
	≥2	30.0%	0.44 (0.18, 1.09)	**0.25 (0.07, 0.80)**[c]	**0.02**[c]
Vaccination	Full	29.6%	0.60 (0.22, 1.50)	0.34 (0.10, 1.08)	0.07
	Incomplete	44.0%	1.12 (0.44, 2.78)	0.66 (0.21, 2.05)	0.48
	No	41.3%	Ref	Ref	
Origin of specimen	From a public center	42.7%	Ref	Ref	
	From a private center	35.0%	0.73 (0.36,1.43)	**0.36 (0.13,0.93)**[c]	**0.04**[c]
Antibiotics last month	Yes	54.5%	**2.23 (1.01, 5.01)**[c]	**3.00 (1.15, 8.17)**[c]	**0.02**[c]
	No	35.9%	Ref	Ref	
Antibiotics last trimester	Yes	51.5%	**2.66 (1.32, 5.47)**[c]	**3.78 (1.56, 9.80)**[c]	**< 0.01**[c]
	No	30.0%	Ref	Ref	

[a]Strains with intermediate and full resistance to erythromycin are included
[b]Ref means a reference group
[c]Statistically significant associations are marked in bold
[d]Adjusted for gender, age, nationality, breastfeeding, exposure to smoking, day care attendance, siblings, vaccination, origin of specimen and antibiotic use the last month
[¶]*p*-values for multiple logistic regression model

Female gender has also been found as an independent protective factor against carriage of penicillin drug resistant strains in comparison to males. Higher frequency of carriage with penicillin drug resistant pneumococcal isolates in boys was also detected in other studies however, no specific explanation has been identified [26]. Nevertheless, the frequency of pneumococcal infections in boys has also been reported to be higher than those in girls in various studies [27–29].

In our study, obtaining the specimen from a child who visited the private sector has been found to be an independent protective factor for carriage of either penicillin or erythromycin drug resistant isolates. This may reflect the dual health care system in Cyprus. It is possible that it could be explained by the difference in socioeconomic level between the two categories of children attending the private versus the public sector. The children visiting paediatricians in the private sector usually come from a higher socioeconomic status. In previous studies, higher socioeconomic level was also associated with lower carriage of pneumococci resistant to penicillin [18].

Our sample of children enrolled in this study, despite being a convenience sample, is largely representative of the general population of this age group. Children enrolled in the study come from the public and the private sector, therefore children from a broad socioeconomic spectrum participated in the study. Further to the above, children who attended a great number of day care centers and many others who were cared for at home are also represented. We believe that this broad representation prevented the cluster effect that would occur if we had included children from only a small number of day care centers.

High immunization coverage with PCV vaccines has been shown to decrease the frequency of invasive infections in general as well as by drug resistant isolates. This phenomenon is attributed to the significant decrease in the presence of pneumococcal serotypes included in the vaccine as many of these serotypes are characterized by significant resistance to antimicrobials [6]. As it has been shown in our published study, two of the most frequent serotypes colonizing Cypriot children, specifically 6B and 19F, are vaccine serotypes and demonstrated a high percentage of resistance to both penicillin and erythromycin [13]. In Cyprus, coverage with the PCV7 vaccine at the time of the study was relatively low [12]. In addition, antibiotic consumption in Cyprus is one of the highest in Europe [30] and antimicrobial resistance of *S. pneumoniae* to the main classes of antimicrobials in Cyprus has been found to be relatively high. In this study, multi-variable analyses revealed recent antibiotic use as the most consistent independent risk factor associated with increased risk of carriage for drug resistant pneumococcal strains to both penicillin and erythromycin. A campaign targeting the prudent use of antibiotics by physicians and the population in general, in combination with a vaccination campaign to increase the coverage of children by the available pneumococcal conjugate vaccines, may be the most important interventions towards the reduction of resistance of *S. pneumoniae* to anti-microbials and the lowering of the burden of these infections in Cyprus.

Conclusions

Prudent use of antibiotics especially for upper respiratory tract infections in children as well as increased vaccination coverage by the pneumococcal conjugate vaccines could prove effective in reducing levels of colonization by non susceptible pneumococcal strains.

Abbreviations

CI: Confidence Intervals); CLSI: Clinical and Laboratory Standards Institute); EU: European Union); MIC: Minimum Inhibitory Concentration); OR: Odds Ratio); PCV7: Pneumococcus 7-valent conjugate vaccine)

Acknowledgements

We would like to express our gratitude to the health visitors at Arch. Makarios III Hospital and various primary care/immunization centers who supported the collection of nasopharyngeal specimens.

Funding

This research study was partly funded by the A. G. Leventis Foundation and the Radiomarathonios non Governmental non Profit organization in Cyprus. The funding bodies had no role in the design of the study, collection, analysis, and interpretation of data and had no role in the writing of the manuscript.

Authors' contributions

MGK and ESS conceived of the idea for the project and designed the study. KA worked in the collection of data by completing the questionnaires, processed the specimens by culturing, performing sensitivity testing and serotyping of the isolates and formed the electronic database. MGK, PI and CE collected the specimens and data for the questionnaires. MGK also processed specimens by culturing, by performing sensitivity testing and by putting data on the electronic database. MGK, DL and GL analysed the data by statistical methods and created the tables. MGK and ESS wrote the first draft of the manuscript. All authors contributed to the preparation of final manuscript. All authors read and approved of the final manuscript.

Competing interests

The authors declare that they have no competing interests.

Author details

[1]Department of Paediatrics, Archbishop Makarios III Hospital, Nicosia, Cyprus. [2]School of Medicine, University of Cyprus, Nicosia, Cyprus. [3]Cyprus Institute of Biomedical Sciences (CIBS), Nicosia, Cyprus. [4]The Hull IVF Unit, Hull, UK. [5]Department of Health Sciences, School of Sciences, European University Cyprus, Nicosia, Cyprus. [6]Private practice, Nicosia, Cyprus. [7]Harvard School of Public Health, Department of Environmental Health, Environmental and Occupational Medicine and Epidemiology (EOME), Boston, USA.

References

1. Musher DM. Infections caused by *Streptococcus pneumoniae*: clinical spectrum, pathogenesis, immunity, and treatment. Clin Infect Dis. 1992;14(4/Apr):801–7.
2. Givon-Lavi N, Fraser D, Porat N, Dagan R. Spread of *Streptococcus pneumoniae* and antibiotic-resistant *S. pneumoniae* from day-care center attendees to their younger siblings. J Infect Dis. 2002;186(11):1608–14.
3. Bogaert D, De Groot R, Hermans PWM. *Streptococcus pneumoniae* colonisation: the key to pneumococcal disease. Lancet Infect Dis. 2004;4(3/Mar):144–54.
4. Kellner JD, McGeer A, Cetron MS, Low DE, Butler JC, Matlow A, et al. The use of *Streptococcus pneumoniae* nasopharyngeal isolates from healthy children to predict features of invasive disease. Pediatr Infect Dis J. 1998;17(4):279–86.
5. Linares J, Ardanuy C, Pallares R, Fenoll A. Changes in antimicrobial resistance, serotypes and genotypes in *Streptococcus pneumoniae* over a 30-year period. Clin Microbiol Infect. 2010;16(5/May):402–10.
6. Kyaw MH, Lynfield R, Schaffner W. Effect of introduction of the pneumococcal conjugate vaccine on drug-resistant *Streptococcus pneumoniae*. N Engl J Med. 2006;354:1455–63.
7. Miller E, Andrews NJ, Waight PA, Slack MP, George RC. Herd immunity and serotype replacement 4 years after seven-valent pneumococcal conjugate vaccination in England and Wales: an observational cohort study. Lancet Infect Dis. 2011;11(10/Oct):760–8.
8. Huang SS, Finkelstein JA, Rifas-Shiman SL, Kleinman K, Platt R. Community-level predictors of pneumococcal carriage and resistance in young children. Am J Epidemiol. 2004;159(7):645–54.
9. Principi N, Marchisio P, Schito GC, Mannelli S. Risk factors for carriage of respiratory pathogens in the nasopharynx of healthy children. Ascanius project collaborative group. Pediatr Infect Dis J. 1999;18(6/Jun):517–23.
10. Katsarolis I, Poulakou G, Analitis A, Matthaiopoulou I, Roilides E, Antachopoulos C, et al. Risk factors for nasopharyngeal carriage of drug-resistant *Streptococcus pneumoniae*: data from a nation-wide surveillance study in Greece. BMC Infect Dis. 2009;9(Jul):120.
11. HY T, Lauderdale TL, Wang JT, Chen YS, Liu JW, Huang JH, Hu BH, Yang CJ, Lu DC, Chang SC. Updated antibiotic resistance and clinical spectrum of infections caused by *Streptococcus pneumoniae* in Taiwan: emphasis on risk factors for penicillin nonsusceptibilities. J Microbiol Immunol Infect. 2013;(Oct;46(5):345–51.
12. Vaccination Coverage in toddlers 17-24 months old, 2009. Unit for surveillance and control of communicable diseases, Medical and public health services. Cyprus: Ministry of Health.
13. Koliou MG, Andreou K, Lamnisos D, Lavranos G, Iakovides P, Economou C,

Soteriades ES. Serotypes and antimicrobial resistance of *S. pneumoniae* nasopharyngeal carriage in children from Cyprus: a country with relatively low coverage with the seven-valent pneumococcal conjugate vaccine. J Epidemiological Res. 2017;3(2):51–7.
14. Ruoff KL. Streptococcus. In: Murray PR, Baron EJ, Pfaller MA, Tenover FC, Yolken RH, editors. Manual of clinical microbiology. 6th ed. Washington, DC: Americal Society for Microbiology; 1995. p. 299–307.
15. Jacobs MR, Bajaksouzian S, Appelbaum PC, Bolmström A. Evaluation of the E-test for susceptibility testing of pneumococci. Diagn Microbiol Infect Dis. 1992;15(5):473–8.
16. Clinical and Laboratory Standards Institute. Performance Standards for Antimicrobial Susceptibility Testing. Pa, USA: Wayne; 2009. p. M100–S19.
17. Huang SS, Finkelstein JA, Lipsitch M. Modeling community- and individual-level effects of child-care center attendance on pneumococcal carriage. Clin Infect Dis. 2005;40(9/May):1215–22.
18. Jourdain S, Smeesters PR, Denis O, Dramaix M, Sputael V, Malaviolle X, et al. Differences in nasopharyngeal bacterial carriage in preschool children from different socio-economic origins. Clin Microbiol Infect. 2011;17(6/Jun):907–14.
19. Volonakis K, Souli M, Kapaskelis A, Baziaka F, Grammelis V, Ziakas PD, et al. Evolution of resistance patterns and identification of risk factors for *Streptococcus pneumoniae* colonisation in daycare Centre attendees in Athens, Greece. Int J Antimicrob Agents. 2006;28(4/Oct):297–301.
20. Chiu SS, Ho PL, Chow FK, Yuen KY, Lau YL. Nasopharyngeal carriage of antimicrobial-resistant *Streptococcus pneumoniae* among young children attending 79 kindergartens and day care centers in Hong Kong. Antimicrob Agents Chemother. 2001;45(10/Oct):2765–70.
21. Bergman M, Huikko S, Huovinen P, Paakkari P, Seppala H. Finnish Study Group for Antimicrobial Resistance (FiRe Network). Macrolide and azithromycin use are linked to increased macrolide resistance in *Streptococcus pneumoniae*. Antimicrob Agents Chemother. 2006;50(11/Nov):3646–50.
22. Riedel S, Beekmann SE, Heilmann KP, Richter SS, Garcia-De-Lomas J, Ferech M, et al. Antimicrobial use in Europe and antimicrobial resistance in *Streptococcus pneumoniae*. Eur J Clin Microbiol Infect Dis. 2007;26(7/Jul):485–90.
23. Van Eldere JJ, Mera RM, Miller LA, Poupard JA, Amrine-Madsen H. Risk factors for development of multiple-class resistance to Streptococcus pneumoniae strains in Belgium over a 10-year period: antimicrobial consumption, population density, and geographic location. Antimicrob Agents Chemother. 2007;51(10/Oct):3491–7.
24. Henderson-Begg SK, Livermore DM, Hall LM. Effect of subinhibitory concentrations of antibiotics on mutation frequency in Streptococcus pneumoniae. J Antimicrob Chemother. 2006;57(5):849–54.
25. Cerdá Zolezzi P, Laplana LM, Calvo CR, Cepero PG, Erazo MC, Gómez-Lus R. Molecular basis of resistance to macrolides and other antibiotics in commensal viridans group streptococci and Gemella spp. and transfer of resistance genes to Streptococcus pneumoniae. Antimicrob Agents Chemother. 2004;48(9):3462–7.
26. Melander E, Mölstad S, Persson K, Hansson HB, Söderström M, Ekdahl K. Previous antibiotic consumption and other risk factors for carriage of penicillin-resistant Streptococcus pneumoniae in children. Eur J Clin Microbiol Infect Dis. 1998;(12):834–8.
27. Klein JO. The epidemiology of pneumococcal disease in infants and children. Rev Infect Dis. 1981;3(2/Mar-Apr):246–53.
28. Scott JA, Hall AJ, Dagan R, Dixon JM, Eykyn SJ, Fenoll A, et al. Serogroup-specific epidemiology of Streptococcus pneumoniae: associations with age, sex, and geography in 7,000 episodes of invasive disease. Clin Infect Dis. 1996;(6):973–81.
29. Burman LA, Norrby R, Trollfors B. Invasive pneumococcal infections: incidence, predisposing factors, and prognosis. Rev Infect Dis. 1985;Mar-Apr7(2):133–142.
30. Adriaenssens N, Coenen S, Versporten A, Muller A, Minalu G, Faes C, et al. ESAC Project Group. European Surveillance of Antimicrobial Consumption (ESAC): outpatient antibiotic use in Europe (1997–2009). J Antimicrob Chemother. 2011;(Suppl):6:vi3–12.

14

Are one-stop centres an appropriate model to deliver services to sexually abused children in urban Malawi?

Yabwile Mulambia[1*], Aaron J. Miller[2], Geraldine MacDonald[3] and Neil Kennedy[1,4]

Abstract

Background: The Republic of Malawi is creating a country-wide system of 28 One-Stop Centres (known as 'Chikwanekwanes' - 'everything under one roof') to provide medical, legal and psychosocial services for survivors of child maltreatment and adult intimate partner violence. No formal evaluation of the utility of such services has ever been undertaken. This study focused on the experiences of the families served at the country's first Chikwanekwane in the large, urban city of Blantyre.

Methods: One hundred seven families were surveyed in their home three months after their initial evaluation for sexual abuse at the Blantyre One Stop Centre, and 25 families received a longer interview. The survey was designed to inquire what types of initial evaluation and follow-up services the children received from the medical, legal and social welfare services.

Results: All 107 received an initial medical exam and HIV testing, and 83% received a follow-up HIV test by 3 months; 80.2% were seen by a social welfare worker on the initial visit, and 29% had a home visit by 3 months; 84% were seen by a therapist at the initial visit, and 12% returned for further treatment; 95.3% had an initial police report and 27.1% ended in a criminal conviction for child sexual abuse. Most of the families were satisfied with the service they received, but a quarter of the families were not satisfied with the law enforcement response, and 2% were not happy with the medical assessment. Conclusions: Although a perception of corruption or negligence by police may discourage use of service, we believe that the One-Stop model is an appropriate means to deliver high quality care to survivors of abuse in Malawi.

Keywords: Child sexual abuse, Treatment, Program development, Law enforcement, Prosecution

Background

With ratification of the new United Nations Sustainable Development Goals, greater attention is being focused on how the medical, legal and social welfare systems should respond in order to ensure the health and safety of these children. Child sexual abuse is increasingly recognized as a public health problem in Sub-Saharan Africa. Of 4412 school children interviewed in a 2005 study in Malawi, 23.8% of children said they had been forced to have sex against their will, 14% reported having been touched on their genitals or breasts against their will, and 3.9% of children over 13 years reported having been forced to engage in some form of oral sex [1]. The Violence Against Children and Young Women Survey in Malawi in 2013 found that 21.8% of girls and 14.8% of boys age 18–24 had experienced sexual abuse prior to age 18; and 37.7% of girls and 9.8% boys age 18–24 said that their first sexual experience before age 18 was unwanted [2]. Services for these children are lacking. Two thirds of sexual assault survivors reported the incident to an authority figure, but only 10% received any professional assistance.

Prior to 2010 in Malawi, the medical, legal and social welfare agencies did not work together to assist survivors of child sexual abuse. Parents would bring their child to police who had not been trained in forensic interviewing or the need for appropriate medical examination. Some of the families were then referred to the

* Correspondence: yabwile@gmail.com
[1]The College of Medicine, University of Malawi, Chichiri, Blantyre 3, Malawi
Full list of author information is available at the end of the article

hospital for an examination, where only 24% of the doctors could correctly interpret genital findings [3]. In most hospitals they had to wait in separate lines for treatment, HIV testing and emergency contraception. Then they were told to go back to the police with their completed form. The poor linkages between departments led to poor case management and children being lost to follow-up [4–7].

Several countries have developed one-stop centres where medical, legal, social welfare, and counseling services take place under one roof [6, 8]. In the United States, these *child advocacy centers* (CACs) have been shown in prospective, controlled studies to increase police involvement in social welfare cases, increase the number of agencies present during interviews, increase the number of children receiving forensic medical exams, increase the non-offending parent satisfaction with the investigation process, and decrease the percentage of children who are very scared and uncomfortable during the interviewing [6, 7, 9].

In Blantyre, Malawi, the Queen Elizabeth Central Hospital (QECH) is home to the country's first one-stop centre, referred to as a Chikwanekwane ("everything under one roof"). Building on the work of a multidisciplinary team which has been operating in Blantyre since 2010 [5, 10], the centre was established by funding from DFID with the support of the Ministries of Health, Social Welfare and UNICEF [11]. The team comprises paediatricians, nurses, social workers, police victim support officers and volunteer counselors working together to provide the best care possible for child survivors. Currently, police Victim Support Units (VSU) are the main referral agents, though self-referral is promoted and welcomed. VSU police officers are trained in the provision of counseling and support to victims. At QECH, experienced doctors examine the child and document findings in a medico-legal report. An HIV test and post-exposure prophylaxis is offered, along with follow-up tests at 3 and 6 months after the incident. Sexually transmitted infection management and emergency contraceptives are given when indicated. Social workers and counselors located within QECH offer safety and psychological support respectively. Counselors have longer contact with the victim than any other provider of the service, and arrange to see families weekly as required. Police and social welfare workers then continue their investigation and visit the victim at home to assess the safety of the child.

The anecdotal experience of staff involved in this centre was that it improved client satisfaction and outcomes. As a result, the government of Malawi has rolled out the 'Chikwanewane' model to establish 4 other large and 23 smaller centres throughout the country. However, no formal evaluation of the impact of these centres has ever been published from Malawi or, to our knowledge, from Sub-Saharan Africa.

The purpose of this study was two-fold: to explore the experiences of children and families who were provided services at the QECH One-Stop Centre, and to assess the proportion of these families that received medical, legal, and social welfare services according to national guidelines.

Methods

The participants were families who had received treatment at the Blantyre One-Stop Centre at Queen Elizabeth Central Hospital. QECH is the largest government hospital in Blantyre offering free care to children from the city and Southern Malawi. All children evaluated for sexual abuse during the study period – August 1, 2012 to June 30, 2013 – were eligible. The children's guardian was the person enrolled in the study and interviewed about their experiences.

The study was introduced to guardians on the day of presentation to the hospital. Guardians were given a brief introductory leaflet explaining the research and contacted 3 months later to determine if they were still willing to be involved in the study. Written consent was obtained. The scope of the questions was designed to assess whether the families had received the medical, legal and social welfare services as required in the Malawi *National Guidelines for Provision of Services for Physical and Sexual Violence* [12]. All interviews took place in the family home 3 months after their evaluation at the One-Stop Centre. All the families received a questionnaire administered in person during this visit (see Additional file 1: Appendix 1). The questionnaire was administered verbally in Chichewa to all the participants; from this cohort, semi-structured interviews were then conducted with 25 guardians who were representative of the study population in terms of age of the victim and gender. With the permission of the respondent, a voice recorder was used to collect the information. The interviews were transcribed. After familiarization of the data in the preliminary analysis, a thematic framework was developed and themes coded. The researchers were blinded to the child protection services outcomes at the time of the visit. The child's guardian was interviewed in order to prevent secondary victimization of the survivor.

Inclusion criteria: Participation in this study was offered to the guardians of all children age 0–14 years who, in the opinion of the medical staff, had been sexually abused and who gave consent to be in the study. From this cohort of participants, a representative subset of 25 guardians were chosen to also participate in the semi-structured interview. Exclusion criteria: cases in which the guardian did not give consent, or in which the final diagnosis was not sexual abuse.

Results

In total, 262 patients were evaluated at the Queen Elizabeth Central Hospital One-Stop Centre between August 1, 2012 and June 30, 2013 (see Fig. 1). Ten cases of physical assault were removed from analysis. An additional 24 cases were removed as the allegation of abuse was not substantiated, and the presentation was unrelated to child sexual abuse. Of the remaining 228 child abuse survivors and their guardians, 59 were lost to follow up and 62 did not give consent, leaving 107 participants who completed the questionnaire. Semi- structured interviews (SSI) were held with 25 guardians in their homes and with 10 service providers representing all the agencies involved in the child protection service.

Three of the questionnaires were conducted either at the centre or another site other than home because the perpetrator or relatives of the perpetrator where at home and guardians felt the environment was unsafe. Ninety-nine per cent of the children were girls, average age 9 years (see Table 1).

How was the abuse discovered, and why did people come?

Most of the children in this sample (57.9%) disclosed the sexual abuse on their own ("spontaneously") without being prompted or having the abuse witnessed by a concerned 3rd party (see Table 2).

Most of the semi-structured interview participants (19 of 25) sought care for their children due to the fear of HIV infection (see Table 3). Other reasons included the desire to "verify" if the child was raped (5 of 25), the desire for justice (3 of 25), for counseling (2 of 25), pregnancy (1 of 25), and just because they were referred by police (1 of 25). Most participants expected an HIV test, physical examination, HIV Post-Exposure Prophylaxis (PEP) and justice. Very few mentioned counseling services and none mentioned social services as a reason for seeking help.

Performance according to the Malawi National Guidelines for provision of services to survivors of violence

Seventy-two of 107 survivors (67.3%) arrived within 72 h in time to start HIV Post-Exposure Prophylaxis (PEP). All received appropriate medical services. 80% had a follow up visit for a second HIV test at 3 months (see Table 4). The requirement for Social Welfare is for an initial assessment at the Chikwanekwane, followed by a home visit within 3 months. The initial assessment by Social Welfare was performed in 80% of the cases during the initial visit at the One-Stop Centre, but only 29% of

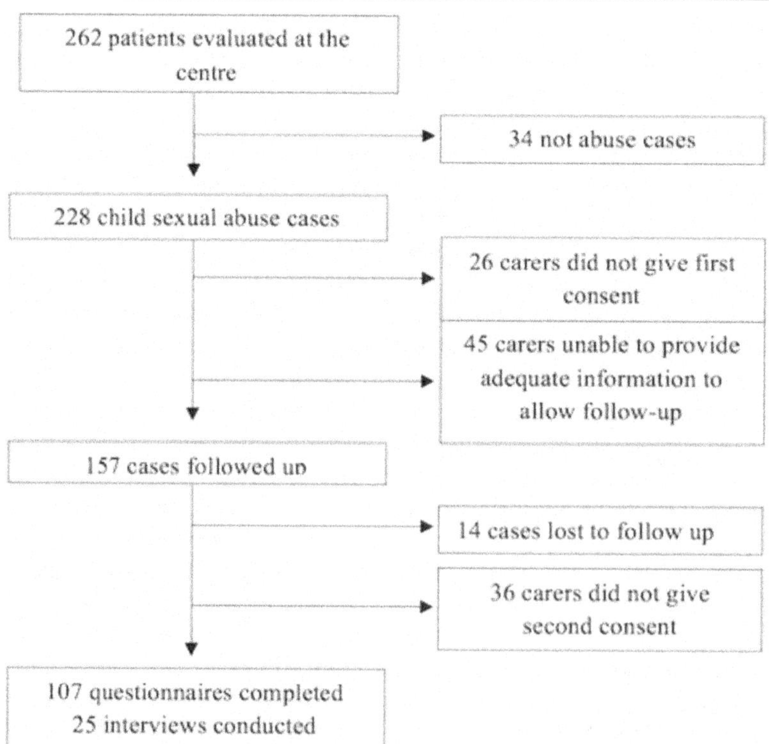

Fig. 1 Consort diagram of Study Participants

Table 1 Participant Demographic Data, $n = 107$

Children Characteristics	Frequency
Female	99.1%
Mean Age (SD)	9.4(3.9)
Guardian Characteristics	Frequency
Female	75.7%
Mean Age (SD)	36.1(9.8)
Average Household size	5.8
Level of Education	
No Education	8.4%
Primary School	43.9%
Secondary School	37.4%
Tertiary	10.3%

the children had a home visit due to a lack of transport. Eighty-four percent of children received psychological support during the initial visit, In 95% of cases there was some form of police investigation with 27.1% of the cases resulting in criminal conviction (Fig. 2).

Overall, 18% of the child abuse cases received all the services required according to the national guidelines.

Of the 107 families, 79 (73.8%) were satisfied with the services provided, and 28 (26.2%) were not satisfied (see Table 5 and Table 6). The commonest reason was dissatisfaction with police with concerns regarding perceived corruption and negligence.

No statistically significant associations were found between client satisfaction levels, and receipt of services (health, social welfare, police or counseling) or outcomes of the case (case referred to court or conviction of the perpetrator) (Table 7).

Impact of child sexual abuse on the child and family

The psychological impact of child sexual abuse was evident to guardians with older children. The semi-structured interview participants expressed feelings of frustration, fear and disbelief (never imagined it would happen to their child). Furthermore, the problem of stigma came up with participants concerned about community perspectives of child sexual abuse, which was often misinterpreted as consensual sex especially if the child involved is older (see Table 8).

Table 2 Pattern of Disclosure

Pattern of disclosure	Frequency	Percentage
Spontaneous	62	57.9
Witnessed assault	25	23.4
Prompted	12	11.2
Informed by witness	8	7.5

Table 3 Sample quotes from semi-structured interview participants on why they sought services at the one-stop centre

Risk of HIV infection: "What we really wanted to find out was the HIV status of the child since there is HIV/AIDS because this is what we fear the child has contracted."
Justice: "Having justice done would have been a lesson to other people."
Psychological support: "This was affecting her, she was depressed and not eating. After school she went straight to her bedroom and wanted to be alone… I found it abnormal."
Fear of pregnancy: "First of all, I feared she could be pregnant; she could fall unexpectedly. Secondly, there are sexually transmitted diseases..."

The child is perceived as immoral and discriminated in the community. Disruption of family relationships was reported when the perpetrator was a family member with some reporting mothers neglecting their child's welfare to save their marriage when the perpetrator was the breadwinner.

Discussion

This is the first study from within the region or a low-income setting to evaluate and report the services provided by a one-stop centre for survivors of child sexual abuse. Building the one-stop centre at Queen Elizabeth Central Hospital in 2012 was associated with nearly tripling the number of children receiving services of sexual abuse each year: from 121 to 168 per year (2006–2011) to 356 in 2014. The majority of clients received the services they needed at presentation, but follow-up by social welfare was hindered by lack of funding. Overall, we found very high levels of client satisfaction, particularly with medical and social welfare services. Despite over half of cases resulting in a court case, and 27% in a successful prosecution, the commonest reason for reporting dissatisfaction was concerns regarding the performance of police. Satisfaction levels were not significantly associated with receipt of services or the outcome of the case. This may be a reflection of the sample size, or because receipt of one service compensated for the lack of receipt of another.

We do not know who referred each child to the one-stop centre, but the fact that 67% of the children arrived

Table 4 Performance by Each Agency, $n = 107$

Adequately handled cases (Indicator)	At Presentation %	By 3 months (%)
Health Examination, HIV 0-3 months)	100	82
Social (Initial assessment, home visit by 3 months	80.2	29
Psychological (Support offered to all clients)	84	12 more than one visit
Justice (Investigation,referral to court)	95.3	53.8

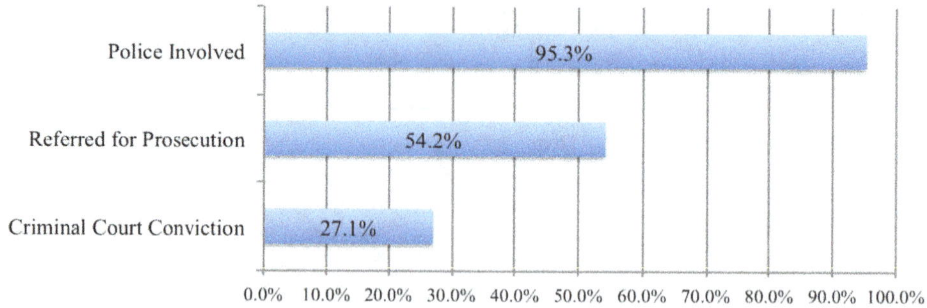

Fig. 2 Law Enforcement Outcomes, *n* = 107

in time for HIV post-exposure prophylaxis is encouraging and worth further study. Fear of HIV was the strongest motivator for seeking services (76%), and the hospital had the highest follow-up rate (82%) of all the agencies. In a country with a high HIV prevalence of 10. 0% [13], the one-stop centre system could be an effective point for HIV prevention, which not only saves the survivor from a life of uncertainty and stigma, but also saves the healthcare system the future costs of HIV care.

A high proportion of our clients in this sample were female, reflecting the profile of service users at the time of the study. In a country where homosexuality remains illegal, male survivors of sexual violence face significant stigma that limits disclosure.

We found a relatively high prosecution rate (27.1%). Past research in industrialized countries has also demonstrated increased prosecution rates and quicker case resolution in districts where medical, legal and social welfare are co-located together [14, 15]. Our study was not designed to assess how the 58 cases referred for prosecution were different than the 49 cases which were not referred for prosecution; nor did we attempt to assess what case characteristics were associated with conviction versus acquittal. The 3-month time frame was deemed adequate to assess whether criminal court cases would reach conclusion based on discussions with local magistrates, prosecutors and police who stated that most cases are resolved – either dropped or move forward - within a few weeks. Very few respondents have attorneys to represent them in court, and almost all cases are closed in less than 3 months.

We acknowledge several limitations to our study: of the 228 children diagnosed with sexual abuse, 60 of the families (26.3%) did not agree to be part of the study, which may represent dissatisfaction with services; we did not interview the child (which may have yielded different answers); and self-report surveys, in general, provide only the participants' perceptions – it is unknown if there were 9 actual cases of police corruption or whether there was a valid reason the case did not move forward which was not communicated to the family. Furthermore, our study was limited to an urban area and the findings can not necessarily be generalized to rural settings.

Our study also had several strengths. It is a relatively large series of client responses from this type of service and provides valuable insight into the experience of families involved. In addition, to a large extent the results obtained from both the qualitative and quantitative

Table 5 Evaluation of Service Satisfaction

26.2% (28/107) were not satisfied with the service	Total
Police	
Perceived corruption (9)	21
Perceived Negligence (3)	
Court: Prison sentence too short	4
Medical Services	
HIV post-exposure prophylaxis not provided (1)	2
Medical exam took too long (1)	
Counseling: Wanted more sessions	1

Table 6 Sample quotes from semi-structured interview participants on their dissatisfaction with one-stop centre services

Perceived inaction of police: "Then they (the police) said if you can manage to catch the perpetrator, bring him here but if you don't have a means of doing that we will see what we can do."
Lack of professionalism and capacity: "The first hearing in court, the prosecutor did not come. Other police officers said he was on leave then. We were told to come on another date. The next scheduled court hearing, he didn't show up again. They said he was sorting out his family issues."
HIV post-exposure prophylaxis not given: "Nothing! We were not given anything…I really hope she continues to remain HIV negative"
Family member perpetrator: The reason the case was not taken to court was that, I am the last born in our family and my elder sister's son is the one who did this...There is no peace in our family now.

Table 7 Caregiver satisfaction according to receipt of services provided ($n = 107$)

		Expressed satisfaction with the overall service	Expressed dissatisfaction with the overall service	Fishers exact test
Agency involvement at presentation	Health – got HIV test and PEP at presentation	52	17	0.81
	Health – did not get HIV test *OR* got HIV test but not PEP at presentation	25	9	
	Justice-got service	30	8	0.64
	Justice-did not get service	49	18	
	Social –got service	64	20	0.77
	Social –did not get service	15	6	
	Psychological –got service	66	22	1.00
	Psychological-did not get service	13	4	
Case outcomes	Perpetrator convicted	25	4	0.13
	Perpetrator not convicted	54	22	
	Case referred to court	43	14	1.00
	Case not referred to court	36	12	

components concurred with each other, suggesting that they were reliable.

With our new understanding of the numerous deleterious short and long-term effects of abuse, and how it leads to a high disease burden on society [16], it was essential that 6 of the new subgoals in the UN Sustainable Development Goals address violence against children and intimate partner violence. Bringing together medical, legal and social welfare agencies - and continuing to develop their capacity - will be key components to ensuring that we interrupt the cycle of violence as early as possible and that we work toward effective solutions for primary and secondary prevention of violence so that every child can grow up with safe, stable, nurturing relationships. We believe that the one-stop centre approach offers a useful model for providing such services in a low-income urban setting.

Table 8 Sample quotes from semi-structured interview participants on the effects of child sexual abuse on the family

Emotional and psychological impact
"After the incident, she now wets and soils the bed…where she sleeps is a sorry sight." Guardian (*mum shedding tears*)
Stigma
"The challenges that she is mainly facing is that she is being discriminated. For example, she will go to her friend's place and her friend's mother says to her you should not be chatting with my child because you have immoral behaviour" Guardian
Effects on family relationships
"She was being abused by her step father…she told her mum first but she did nothing. She accused her of trying to break her marriage…. She (victim) last saw her mother in court. Until today, her mother has no interest in the welfare of the child." Guardian

Conclusion

One-stop centres where health practitioners, police and social workers coordinate closely, was an effective strategy to improve the health, safety and well-being of survivors of sexual and physical violence in an urban setting in Malawi. Longer term evaluation studies which listen to the voice of survivors in this and other urban African settings are needed. Effective service models for rural survivors of violence are required.

Abbreviations

HIV: Human Immunodeficiency Virus; OSC: One Stop Centre; PEP: Post-Exposure Prophylaxis; QECH: Queen Elizabeth Central Hospital; SD: Standard Deviation; SSI: Semi-structured Interview; UN: United Nations; UNICEF: United Nations Children's Emergency Fund; VSU: Victim Support Unit

Acknowledgements

We would like to thank the Association of Physicians in Britain and Ireland with providing a portion of the funding to YM needed to conduct this study, though they were not involved in any portion of conceiving, designing, conducting, analyzing, writing this paper or deciding to publish.

Funding

This study was partially funded by the Association of Physicians in Britain and Ireland. The funder was not involved in the design of the study, data collection, analysis or interpretation of data.

Authors' contributions

YM conceived this study, wrote the survey, enrolled participants, interviewed them in their homes, and helped write the manuscript. AM provided the initial medical training for the Blantyre One Stop Centre, helped analyze the data, and wrote much of the manuscript. GM helped design the study and review the data, and NK worked closely with YM from the beginning in designing the study, analyzing the data, and writing the manuscript. All four authors read and approved the final manuscript.

Ethics approval and consent to participate

Ethical approval to consent and participate was obtained from the College of Medicine Research Ethics Committee, University of Malawi. The study was introduced to the child's guardian on the day of presentation to the hospital. Guardians were given a brief introductory leaflet explaining the research and contacted 3 months later to determine if they were still willing to be involved in the study. Written consent was obtained. All interviews took place in the family home 3 months after their evaluation at the One-Stop Centre. With the permission of the respondent, a voice recorder was used to collect the information. The interviews were transcribed. The researchers were blinded to the child protection services outcomes at the time of the visit. The child's guardian was interviewed in order to prevent secondary victimization of the survivor.

Research on this topic risks causing distress to guardians as they recall traumatic events. This was mitigated by informing all potential participants early in the process and providing several opportunities for them to withdraw from the study. The consent form included information about the purpose of the study and assured confidentiality. It also indicated that if the child was still at risk of abuse, the information will have to be shared with law enforcers for the safety of the child. Written consent was sought from the guardian to enroll in the study. We kept the information obtained confidential and anonymous.

The questionnaire was not conducted during the initial visit in order to prevent any families from feeling pressure to give a positive evaluation if they thought this necessary to receive further services. During data collection, participants who had stopped attending for counseling, but who still required psychological support were re-referred to QECH for counselors to provide assistance accordingly. When information was revealed which indicated the child was still at risk, appropriate measures were taken to protect the child and reveal information appropriately especially to the family and involved social worker.

All data were treated as confidential and coded, locked in a cabinet. Electronic data were password protected. Following transcription, digital recordings of the interviews were stored as password protected audio files.

Competing interests

Aaron Miller worked as a paid consultant for UNICEF Malawi 2014–2016 to develop trainings for the One Stop Centres. Neither UNICEF nor any of the authors have any competing interests, nor do any of them earn any money from the operation of Malawi's One Stop Centres.

Author details

[1]The College of Medicine, University of Malawi, Chichiri, Blantyre 3, Malawi. [2]Building Regional Alliances to Nurture Child Health, 2 Gold St, New York, NY 10038, USA. [3]Institute of Child Care Research, Queen's University, University Rd, Belfast BT7 1NN, UK. [4]Centre for Medical Education, Queens's University Belfast, University Rd, Belfast BT7 1NN, UK.

References

1. Burton P. Suffering at school: the results of the Malawi gender-based violence in schools survey. Pretoria: Institute for Security Studies; 2005.
2. Violence against children and young women in Malawi. Findings from a national survey. Ministry of Gender. Lilongwe: Children, Disability and Social Welfare; 2014.
3. Miller A, Toombs K. Educating physicians internationally in the diagnosis of child sexual abuse: Evaluation of a brief educational intervention in Malawi. J Child Sex Abus: Research, Treatment, & Program Innovations for Victims, Survivors, & Offenders. 2009;23(3):247–55. https://doi.org/10.1080/10538712.2014.888120
4. Richter L, Dawes A, Higson-smith C. Sexual abuse of young children in Southern Africa. Cape Town: HRSC press; 2005.
5. Chesshyre ELD, Molyneux EM. Presentation of child sexual abuse cases to queen Elizabeth central hospital following the establishment of an HIV post-exposure prophylaxis program. Malawi Med J. 2009;2:54–8. 2035004
6. Jones LM, Cross TP, Walsh WA, Simone M. Do Children's advocacy centers improve families' experiences of child sexual abuse investigations? Child Abuse Negl. 2007;31(10):1069–85. https://doi.org/10.1016/j.chiabu.2007.07.003.
7. Walsh WA, Cross TP, Jones LM, Simone M, Kolko DJ. Which sexual abuse victims receive a forensic medical examination? The impact of Children's Advocacy Centers. Child Abuse & Neglect. 2007;31(10):1053–68. https://doi.org/10.1016/j.chiabu.2007.04.006.
8. Allnock D, et al. Sexual abuse and therapeutic services for children and young people: the gap between provision and need. London: NSPCC; 2009. Available at: https://www.nspcc.org.uk/globalassets/documents/research-reports/sexual-abuse-therapeutic-services-children-young-people-summary.pdf.
9. Cross TP, Jones LM, Walsh WA, Simone M, Kolko D. Child forensic interviewing in Children's advocacy centers: empirical data on a practice model. Child Abuse Negl. 2007;31(10):1031–52. https://doi.org/10.1016/j.chiabu.2007.04.007.
10. Mtibo C, Kennedy N, Umar E. Explanations for child sexual abuse given by convicted offenders in Malawi: no evidence for "HIV cleansing". Child Abuse Negl. 2011 Feb;35(2):142–6. https://doi.org/10.1016/j.chiabu.2010.10.001.
11. Molyneux EM, Kennedy N, Dano A, Mulambia Y. Sexual abuse of children in low-income settings: time for action. Paediatrics and International Child Health. 2013;33(4):239–46. https://doi.org/10.1179/2046905513Y.0000000087.
12. National Guidelines for Provision of Services for Physical and Sexual Violence. Malawi ministries of health, Gender. Lilongwe: Police and Judiciary; 2015.
13. UNAIDS. http://www.unaids.org/en/regionscountries/countries/malawi. Accessed on 25 Nov 2015.
14. Miller A, Rubin D. The contribution of children's advocacy centers to criminal prosecutions of child sexual abuse. Child Abuse & Neglect: The International Journal. 2009;33(1):12–8. https://doi.org/10.1016/j.chiabu.2008.07.002.
15. Walsh WA, Lippert T, Cross TP, Maurice DM, Davison KS. How long to prosecute child sexual abuse for a community using a children's advocacy center and two comparison communities? Child Maltreatment. 2008;13(1): 3–13. https://doi.org/10.1177/1077559507307839.
16. Reza A, et al. Sexual violence and its health consequences for female children in Swaziland: a cluster survey study. Lancet. 2009;373:1966–72. https://doi.org/10.1016/S01406736(09)60247-6.

Leisure time physical activity in 9- to 11-year-old children born moderately preterm

M. Nordvall-Lassen[1*], H. K. Hegaard[1,2,3,4], C. Obel[5], M. S. Lindhard[6], M. Hedegaard[3] and T. B. Henriksen[6]

Abstract

Background: Physical activity is one of the best documented activities with impacts on health in children and adults. Children born preterm show reduced physical and psychosocial function compared to children born at term. This may influence their level of physical activity. Reports on moderately preterm children's physical activities during childhood are limited. Thus, the aim of this study was to compare the leisure time physical activity at age 9-11 years of moderately preterm children with that of children born at term.

Methods: Data from 4941 mother-child pairs from the Aarhus Birth Cohort (1989-91) were used. The cohort gathered clinical information, including gestational age at delivery. Information about parental socio-demographic and lifestyle factors was obtained from questionnaires completed during the second trimester of pregnancy. Information about children's physical activities was reported in a 9- to 11-year follow-up questionnaire completed by parents detailing how many times per week their child participated in sports activities outside of school, hours spent per week playing outside, and hours per week engaged in sedentary activities. Data were analysed using multiple logistic regression with the lowest activity group as a reference group.

Results: A total of 158 children (3.2%) were born moderately preterm, i.e., between 32 and 36 completed weeks. Children born moderately preterm participated in sports activities as often as their peers born at term; they also participated in frequent sports activities (≥ 4 times per week) as often as their peers. There were no differences in hours per week spent playing outside or in sedentary activities between the two groups.

Conclusions: Nine- to 11-year-old moderately preterm children participated in sports activities outside school to a similar extent as their peers and engaged in outdoor activities and sedentary activities for the same duration of time per week as their peers born at term.

Keywords: Preterm birth, Leisure time physical activity, Moderately preterm, School age children

Background

Preterm delivery, defined as birth before 37 weeks of gestation [1], is strongly associated with neonatal morbidity and mortality [2] and with long-term sequelae [3–6]. Due to advances in neonatal intensive care, the survival of preterm children has increased considerably [7–10]. Preterm children are predisposed to difficulties with cognitive, behavioural, social, psychological, and motor functions [7, 11–16]; even moderately preterm (32-36 weeks) children are at an increased risk for developmental delay, neurologic impairments and learning problems [17, 18], which may contribute to difficulties participating in physical activities. Many studies have focused on these functional parameters, but little is known about normal everyday life functions, such as physical activity levels. Studies on adults with a birth weight of less than 1500 g have shown that they engage less frequently in leisure time physical activity [19, 20].

However, few studies have focused on physical activity in children born moderately preterm, even though this group makes up 80% of all premature births [17]. Physical inactivity is a risk factor for obesity, cardiovascular

* Correspondence: Nordvall_maria@hotmail.com
[1]The Research Unit of Women's and Children's Health, section 7821, The Juliane Marie Centre, Copenhagen University Hospital, Rigshospitalet, Blegdamsvej 9, DK-2100 Copenhagen, Denmark
Full list of author information is available at the end of the article

disease, type-2 diabetes, metabolic syndrome, and several other diseases [21, 22]. Adults born preterm have higher levels of risk factors for these diseases, such as high blood pressure [23], impaired glucose regulation [24, 25] and lower bone mineral density [26]. Cardiovascular disease risk factors have been reported to be reduced by regular physical activity, particularly in subjects with a low birth weight [27].

Research has shown that there is a life-trajectory of physical activity that begins early in life [28]. It is therefore important to investigate the level of physical activity in school-aged children who were born preterm without evident morbidity and who attend the same schools as children born at term. Do these children require special intervention to attain an adequate level of physical activity? Physical activity is quite possibly one of the best documented healthy activities for children [29]. The Danish National Board of Health has recommended a daily minimum of 60 min of moderate to high intensity physical activity and high intensity physical activity for a minimum 30 min at least three times a week for children [29].

Accordingly, we compared the leisure time physical activity of 9- to 11-year-old former moderately preterm children with their peers born at term using a birth cohort with a decade of follow-up. Moderately preterm delivery is defined as children born between 32 and 36 completed gestational weeks.

Methods

We used data from the Aarhus Birth Cohort. The cohort was established at the Department of Obstetrics at Aarhus University Hospital in August 1991 [30] The obstetrics department was the only maternity unit in the community of Aarhus and served a well-defined geographic area with a population of approximately 250,000 inhabitants. Antenatal care is free of charge in Denmark, and almost all (> 97%) women participated in the programme.

Briefly, all women attending routine antenatal care at Aarhus University Hospital in the period beginning in August 1989 and ending in September 1991 were invited to participate in the study. At enrolment, women at approximately 16 weeks' gestation were asked to complete a clinical questionnaire providing information about their medical and obstetrics histories, as well as information about their ages, heights, pre-pregnancy weights, levels of alcohol consumption, and smoking habits, as well as a second questionnaire (the research questionnaire) about socio-demographic characteristics and leisure time physical activities [31] The clinical questionnaire provided information included in each pregnant woman's obstetrical records. Following delivery, the attending midwife completed a structured birth registration form with information about the course of delivery and the condition of the newborn.

The present follow-up study is based on children from the cohort who were born between January 1990 and June 1992. During this period, 8643 women completed the clinical questionnaire, and 6782 women completed both questionnaires. Women who experienced foetal death ($n = 2$), delivered twins and triplets ($n = 165$) and delivered singletons without a valid gestational age ($n = 15$) were excluded, resulting in a study population of 6600 women.

In 2001, (January – December), the parents of these children were identified using the civil registration system [32], and they were invited to complete a parent-administered questionnaire concerning their child's behaviour, physical activity, health, and development. A total of 5147 questionnaires were returned. From this population we excluded children whose parents did not provide information on sports activities per week ($n = 78$). Children with significant physical handicaps, chromosome abnormalities, autism, Asperger syndrome, cerebral palsy, mental retardation, severe chronic diseases, blindness, severe hearing loss and deafness, and severe heart defects were also excluded ($n = 113$) as well as children born before 32 completed gestational weeks ($n = 15$), leaving 4941 singleton infants born at term and moderately preterm, available for analysis.

Exposure

Moderately preterm delivery was defined as delivery between 32 and 36 completed gestational weeks. Gestational age was estimated by ultrasound measurements before 21 completed weeks of gestation in 86% of cases. In 8% of cases, gestational age was estimated using the date of a valid last menstrual period (LMP), corrected to a cycle length of 28 days: in 6%, gestational age was estimated by the midwife using a less reliable LMP (primarily an LMP without information regarding specific cycle length) or ultrasound measurements taken after 21 weeks [33].

Outcome

Information regarding each child's leisure time physical activity level was obtained from the parent-administered questionnaires completed when each child was between 9 and 11 years of age. They were asked how many times per week their child participated in sports activities outside of school, how many hours a week after school their child was active outdoors, how many hours a week their child watched television, how many hours a week (in addition to schoolwork) their child read, including comic books, and how many hours a week (in addition to schoolwork) the child used a computer or played videogames. We created a category for children with very low physical activity levels whose parents reported that they did not participate in sports activities outside of school and engaged in fewer than four weekly hours of outdoor activities. The following characteristics were categorized as described in Table 1: whether the child's parents cohabited; maternal pre-existing chronic maternal disease; maternal smoking before, during and after pregnancy; partner's smoking during and after pregnancy; maternal alcohol consumption during pregnancy; maternal leisure time physical activity during pregnancy; and parental education level.

The children's heights and weights were described by a mean and SD (standard deviation). The parents were asked if a medical doctor had ever diagnosed their child with asthma.

Statistical analysis

An initial Chi-square test for independence within contingency tables was used. Testing for trends and t-tests were carried out where appropriate. In a multivariate logistic regression analysis, the relation between preterm birth (gestational age, 32-36 completed weeks gestation vs. ≥ 37 weeks gestation) and physical activity levels in children aged 9 to 11 was tested. A priori, we chose to include the following covariates in the analysis: maternal leisure time physical activity during pregnancy, maternal education level, paternal education level, maternal and paternal smoking habits after delivery, and the sex of the child, given previously demonstrated associations between preterm delivery as well as the child physical activity level [19, 34]. We repeated all analyses in a sub analysis comparing the children born 32-36 weeks to those born 39-40 weeks. Furthermore, we repeated all analyses stratified by sex and after excluding children with asthma. We presented adjusted odds ratios with 95% confidence intervals (CIs). Statistical significance was defined as a two-sided *P* value less than 0.05. We used SPSS 20.0 software (IBM) for all statistical analyses.

Results

Table 1 shows the proportion of children born moderately preterm and at term in relation to prenatal, parental and offspring characteristics at birth and 9 to 11 years later. In total, 158 infants (3.2%) were born moderately preterm. Moderately preterm birth was associated with pre-existing maternal chronic diseases; maternal smoking before, during and after pregnancy; paternal smoking during pregnancy; less maternal leisure time physical activity during pregnancy and fewer years of parental education. Furthermore, children born moderately preterm had the same height and weight by ages 9 to 11 as children born at term. Children born moderately preterm had a higher frequency of asthma, as 19% of moderately preterm children had asthma compared to 8.3% of children born at term (Table 1).

In our study population, 82% ($n = 4069$) of children participated in sports outside of school on a weekly basis. Only 28% of school-aged children in our population participated in sports activities 3 times per week or more, as recommended by the national health guidelines for children [29]. More than half of the children reported participating in outdoor activities for more than 7 h a week. Eleven percent of the children reported participating in sedentary activities for 7 h or less per week. Less than half of the children reported participating in 15 h or more of sedentary activities per week (Table 2). No differences were observed between children born moderately preterm and children born at term.

The adjusted multivariate analysis showed that children born moderately preterm participated in sports activities as often as their peers born at term (OR = 1.03, 95% CI (0.67-1.58)) and participated in sports activities 3 times per week and ≥ 4 times per week as often as their peers born at term (Table 2). Similarly, children born moderately preterm played outside as often as their peers born at term. Furthermore, children born moderately preterm had the same level of very low physical activity as their peers born at term (OR = 1.36, 95% (0.59-3.2)). Multiple logistic regression analyses showed that infants born moderately preterm participated in sedentary activity (watching television, using a computer, playing videogames, reading books and comics) as often as their peers born at term (Table 2). Sub-analyses showed similar results when we compared the children born moderately preterm with the children born in weeks 39-40.Additional sub-analyses showed that results were similar for boys and girls and that the results remained essentially unchanged after excluding 429 children diagnosed with asthma (data not shown).

Discussion

Due to the well-established higher risk of physical disadvantages, one may expect that children born preterm would be less leisure time physically active than their peers born at term. However, our data showed no differences in the activity levels of term and moderately preterm children aged 9 to 11 years. Parents of children born moderately preterm reported that their children were involved in leisure time sports activities to the same extent as children born at term. The same proportion of children in both groups followed the recommendation of high intensive physical activity by the Danish National Board of Health [29].

Additionally, there were no differences between children born moderately preterm and children born at term, considering hours spent participating in outdoor activities per week. Nor were there any differences in hours spent participating in sedentary activities—watching television, playing videogames, using a computer and reading.

Table 1 Parental and offspring ($N = 4941$) characteristics at birth and 9-11 years after moderately preterm birth (32-36 completed weeks). The Aarhus Birth Cohort, Denmark 1989-2001

	Moderately preterm birth n[a] (%)	Term birth n (%)	*p*-value
Total	158 (3.2)	4783 (96.8)	
Prenatal maternal and paternal factors			
Cohabiting *Missing data (67)*	151 (96.2)	4583 (97.2)	0.46
Pre-existing chronic disease *Missing data (173)*	13 (8.5)	179 (3.9)	0.01
Smoking before pregnancy *Missing data (11)*	85 (53.8)	1857 (38.9)	< 0.001
Smoking during pregnancy *Missing data (96)*	66 (42.3)	1311 (28.0)	< 0.001
Partner smoking during pregnancy *Missing data (96)*	81 (63.3)	1875 (47.5)	0.001
Alcohol during pregnancy (units per week)			0.99
< 1	94 (59.9)	2786 (59.5)	
1-2	43 (27.4)	1287 (27.5)	
3+ *Missing data (98)*	20 (12.7)	613 (13.1)	
Leisure time physical activity during pregnancy			0.005
Sedentary	80 (52.6)	1867 (40.9)	
Light activity	68 (44.7)	2382 (52.2)	
Moderate to heavy activity *Missing data (225)*	4 (2.6)	315 (6.9)	
Offspring at 9-11 years			0.52
Girl	74 (46.8)	2379 (49.7)	
Boy	84 (53.2)	2404 (50.3)	
Height, mean (SD)	142 (8.1)	142 (8.0)	0.74
Weight, median (min-max) *Missing data (0)*	35 (7.3)	34.5 (7.1)	0.34
Asthma diagnosed by a medical doctor			< 0.001
Yes	30 (19)	399 (8.3)	
No	127 (80.4)	4348 (90.9)	
Do not know *Missing data (0)*	1 (0.6)	36 (0.8)	
Maternal smoking after delivery *Missing data (12)*	85 (53.8)	1926 (40.6)	0.001
Paternal smoking after delivery *Missing data (149)*	95 (61.3)	2063 (44.5)	< 0.001
Maternal professional education			0.07
No education (after secondary schools +/− high schools)	12 (7.6)	354 (7.5)	
Currently studying	10 (6.3)	104 (2.2)	
1-2 years of education (after secondary schools +/− high schools)	44 (27.8)	1295 (26.4)	
3-4 years of education (after secondary schools +/− high schools)	75 (47.5)	2271 (47.9)	
4 + years of education (after secondary schools +/− high schools) *Missing data (40)*	17 (10.8)	763 (16.1)	
Paternal professional education			0.022
No education (after secondary schools +/− high schools)	25 (16.3)	487 (10.5)	
Currently studying	1 (0.7)	64 (1.4)	

Table 1 Parental and offspring ($N = 4941$) characteristics at birth and 9-11 years after moderately preterm birth (32-36 completed weeks). The Aarhus Birth Cohort, Denmark 1989-2001 *(Continued)*

	Moderately preterm birth n[a] (%)	Term birth n (%)	*p*-value
1-2 years of education (after secondary schools +/− high schools)	19 (12.4)	553 (12.0)	
3-4 years of education (after secondary schools +/− high schools)	79 (51.6)	2163 (46.8)	
4 + years of education (after secondary schools +/− high schools) *Missing data (167)*	29 (19.0)	1354 (29.3)	

[a]Total differs due to missing values

Previous studies of physical activity and the exercise capacity of preterm children showed diverging results. Consistent with the results of our study, some studies of preschool- and school-aged children reported no differences in the levels of physical activity of preterm and term children [9, 35–37]. Other studies showed that young adults who were born preterm reported less exercise than control subjects [19, 38, 39]. This disparity may reflect real differences between the populations studied but may also be due to differences in the measurements of physical activity used for each of the studies. In our study, we measured each child's leisure time physical activity level based both on the frequency of sports activities per week and hours of outdoor activities per week, but we did not measure the performance level of each child.

Most previous studies included only children with very low birthweights (1000-1500 g) or extremely low birthweights (< 1000 g) [9, 17–19, 35, 37, 38]. This may increase the likelihood of observing differences in the activity levels of children born preterm and children born at term due to the much higher overall

Table 2 Moderately preterm birth (32-36 completed weeks) and levels of sports activity, outdoor activity and sedentary activity at 9-11 years of age. The Aarhus Birth Cohort, Denmark 1989-1991, N = 4941

	Moderately preterm birth n (%) 158 (3.2)	Total n[a] 4941	OR	OR 95% CI
Participating in sports during the week				
No	29 (3.3)	872	1.00 (ref)	1.00 (ref)
Yes	129 (3.2)	4069	0.95	1.03 (0.67-1.58)
Sports activity: number of days per week				
0	29 (3.3)	872	1.00 (ref)	1.00 (ref)
1	29 (2.6)	1116	0.78	1.26 (0.60-2.65)
2	51 (3.3)	1559	0.98	1.02 (0.49-2.16)
3	36 (3.8)	947	1.15	1.37 (0.68-2.75)
≥ 4	13 (2.9)	447	0.87	1.63 (0.80-3.35)
Outdoor activity: hours per week				
0-3	23 (2.8)	812	1.00 (ref)	1.00 (ref)
4-6	37 (3.2)	1162	1.13	1.01(0.59-1.74)
7-13	55 (3.2)	1704	1.14	1.02 (0.61-1.70)
14-20	27 (3.3)	830	1.15	0.93 (0.52-1.67)
21-60	7 (3.4)	207	1.20	0.88(0.35-2.22)
Children with very low level physical activity levels				
Yes	6 (2.4)	247	1.00 (ref)	1.00 (ref)
No	152 (3.2)	4694	1.34	1.36 (0.59-3.2)
Sedentary activities: hours per week[b]				
0- 7	14 (2.5)	569	1.00 (ref)	1.00 (ref)
8-14	73 (3.5)	2083	1.44	1.35 (0.74-2.49)
15-21	50 (3.5)	1412	1.46	1.38 (0.73-2.62)
22-28	11 (2.0)	549	0.81	0.68 (0.30-1.57)
29+	6 (2.6)	233	1.05	0.81 (0.28-2.36)

[a] Total differs due to missing values
[b] Watching television, using a computer, playing video games and reading books and comics
OR Odds ratio, *CI* Confidence interval

morbidity observed in this newborn population [9]. However, moderately preterm infants account for 80% of premature births [17]. Therefore, it is important to focus on this large group, particularly because there is increasing evidence that these patients are also at increased risk for developmental and behavioural morbidities [17, 18]. To the best of our knowledge, our study is the first to investigate a group of moderately preterm infants regarding leisure time physical activity.. By excluding multiple births and all children with handicaps that may influence their ability related to physical activity our results can only be generalized to singletons without a moderate to severe physical handicap born moderately preterm.

Our moderately preterm population had a significantly higher prevalence of asthma (19%) than children born at term (8.3%), which has also been demonstrated in other populations [40]. However, there was no difference in the amount of time spent engaged in physical activity. One explanation may be that the parents of children born preterm who suffer from asthma may be more motivated to enrol their child in sports activities. Another reason could be that most Danish children have well controlled asthma or that parents with children born preterm reported that their children suffer from asthma more often than other parents. The results of our subanalysis demonstrated that the results remained essentially unchanged after excluding children diagnosed with asthma.

We conducted a population-based cohort study using prospective data from a single prenatal care setting and obstetrics department in the second largest city in Denmark, where prenatal care and hospital delivery are free of charge; therefore, the cohort represents all socio-demographic groups. We excluded children with severe mental and physical health problem, twins and triplets to enhance comparability between the two groups of children. A self-administered questionnaire was used to collect information about the children's physical activities; this could potentially introduce inaccuracy. The questionnaire used to assess physical activity resulted in a mere description of duration and type of leisure time activity rather than intensity. The type and duration should be simple for parents to reconstruct since many children attend sports on specific weekdays for a well-defined number of hours that the parents will pay for. Differential misclassification of children's physical activity would impact our results. However, we have no reason to believe that parents of preterm children would report their activity differently than parents of children born at term. Another way to measure physical activity is with an objective form of measurement, such as an accelerometer, as seen elsewhere [9]. Objective measurements may introduce selection biases into the study due to compliance problems while obtaining measurements or due to a lack of willingness to participate in the assessment. The care of children born after 32 weeks has essentially remained unchanged over the last decades. Accordingly, we believe that our results may be extrapolated to more recent time.

The fraction of moderately preterm children was similar in children followed up to that among children lost to follow up (3.2% vs 4.2%). However, if the families with more physical active children were more prone to participate if the child was preterm than if they were term, this may have introduced bias towards a more favorable physical profile for preterm compared to term children. However, we consider this explanation for our results unlikely.

The proportion of healthy children born moderately preterm among participants is comparable to the proportion of preterm delivery in the Danish national birth register at that time [41]. This indicates that selection biases may not be a major issue. The overall rate of preterm delivery in Denmark is rather low compared to other industrialized countries such as United States [42]. However, we have no reason to believe that the results of this study cannot be found in populations in other countries.

Physical inactivity is associated with a higher risk of obesity, and children and adolescents are becoming more sedentary [21, 22]. It may be even more important for infants born preterm to follow the guidelines for physical activity, as studies have indicated that preterm delivery is associated with a higher risk of stroke [43] and type 2 diabetes [24] in adulthood. These diseases are associated with lower levels of physical activity, and there is evidence that physical activity may prevent them [21, 22].

Conclusions

In this study of 9- to 11-year-old children, we found no differences in leisure time activities as weekly number of sports activities outside school, hours spent on outdoor activity and hours spent on sedentary activity between children born moderately preterm and children born at term. This finding is reassuring as physical activity is a fundamental element of a normal childhood and is important for long-term development [44]. Only one-third of school-aged children regardless of gestational age at birth in our study were as physically active as recommended by the national health guidelines for children [29]; thus, a focus on the factors that increase physical activity of all children is necessary.

Abbreviations

CI: Confidence intervals; LMP: Last menstrual period; OR: Odds Ratio; SD: Standard deviation

Funding

The Augustinus Foundation and the Lundbeck Foundation. The funding bodies had no influence on study design and have no role in data acquisition, data analyses and interpretation or manuscript preparation.

Authors' contributions

MNL, HKH, MSL and TBH conceptualized the idea and design of the study. TBH, MH, CO, and MSL were responsible for acquisition of data. MNL and HKH were responsible for data analyses and they drafted the first version of the manuscript. All authors have been involved in revising the manuscript critically for important intellectual content and have given final approval of the version to be published. In addition, all authors have agreed to be accountable for all aspects of the work in ensuring that questions related to the accuracy or integrity of any part of the work are appropriately investigated and resolved.

Competing interests

The authors declare that they have no competing interests.

Author details

[1]The Research Unit of Women's and Children's Health, section 7821, The Juliane Marie Centre, Copenhagen University Hospital, Rigshospitalet, Blegdamsvej 9, DK-2100 Copenhagen, Denmark. [2]Faculty of Health and Medical Sciences, University of Copenhagen, Copenhagen, Denmark. [3]Obstetric Clinic, The Juliane Marie Centre, Rigshospitalet, Copenhagen University Hospital, Copenhagen, Denmark. [4]Child, Family and Reproductive Health, Department of Health Science, Faculty of Medicine, Lund University, Lund, Sweden. [5]Institute of General Medical Practice, Department of Public Health, Aarhus University, Aarhus, Denmark. [6]Perinatal Epidemiology Research Unit, Department of Paediatrics, Aarhus University Hospital, Skejby, Aarhus, Denmark.

References

1. WHO: recommended definitions, terminology and format for statistical tables related to the perinatal period and use of a new certificate for cause of perinatal deaths. Modifications recommended by FIGO as amended October 14, 1976. Acta Obstet Gynecol Scand. 1977;56:247–53.
2. Slattery MM, Morrison JJ. Preterm delivery. Lancet. 2002;360:1489–97.
3. Anderson P, Doyle LW. Neurobehavioral outcomes of school-age children born extremely low birth weight or very preterm in the 1990s. JAMA. 2003; 289:3264–72.
4. Moss TJ. Respiratory consequences of preterm birth. Clin Exp Pharmacol Physiol. 2006;33:280–4.
5. Taylor HG, Minich NM, Klein N, Hack M. Longitudinal outcomes of very low birth weight: neuropsychological findings. J Int Neuropsychol Soc. 2004;10: 149–63.
6. Hack M, Flannery DJ, Schluchter M, Cartar L, Borawski E, Klein N. Outcomes in young adulthood for very-low-birth-weight infants. N Engl J Med. 2002; 346:149–57.
7. Moster D, Lie RT, Markestad T. Long-term medical and social consequences of preterm birth. N Engl J Med. 2008;359:262–73.
8. Wilson-Costello D, Friedman H, Minich N, Fanaroff AA, Hack M. Improved survival rates with increased neurodevelopmental disability for extremely low birth weight infants in the 1990s. Pediatrics. 2005;115:997–1003.
9. Welsh L, Kirkby J, Lum S, Odendaal D, Marlow N, Derrick G, et al. The EPICure study: maximal exercise and physical activity in school children born extremely preterm. Thorax. 2010;65:165–72.
10. Ekeus C, Lindstrom K, Lindblad F, Rasmussen F, Hjern A. Preterm birth, social disadvantage, and cognitive competence in Swedish 18- to 19-year-old men. Pediatrics. 2010;125:e67–73.
11. Hille ET, den Ouden AL, Saigal S, Wolke D, Lambert M, Whitaker A, et al. Behavioural problems in children who weigh 1000 g or less at birth in four countries. Lancet. 2001;357:1641–3.
12. Bhutta AT, Cleves MA, Casey PH, Cradock MM, Anand KJ. Cognitive and behavioral outcomes of school-aged children who were born preterm: a meta-analysis. JAMA. 2002;288:728–37.
13. Saigal S, den OL, Wolke D, Hoult L, Paneth N, Streiner DL, et al. School-age outcomes in children who were extremely low birth weight from four international population-based cohorts. Pediatrics. 2003;112:943–50.
14. Hack M, Taylor HG, Drotar D, Schluchter M, Cartar L, Andreias L, et al. Chronic conditions, functional limitations, and special health care needs of school-aged children born with extremely low-birth-weight in the 1990s. JAMA. 2005;294:318–25.
15. Litt J, Taylor HG, Klein N, Hack M. Learning disabilities in children with very low birthweight: prevalence, neuropsychological correlates, and educational interventions. J Learn Disabil. 2005;38:130–41.
16. Marlow N, Wolke D, Bracewell MA, Samara M. Neurologic and developmental disability at six years of age after extremely preterm birth. N Engl J Med. 2005;352:9–19.
17. Vohr B. Long-term outcomes of moderately preterm, late preterm, and early term infants. Clin Perinatol. 2013;40:739–51.
18. McGowan JE, Alderdice FA, Holmes VA, Johnston L. Early childhood development of late-preterm infants: a systematic review. Pediatrics. 2011; 127:1111–24.
19. Kajantie E, Strang-Karlsson S, Hovi P, Raikkonen K, Pesonen AK, Heinonen K, et al. Adults born at very low birth weight exercise less than their peers born at term. J Pediatr. 2010;157:610–6. 616
20. Kaseva N, Wehkalampi K, Strang-Karlsson S, Salonen M, Pesonen AK, Raikkonen K, et al. Lower conditioning leisure-time physical activity in young adults born preterm at very low birth weight. PLoS One. 2012;7: e32430.
21. Hu FB. Sedentary lifestyle and risk of obesity and type 2 diabetes. Lipids. 2003;38:103–8.
22. Pedersen BK: Fysisk aktivitet - håndbog om forebyggelse og behandling. 2003.
23. Doyle LW, Faber B, Callanan C, Morley R. Blood pressure in late adolescence and very low birth weight. Pediatrics. 2003;111:252–7.
24. Kaijser M, Bonamy AK, Akre O, Cnattingius S, Granath F, Norman M, et al. Perinatal risk factors for diabetes in later life. Diabetes. 2009;58:523–6.
25. Hofman PL, Regan F, Jackson WE, Jefferies C, Knight DB, Robinson EM, et al. Premature birth and later insulin resistance. N Engl J Med. 2004; 351:2179–86.
26. Hovi P, Andersson S, Jarvenpaa AL, Eriksson JG, Strang-Karlsson S, Kajantie E, et al. Decreased bone mineral density in adults born with very low birth weight: a cohort study. PLoS Med. 2009;6:e1000135.
27. Laaksonen DE, Lakka HM, Lynch J, Lakka TA, Niskanen L, Rauramaa R, et al. Cardiorespiratory fitness and vigorous leisure-time physical activity modify the association of small size at birth with the metabolic syndrome. Diabetes Care. 2003;26:2156–64.
28. Telama R, Yang X, Viikari J, Valimaki I, Wanne O, Raitakari O. Physical activity from childhood to adulthood: a 21-year tracking study. Am J Prev Med. 2005;28:267–73.
29. SST. Anbefalinger om fysisk aktivitet til børn og unge (5-17 år). 2004. Ref Type: Online Source.
30. Larsen PS, Kamper-Jorgensen M, Adamson A, Barros H, Bonde JP, Brescianini S, et al. Pregnancy and birth cohort resources in europe: a large opportunity for aetiological child health research. Paediatr Perinat Epidemiol. 2013;27: 393–414.
31. http://dda.dk/catalogue/9185?lang=en Ref Type: Online Source.
32. Pedersen CB, Gotzsche H, Moller JO, Mortensen PB. The Danish civil registration system. A cohort of eight million persons. Dan Med Bull. 2006; 53:441–9.
33. Hedegaard M, Henriksen TB, Sabroe S, Secher NJ. Psychological distress in pregnancy and preterm delivery. BMJ. 1993;307:234–9.
34. Dahan-Oliel N, Mazer B, Majnemer A. Preterm birth and leisure participation: a synthesis of the literature. Res Dev Disabil. 2012;33:1211–20.
35. Keller H, Bar-Or O, Kriemler S, Ayub BV, Saigal S. Anaerobic performance in 5- to 7-yr-old children of low birthweight. Med Sci Sports Exerc. 2000;32: 278–83.
36. Svien LR. Health-related fitness of seven- to 10-year-old children with histories of preterm birth. Pediatr Phys Ther. 2003;15:74–83.
37. Kriemler S, Keller H, Saigal S, Bar-Or O. Aerobic and lung performance in

premature children with and without chronic lung disease of prematurity. Clin J Sport Med. 2005;15:349–55.
38. Clemm H, Roksund O, Thorsen E, Eide GE, Markestad T, Halvorsen T. Aerobic capacity and exercise performance in young people born extremely preterm. Pediatrics. 2012;129:e97–e105.
39. Saigal S, Stoskopf B, Boyle M, Paneth N, Pinelli J, Streiner D, et al. Comparison of current health, functional limitations, and health care use of young adults who were born with extremely low birth weight and normal birth weight. Pediatrics. 2007;119:e562–73.
40. Jaakkola JJ, Ahmed P, Ieromnimon A, Goepfert P, Laiou E, Quansah R, et al. Preterm delivery and asthma: a systematic review and meta-analysis. J Allergy Clin Immunol. 2006;118:823–30.
41. Langhoff-Roos J, Kesmodel U, Jacobsson B, Rasmussen S, Vogel I. Spontaneous preterm delivery in primiparous women at low risk in Denmark: population based study. BMJ. 2006;332:937–9.
42. Denney JM, Culhane JF, Goldenberg RL: Prevention of preterm birth. Womens Health (Lond Engl) 2008:4;625–38.
43. Koupil I, Leon DA, Lithell HO. Length of gestation is associated with mortality from cerebrovascular disease. J Epidemiol Community Health. 2005;59:473–4.
44. Waxman A. WHO global strategy on diet, physical activity and health. Food Nutr Bull. 2004;25:292–302.

16

Henoch-Schönlein purpura with acute pancreatitis: analysis of 13 cases

Qin Zhang[1], Qi Guo[1], Ming Gui[1], Zhenhua Ren[2], Bo Hu[1], Ling Lu[1] and Fang Deng[1*]

Abstract

Background: Henoch-Schönlein purpura is a common small vessel vasculitis in children. Acute pancreatitis rarely presents as a complication of Henoch-Schönlein purpura and has not been well characterized.

Methods: We retrospectively reviewed 13 cases of Henoch-Schönlein purpura with acute pancreatitis among 3212 patients who attended our hospital between January 2003 and June 2016 and analyzed their clinical characteristics, laboratory findings, imaging findings, treatment and overall prognosis.

Results: All patients had abdominal manifestations, including significant abdominal pain (13/13), vomiting (9/13), abdominal distension (3/13) and melena (6/13). Serum amylase level significantly increased in all patients, and urine amylase was increased in 7 cases (7/10). However, increased urine lapse was only noted in 2 cases (2/5), and diffuse swelling of the pancreas was seen in 2 cases (2/13) by abdominal ultrasonography. Although all patients had typical skin purpura (13/13), 5 patients (5/13) with acute pancreatitis initially experienced acute abdominal pain in clinical onset of Henoch-Schönlein purpura. Glucocorticoid therapy was effective in alleviating abdominal symptoms of Henoch-Schönlein purpura patients with acute pancreatitis. All patients were in good general condition without any abdominal complications 6–12 months after discharge.

Conclusions: Acute pancreatitis is rarely observed in Henoch-Schönlein purpura children and has no specific clinical features that differentiate it from abdominal manifestations of Henoch-Schönlein purpura. Therefore, in Henoch-Schönlein purpura patients with severe abdominal pain, serum amylase levels should be assessed to confirm the diagnosis of acute pancreatitis. Early diagnose of Henoch-Schönlein purpura with acute pancreatitis and treatment timely was very important for good clinical outcomes.

Keywords: Henoch-Schönlein purpura, Acute pancreatitis, Complication, Children

Background

Henoch-Schönlein purpura (HSP), a systemic small-vessel vasculitis syndrome, typically occurs in children and causes purpuric skin lesions accompanied by various presentations, including gastrointestinal symptoms, arthritis, and nephritis [1]. The severity of symptoms and the order of their appearance differ among patients. Gastrointestinal manifestations occur in two-thirds of patients and vary from mild abdominal pain to colicky features [2].

Acute pancreatitis (AP) has been reported by only a limited number of authors, with different clinical features during the course of HSP. Most cases of HSP pancreatitis are mild in clinical characteristics but can evolve into hemorrhage, necrosis and pseudocyst [3, 4]. As a complication, AP can be diagnosed on the basis of a high level of serum amylase in HSP patients with abdominal pain. In cases with epigastric tenderness, routine serum and urine amylase evaluations may reveal pancreatic involvement in HSP [4]. We herein retrospectively reviewed 13 cases of HSP patients with AP among 3212 HSP patients and analyzed symptoms and signs, laboratory findings, imaging findings, treatment and their prognosis.

* Correspondence: fangdun31123@qq.com
[1]Department of Pediatrics, First Affiliated Hospital of Anhui Medical University, 19th Floor of Medicine and Medical Tech Building, 218 Jixi Road, Hefei 230022, Anhui, China
Full list of author information is available at the end of the article

Methods

All the clinical data used in this study were obtained from the paper and electronic medical records (EMRs) of our hospital. The study protocol was approved by the Research Ethics Commission of the First Affiliated Hospital of Anhui Medical University.

Patients

Children with a final diagnosis of HSP presenting to the Department of Pediatrics, First Affiliated Hospital of Anhui Medical University were prospectively enrolled between January 2003 and June 2016. All patients conformed to the standard established by the European League Against Rheumatism/Paediatric Rheumatology International Trials Organization/Paediatric Rheumatology European Society [5]. All patients had typical skin purpura over the buttocks and lower extremities and exhibited 1 or more of the typical manifestations of the syndrome, including abdominal symptoms, hematuria, or arthritis. The diagnosis of AP was made in patients with two of the following three manifestations: characteristic upper abdominal pain, elevated levels of pancreatic enzymes, or imaging findings suggesting AP [6].

Data collection

We reviewed the age, length of hospital stay, and initial manifestation of HSP patients with AP. The abdominal manifestations of HSP among patients with AP, including abdominal pain, nausea, vomiting, upper gastrointestinal bleeding manifested with tarry stool passage, hematochezia and diarrhea, were analyzed. Laboratory studies including serum and urine amylase levels, hemogram, blood calcium, fecal occult blood, and imaging reports were recorded. The treatment process and outcome were also reviewed.

Results

Clinical features

Three thousand two hundred twelve HSP children, including 1966 males and 1249 females (mean age 6. 7 ± 2.41 years old, absolute range 1.4–15 years), were enrolled in the study. Among the 3212 HSP patients, only 13 patients (0.4%), including 9 males and 4 females (mean age 10.58 ± 2.63 years old, absolute range 6–14 years), had AP as a complication of HSP. Eight cases with AP had typical rash for HSP in the onset (8/13), and the time interval between skin purpura and identification of pancreatic damage was from 2 to 30 days (the average was 9.25 ± 9.65 days). Five cases with AP initially experienced acute abdominal pain (5/13), and skin purpura appeared 4–15 days after disease onset (the average was 7.40 ± 4.83 days). Details regarding age, duration of hospital stay, and initial manifestation are presented in Table 1.

In all HSP patients with AP, we encountered two uncommon cases. They (Case No. 1 and No. 2) initially experienced acute abdominal pain and underwent operations due to the suspicion of acute appendicitis or cholecystitis (Table 1). Their purpuric skin rashes appeared later than the presentation of abdominal pain. HSP was diagnosed after the appearance of a typical rash.

All HSP patients with AP exhibited a palpable purpura rash, and the purpura typically appeared on the buttocks and the extensor surfaces of the arms and legs. However, any area of the body may be involved. As shown in Table 2, significant abdominal pain and tenderness were common abdominal manifestations in HSP patients with AP. The periumbilical area was most common location of abdominal tenderness. Six cases (6/13) exhibited upper gastrointestinal tract bleeding presenting with tarry stool

Table 1 The age, hospital stay time, and initial manifestation in 13 HSP children

case number	Hospital stay (d)	Initial manifestation	Time interval between skin purpura and finding pancreatitis (d)	Time between pancreatitis and skin purpura (d)
1	45	AAp	–	3
2	28	AAp	–	4
3	12	AAp	–	9
4	3	SP	2	–
5	5	SP	5	–
6	15	SP	30	–
7	11	SP	15	–
8	33	AAp	–	15
9	44	SP	3	–
10	24	AAp	–	6
11	25	SP	12	–
12	17	SP	5	–
13	9	SP	2	–

M Male, *F* Female, *SP* skin purpura, *AAp* acute abdominal pain

Table 2 Clinical features of abdominal symptoms among 13 children with Henoch-Schönlein purpura and acute pancreatitis

Clinical features		No. of patients	Percent (%)
Colicky abdominal pain		13	100
Abdominal tenderness		13	100
Abdominal tenderness location	periumbilical area	6	46
	upper abdomen	1	7.7
	whole abdomen	3	23
	No definite position	3	23
Abdominal distension		3	23
Abdominal wall tension		3	23
Nausea and vomiting		9	69
Upper gastrointestinal tract bleeding		6	46
Melena		6	46
Hematemesis		1	7.7
Diarrhea		1	7.7
Arthritis		7	54
nephritis		10	77

passage (Table 2). In addition, arthritis involvement was noted in 7 patients (7/13), and nephritis presenting with proteinuria occurred in 10 patients (10/13).

Laboratory studies

Laboratory values are presented in Table 3. Of note, serum amylase was elevated in all patients with AP. Moreover, urine amylase levels increased in 7 cases (7/10), and serum lipase levels only increased in 2 cases (2/5). As shown in Table 3, all patients with AP had an abnormal hemogram. None of the patients had a bleeding tendency or coagulopathy. Other examinations, including imaging examination, electrocardiogram, myocardial enzymes and liver function, were performed in some HSP patients with AP. Their results are depicted in Table 4.

Treatment

Methyl prednisolone pulse therapy was used for HSP patients presenting with AP. The patients were treated with methyl prednisolone (10–15 mg/kg/day) every other day 3 times during a treatment course, and one or two additional treatment courses were considered depending on the conditions of the patients. Moreover, for the treatment of AP, H2 receptor antagonists or proton pump inhibitors are used to inhibit the secretion of gastric acid. The anti-secretory agents (octreotide) and anti-

Table 3 The Laboratory values in 13 HSP children

case number	Serum amylase (< 110 IU/L)	Urine amylase (< 900 U/L)	Serum lipase (< 300 U/L)	White blood cell count (< 10 × 10^9/L)	Neutrophil ratio (< 70%)	Blood calcium (> 2.03 mmol/L)	Occult blood (+)
1	132	–	–	22	78	1.6	2(+)
2	382	8687	845	17	78	2.3	1(+)
3	182	2600	–	16	67	2.6	(–)
4	365	80	–	21	88	–	(–)
5	222	775	–	10	60	2.4	–
6	546	4411	32	29	88	2.5	(–)
7	143	941	–	20	80	2.6	(–)
8	174	1210	–	15	79	1.9	2(+)
9	325	1330	258	22	83	2.0	3(+)
10	162	–	–	18	86	2.0	2(+)
11	193	3524	548	12	83	2.4	(+)
12	121	–	–	20	67	2.3	–
13	175	446	61	19	81	2.3	(+)

(+): positive; (–): Negative; –-: No test

Table 4 Additional examinations in 13 children with Henoch-Schönlein purpura and acute pancreatitis

case number	Abdominal radiograph	Abdominal ultrasonography	CT	ECG	Myocardial enzymes
1	BD	PE	–	AN	AN
2	N	N	–	N	N
3	–	N	–	N	N
4	–	PE	N	N	N
5	N	N	N	AN	AN
6	–	N	–	N	N
7	–	N	–	N	N
8	BD	PDS	–	N	N
9	–	PE	–	AN	AN
10	N	PE	–	N	N
11	N	N	N	N	N
12	–	PDS	–	N	N
13	–	N	PDS	N	N

CT Computerized tomography, *ECG* Electrocardiogram, *BD* Bowel dilatation, *PDS* Pancreatic diffuse swelling, *PE* Peritoneal effusion, *AN* Abnormality, *N* Normal; —: No test

inflammatory drugs (amoxicillin and clavulanate potassium) were used to prevent pancreatic enzyme secretion and anti-bacterial infection, respectively. According to the available guidelines for the treatment of AP, supportive care was pivotal. In addition, pain management should be mentioned when caring for a patient with AP.

After methyl prednisolone pulse therapy, the symptoms of abdominal pain were alleviated, and serum and urine amylase levels returned to normal. Then, prednisolone (1 mg/kg/day) was administered orally until urine test were normal and the symptoms had completely disappeared. The average duration of treatment of the HSP patients with methyl prednisolone and prednisolone was 18.56 ± 8.18 days, and the total course of treatment ranged from 3 to 45 days.

Outcome and follow-up

After methyl prednisolone pulse therapy and the treatment of AP, purpuric skin rashes and gastrointestinal symptoms disappeared in all HSP children with AP. Serum amylase recovered to normal levels from 3 to 6 days after treatment, and urine amylase levels returned to normal in 3–13 days.

In the follow-up period of 6–12 months, no recurrence of AP or pancreatic cyst formation was observed in any of the HSP children. However, the recurrence of abdominal pain was noted in 4 children (1 episode in 3 patients and 2 episodes in 1 patient). The interval between the first episode and recurrence ranged from 12 to 44 days with a mean time of 19.3 days. All of these patients with recurrence were treated with corticosteroids. Three patients developed Henoch–Schönlein purpura nephritis (HSPN).

Discussion

Henoch–Schönlein purpura (HSP) is a systemic vasculitis that is characterized by the deposition of IgA-containing complex and complement component 3 (C3) on arterioles, capillaries, and venules [7]. Clinical manifestations observed in HSP, including skin purpura, abdominal pain, arthritis, and glomerulonephritis, are typically attributed to widespread vasculitis in the small vessels, which causes an increase in vascular permeability and fragility [8].

HSP complicated by acute pancreatitis (AP) occurs rarely, and the exact cause is unknown. The pathophysiologic mechanism of AP is thought to be vasculitic involvement of the capillaries, small arteries and small veins within pancreatic tissues, which increases vascular permeability and leads to pancreatic edema [8–10]. Embolism in the small vessels of the pancreas causes pancreatic ischemia and hypoxia and the abnormal activation of digestive enzymes. These effects lead to inflammation, edema, vascular injury, and even cellular death [11].

AP in HSP was generally recorded as case reports in previous studies [10, 12–15]. Among all HSP complications, the incidence of AP is very low. In a study of 208 patients with HSP, Chen SY et al. report gastrointestinal manifestations and complications of HSP. Among these patients, only one case (0.48%) exhibited highly elevated serum amylase and lipase levels [2]. A recent study reviewed that 50 case reports documented the involvement of the pancreato-biliary system in HSP, and found that only 23 cases among of records in the US National Library of Medicine database from 1977 to 2015 had pancreatitis in HSP [15]. In our study, we identified only 13 children with AP among 3212 HSP patients (0.4%) during the past 14 years. Because serum amylase and lipase levels have not been routinely measured in all HSP cases, the incidence of AP may be higher than our data [16].

To the best of our knowledge, the reported 13 patients represent the biggest retrospective case series hitherto published. The complication of pancreatitis can occur as an initial manifestation of HSP. Frigui et al. analyzed pediatric HSP cases with pancreatitis, and identified AP as an initial manifestation in half of cases [4, 10, 17, 18]. In this study, 5 HSP children among 13 patients (38%) exhibited an onset of abdominal symptoms. The other 8 HSP cases with AP (62%) first presented with the characteristic rash. Elevated serum amylase levels are an early diagnostic finding for HSP pancreatitis [17]. Serum amylase and lipase levels might be more important and should be measured in patients who present with severe abdominal pain as the initial complaint. Ultrasonography or CT signs, such as swollen pancreas, edema and necrosis, are useful to confirm the diagnosis only if pancreatitis is severe. In our study, although serum and urine amylase levels increased significantly in all HSP patients with AP, only 2 cases (15%) exhibited diffuse swelling of the pancreas by ultrasonography.

Pancreatic involvement in HSP is mild in nature and self-limiting. According to Working Group IAP/APA Acute Pancreatitis Guidelines, oral feeding can be initiated as soon as the pain decreases and inflammatory markers are lowering [19]. Octreotide is a synthetic analogue of somatostatin that is effective for the treatment of AP via the inhibition of the release of exocrine secretions of the pancreas [20]. Steroid administration has been controversial in the treatment of AP over the past few decades. The evidence indicates that steroid administration worsened pancreatitis and should not be applied in AP [4]. However, the results of experimental animal models of AP demonstrated that steroids have an inhibitory effect on pancreatic secretion [21] and inhibit the development of AP partly via cytokine release [22]. Steroid therapy can be used in HSP patients with AP and is effective in alleviating symptoms of AP [4, 16, 18]. However, the previous study demonstrated that corticosteroid use was associated with an increased risk of gastrointestinal bleeding and perforation [23]. Therefore, HSP patients, especially children complicated with gastrointestinal bleeding, must be closely followed up during steroid treatment [4]. In our study, all the patients with AP were treated with methyl prednisolone and achieved a good outcome. No patient experienced a gastrointestinal complication during the course of steroid therapy.

Conclusions

HSP patients with severe abdominal pain should be evaluated for pancreatitis. Serum amylase level is a useful tool for the early diagnosis of acute pancreatitis. Although good outcome can be achieved in most HSP patients, supportive treatment for HSP pancreatitis and maybe also steroid therapy might be performed to avoid unnecessary surgical interventions.

Abbreviations

AP: Acute pancreatitis; CT: Computerized tomography; EMR: Electronic medical record; EULAR: European League Against Rheumatism; HSP: Henoch-Schönlein purpura; HSPN: Henoch-Schönlein purpura nephritis; MRI: Magnetic resonance imaging; PReS: Pediatric Rheumatology Society; US: Ultrasonography

Funding

This study was funded by the National Natural Science Foundation of China (81372693) and in part by the Anhui Natural Science Foundation (1308085MH119) and the Youth Training Program of the First Affiliated Hospital of Anhui Medical University (2010KJ17). None of the funders were involved in the study design, data analysis, manuscript preparation, or decision to disseminate and publish the study findings.

Authors' contributions

QZ and QG reviewed the medical records, analyzed and interpreted the data, and drafted the manuscript. ZR interpreted the data and drafted the manuscript. MG analyzed and interpreted the data. LL, FD and BH designed and oversaw the study, interpreted the data, and revised the manuscript. All authors have read and approved the final manuscript for publication.

Competing interests

The authors declare that they have no competing interests.

Author details

[1]Department of Pediatrics, First Affiliated Hospital of Anhui Medical University, 19th Floor of Medicine and Medical Tech Building, 218 Jixi Road, Hefei 230022, Anhui, China. [2]Department of Anatomy, School of Basic Medicine, Anhui Medical University, Hefei 230032, Anhui, China.

References

1. Yang YH, Yu HH, Chiang BL. The diagnosis and classification of Henoch-Schonlein purpura: an updated review. Autoimmun Rev. 2014;13(4–5):355–8.
2. Chen SY, Kong MS. Gastrointestinal manifestations and complications of Henoch-Schonlein purpura. Chang Gung Med J. 2004;27(3):175–81.
3. Bowman P, Quinn M. Question 1: should steroids be used to treat abdominal pain caused by Henoch-Schonlein purpura? Arch Dis Child. 2012; 97(11):999–1000.
4. Soyer T, Egritas O, Atmaca E, Akman H, Ozturk H, Tezic T. Acute pancreatitis: a rare presenting feature of Henoch Schonlein purpura. J Paediatr Child Health. 2008;44(3):152–3.
5. Brogan P, Eleftheriou D, Dillon M. Small vessel vasculitis. Pediatr Nephrol. 2010;25(6):1025–35.
6. Kiriyama S, Gabata T, Takada T, Hirata K, Yoshida M, Mayumi T, Hirota M, Kadoya M, Yamanouchi E, Hattori T, et al. New diagnostic criteria of acute pancreatitis. J Hepatobiliary Pancreat Sci. 2010;17(1):24–36.
7. Rigante D, Castellazzi L, Bosco A, Esposito S. Is there a crossroad between infections, genetics, and Henoch-Schonlein purpura? Autoimmun Rev. 2013; 12(10):1016–21.
8. Pan YX, Ye Q, Shao WX, Shang SQ, Mao JH, Zhang T, Shen HQ, Zhao N. Relationship between immune parameters and organ involvement in children with Henoch-Schonlein purpura. PLoS One. 2014;9(12):e115261.

9. Gow KW, Murphy JJ 3rd, Blair GK, Magee JF, Hailey J. Multiple entero-entero fistulae: an unusual complication of Henoch-Schonlein purpura. J Pediatr Surg. 1996;31(6):809–11.
10. Dinler G, Bek K, Acikgoz Y, Kalayci AG. Acute pancreatitis as a presenting feature of Henoch-Schonlein purpura. Turk J Pediatr. 2010;52(2):191–3.
11. Milnerowicz H, Bukowski R, Jablonowska M, Sciskalska M, Milnerowicz U. The antioxidant profiles, lysosomal and membrane enzymes activity in patients with acute pancreatitis. Mediat Inflamm. 2014;2014:376518.
12. Branski D, Gross V, Gross-Kieselstein E, Roll D, Abrahamov A. Pancreatitis as a complication of Henoch–Schonlein purpura. J Pediatr Gastroenterol Nutr. 1982;1(2):275–6.
13. Garner JA. Acute pancreatitis as a complication of anaphylactoid (Henoch-Schonlein) purpura. Arch Dis Child. 1977;52(12):971–2.
14. Puppala AR, Cheng JC, Steinheber FU. Pancreatitis–a rare complication of Schonlein-Henoch purpura. Am J Gastroenterol. 1978;69(1):101–4.
15. Helbling R, Lava SA, Simonetti GD, Camozzi P, Bianchetti MG, Milani GP. Gallbladder and pancreas in Henoch-Schonlein Purpura: review of the literature. J Pediatr Gastroenterol Nutr. 2016;62(3):457–61.
16. Shin JI, Lee JS. Comment on acute pancreatitis: a rare presenting feature of Henoch-Schonlein purpura. J Paediatr Child Health. 2008;44(11):678–9. author reply 679
17. Frigui M, Lehiani D, Koubaa M, Bouaziz Z, Abid B, Beyrouti I, Mnif Z, Bahloul Z, Jemaa MB. Acute pancreatitis as initial manifestation of adult Henoch-Schonlein purpura: report of a case and review of literature. Eur J Gastroenterol Hepatol. 2011;23(2):189–92.
18. Cheung KM, Mok F, Lam P, Chan KH. Pancreatitis associated with Henoch-Schonlein purpura. J Paediatr Child Health. 2001;37(3):311–3.
19. Working Group IAPAPAAPG. IAP/APA evidence-based guidelines for the management of acute pancreatitis. Pancreatology. 2013;13(4 Suppl 2):e1–15.
20. Wang G, Liu Y, Zhou SF, Qiu P, Xu L, Wen P, Wen J, Xiao X. Effect of somatostatin, Ulinastatin and Gabexate on the treatment of severe acute pancreatitis. Am J Med Sci. 2016;351(5):506–12.
21. Kimura T, Zuidema GD, Cameron JL. Steroid administration and acute pancreatitis: studies with an isolated, perfused canine pancreas. Surgery. 1979;85(5):520–4.
22. Takaoka K, Kataoka K, Sakagami J. The effect of steroid pulse therapy on the development of acute pancreatitis induced by closed duodenal loop in rats. J Gastroenterol. 2002;37(7):537–42.
23. Narum S, Westergren T, Klemp M. Corticosteroids and risk of gastrointestinal bleeding: a systematic review and meta-analysis. BMJ Open. 2014;4(5):e004587.

17

Changing outpatient referral patterns in a small pediatric nephrology practice

Coral Hanevold[1*], Susan Halbach[1], Jin Mou[2] and Karyn Yonekawa[1]

Abstract

Background: We have noted a large number of referrals for abnormal kidney imaging and laboratory tests and postulated that such referrals have increased significantly over time. Understanding changes in referral patterns is helpful in tailoring education and communication between specialists and primary providers.

Methods: We performed a retrospective chart review of new patient referrals to Mary Bridge Children's Nephrology clinic for early (2002 to 2004) and late (2011 to 2013) cohorts. The overall and individual frequencies of referrals for various indications were compared.

Results: The overall number of new visits was similar for early (511) and late (509) cohorts. The frequency of referrals for solitary kidneys and multi-cystic dysplastic kidneys, microalbuminuria and abnormal laboratory results increased significantly (Odds Ratio (OR) and 95% Confidence Interval of OR: 1.920 [1.079, 3.390], 2.862 [1.023, 8.006], 2.006 [1.083, 3.716], respectively) over the time interval while the proportion of referrals for urinary tract infections (UTIs) and vesicoureteral reflux (VUR) decreased by half (OR: 0.472, 95% CI: 0.288, 0.633). Similarly, referrals for urinary tract dilation and hydronephrosis occurred significantly less often (8% versus 6%, OR: 0.737, 95% CI: 0.452, 1.204) with similar changes in referrals for voiding issues (OR: 0.281, 95% CI: 0.137, 0.575). However, these changes were not statistically significant. Frequencies for other indications showed little variation.

Conclusions: Changes in indications for referral likely reflect evolution of practice in management of UTIs and VUR and increased use of imaging and laboratory testing by pediatric providers. These findings have relevance for ongoing education of pediatricians and support the need for collaboration between primary providers and nephrologists to assure the judicious use of resources.

Keywords: Nephrology, Ambulatory referrals, Pediatrics

Background

For most pediatric nephrologists, outpatient care constitutes a significant volume of their clinical work. Primary care providers differ in regard to potential triggers for consultation with a pediatric nephrologist. This variation may be due to differences in training, experience, practice philosophy, patient volume, parental attitudes, among other factors. In turn, access to pediatric nephrologists is influenced by factors such as geography, financial considerations, sub-specialty practice approach, overlap with other specialists or other centers, center volume and availability of pediatric nephrologists [1–3]. Requirements for prior evaluation may vary from none to well-defined criteria, depending on the referral indication [4].

The increased availability and utilization of laboratory testing and imaging have been documented over the last two decades) [5–7]. Clinical guidelines for the evaluation and management of vesicoureteral reflux (VUR) have also changed during this time period [8, 9]. To evaluate how these changing practices may have impacted indications for referral to pediatric nephrology, we compared referral indications over two time periods, 2002–2004 and 2011–2013, to Mary Bridge Children's, a general non-academic pediatric nephrology practice in the Pacific Northwest of the United States (US) with a catchment population of 549,000 children and adolescents under 18 years of age.

* Correspondence: coral.hanevold@seattlechildrens.org
[1]Department of Pediatrics, Division of Nephrology, University of Washington, Seattle, WA, USA
Full list of author information is available at the end of the article

Methods

This study was a retrospective chart review of children referred for outpatient evaluation at the pediatric nephrology practice at Mary Bridge Children's during two 24-month time periods: early cohort (July 2002–June 2004) and late cohort (May 2011–April 2013). All visits were conducted by pediatric nephrologists (two and three for early and late cohorts, respectively) who varied between the two time periods. All new referrals for initial outpatient visits were included as well as a limited number of patients with known renal disease transferring care to our center from other programs. New inpatient consults and hospital follow-up visits were excluded. Patients were identified using the Current Procedural Terminology (CPT) codes: "new visits (99202- 99205) AND outpatient consultations (99242- 99245)" in the electronic medical record system. The primary care provider's indication for referral was determined by reviewing documentation by the pediatric nephrologist and was categorized as shown in Table 1. If more than one problem was noted at the time of referral the primary indication leading to referral was used for classification. The indication for referral provided by referring provider differed at times from the diagnosis of the pediatric nephrologist, but for these analyses only referral indications were considered. Hematuria and proteinuria were considered together as the two conditions frequently occur concomitantly. Urinary tract infections (UTIs) and VUR were considered together and separately on subsequent analysis. Children referred for VUR could have a history of UTIs, but referral was prompted by the imaging finding.

Pearson's chi square tests were used to compare the overall composition and distribution of referrals between the two time periods as well as individual referral categories. Additional comparisons were performed considering referrals for abnormal imaging, using the following categories: solitary kidney/multicystic dysplastic kidney, urinary tract dilation or other abnormal finding (cysts, abnormal echogenicity or size, etc). These sub-analyses were also done using the Pearson's chi square test. Taking the early cohort as the reference, risks for each specific referral reasons in the later cohort were calculated and odds ratio was presented with 95% confidence interval. Data were analyzed using Stata 14 (Stata Corp, College Station, TX). This study was fully approved by the MultiCare Health System Institutional Review Board (MHSIRB, IRB Study Number: 11.29). Due to its retrospective data review feature, no patient consent was requested.

Table 1 Indications for Referral

HBP	Elevated blood pressures/hypertension
HEM/PRO	Hematuria and/or proteinuria
UTI/VUR	Urinary tract infection and/or vesicoureteral reflux
ABN IMAGING	Includes solitary kidney, hydronephrosis, dilation of collecting systems, horseshoe kidney, duplicated collecting systems, isolated simple cysts, multicystic kidney, and other minor abnormalities such as abnormal size or appearance of one or both kidneys
↓GFR	Decreased glomerular filtration rate, acute or chronic, includes hemolytic uremic syndrome
STONES/NC	Stones/nephrocalcinosis and hypercalciuria
MICROALB	Microalbuminuria
GLOM/VAS	Glomerular disease or vasculitis, includes nephrotic syndrome, Henoch Schonlein purpura, hereditary nephritis, acute glomerulonephritis or vasculitis of any type
VOIDING ISSUES	Includes enuresis, urinary frequency or urgency, dysuria, polyuria, daytime incontinence
ABN LABS	Abnormal laboratory studies (urine or blood) excluding hypercalciuria, microalbuminuria
OTHER	Such as tuberous sclerosis, polycystic kidney disease, Bardel Biedel syndrome, Beckwith Wiedeman, prenatal counseling, edema, flank pain, family history of kidney disease

Results

The volume of new patients was similar in the two cohorts (511 in early, 509 in late cohorts respectively). Additionally, the distribution across age groups was consistent between the two time periods (data not shown). A summary of differences in referral indications between the time periods is displayed in Table 2. Overall the composition of the referral indications differed between the two time periods ($p < .001$). Looking at specific indications for referrals, abnormal laboratory results were a more frequent reason for referral in the late cohort as compared to the early cohort. Microalbuminuria was considered as a separate category and showed a significant increase from 1 to 3% though the absolute number of patients referred for this indication was small. Referral for voiding issues occurred much less frequently in the later cohort. Hematuria and/or proteinuria and elevated blood pressure or hypertension were the leading indications for referral in both cohorts and did not differ appreciably between the two time periods.

Referrals for UTIs and VUR when considered together showed a significant decline in the latter cohort as compared to the earlier group (Tables 2 and 3). When considered separately, the change for each indication was similar. UTIs (alone) as the indication for referral decreased from 43 (8%) to 20 (4%) while VUR (alone) referrals decreased from 44 (9%) to 21 (4%) ($p < .001$ for both, data not shown).

Referrals for abnormal imaging findings did not show a significant change overall, though did increase from 15 to 19% of total referrals. The results from sub-group analysis of imaging referrals are shown in Table 3. Referrals for urinary tract dilation occurred less frequently in the

Table 2 Referral Indications for Early and Late Cohorts*

Indication for Referral	Early Cohort (2002–2004) *n* (%)	Late Cohorts (2011–2013) *n* (%)	χ^2, *p*	Odds Ratio‡ [95% CI]
HBP	107 (20.9%)	120 (23.6%)	1.024, 0.311	1.165 [0.867, 1.565
HEM/PRO	108 (21.1%)	105 (20.6%)	0.040, 0.842	0.970 [0.717, 1.312]
UTIs/VUR*	87 (17.0%)	41 (8.1%)	18.698, 0.000	0.472 [0.288, 0.633]
ABN IMAGING	79 (15.5%)	96 (19.1%)	2.311, 0.128	1.287 [0.929, 1.784]
VOIDING ISSUES*	34 (6.7%)	10 (2.0%)	13.583, 0.000	0.281 [0.137, 0.575]
↓GFR	21 (4.1%)	18 (3.5%)	0.228, 0.633	0.855 [0.450, 1.625]
STONES/NC	17 (3.3%)	23 (4.5%)	0.961, 0.327	1.375 [0.726, 2.606]
GLOM/VAS	20 (3.9%)	30 (5.9%)	2.145, 0.143	1.538 [0.861, 2.745]
ABN LABS†	16 (3.1%)	31 (6.1%)	5.080, 0.024	2.006 [1.083, 3.716]
MICROALB†	5 (1.0%)	14 (2.8%)	4.380, 0.036	2.862 [1.023, 8.006]
OTHER	17 (3.3%)	21 (4.1%)	0.454, 0.501	1.250 [0.652, 2.399]

Overall frequencies within categories differed ($p < 0.001$ comparing cohorts)
HBP elevated blood pressure or hypertension, *HEM/PRO* hematuria and/or proteinuria, *UTI/VUR* urinary tract infection/vesicoureteral reflux, *ABN* abnormal, *↓GFR* decreased glomerular filtration rate, *NC* nephrocalcinosis; GLOM/VAS, glomerular disease, vasculitis, *LABS* laboratory studies, *MICROALB* microalbuminuria; OTHER (as defined in Table 1)
*$p < .001$, †$p < .05$, ‡Early cohort as reference

later cohort as compared to the earlier group (not statistically significant), while referrals for solitary kidneys/ multi-cystic dysplastic kidneys increased ($p < 0.05$). Miscellaneous imaging findings generated referrals more often in the recent time period but the difference did not reach significance.

Discussion

There are limited data available on indications for nephrology referrals in the outpatient setting. Previous reports included inpatient as well as outpatient referrals, were limited to earlier decades (1977 to 2002) and categorized referrals based on the diagnosis rendered by the nephrologists rather than the referral indication given by primary care physician [10, 11]. Practice changes have occurred in the interim rendering the information less applicable to the current practice of pediatric nephrology. For example, one of these older analyses encompassed a time period before prenatal ultrasounds were performed or at least before they had become routine [10]. Additionally, with the inclusion of inpatient consultations in these older studies, it is not possible to determine what may have prompted primary care providers to request outpatient nephology consultations, the focus of the current study [10, 11]. There is a more recent study that addressed adherence to waiting time recommendations and reviewed outpatient referral to a single Canadian tertiary pediatric nephrology center during the period of 2007 to 2008 [4]. Their findings showed some similarities to ours with congenital abnormalities of the urinary tract and hydronephrosis (17%), hematuria or proteinuria (combined 22%), UTIs (12%) and elevated blood pressure (12%) accounting for almost 2/3 of the referrals.

Our study differs from these previous reports in that it offers a comparison of referral indications over a decade and focuses solely on the referring providers' perception

Table 3 Referrals for Imaging

	Early cohort (2002–2004)	Late cohort (2011–2013)	
Referral Indication	n (% within cohort, % within category)	n (% within cohort, % within category)	χ [2], *p*; Odds Ratio [95% CI of OR]
Total	79 (15.5%)	96 (18.9%)	2.311, 0.128, 1.287 [0.929, 1.784]
ABN, US, OR CT IMAGING	20 (3.9, 25.0%)	31 (6.1, 32.0%)	2.543, 0.111, 1.592 [0.895, 2.832]
SK OR MCKD*	19 (3.7, 24%)	35 (6.9, 37.0%)	5.072, 0.024, 1.920 [1.079, 3.390]
HYDRO/DILATION UT	40 (7.8, 51.0%)	30 (5.9, 31.0%)	1.492, 0.222, 0.737 [0.452, 1.204]

ABN abnormal, *US* ultrasound, *CT* computed tomography, *SK* solitary kidney, *MCDK* multi-cystic dysplastic kidney, *HYDRO/DILATION UT*, hydronephrosis/dilation of urinary tract
*$p < 0.05$

of the indication for pediatric nephrology input. Interestingly, we found a high rate of referral for abnormal imaging or laboratory results with a combined percentage of 18 and 25% for the early and late time periods, respectively. Comparison of our two cohorts demonstrated an increase in the number of referrals generated due to abnormal imaging in the latter group. These findings were not due to increasing recognition of antenatal hydronephrosis as the number of referrals for urinary tract dilation and hydronephrosis was reduced. Instead, referrals for solitary kidneys/multi-cystic dysplastic kidneys doubled. Referrals for various other abnormalities found on imaging such as isolated renal cysts, abnormal appearance or size of kidneys occurred at an increased frequency but due to our small numbers did not reach significance. Also as clinically suspected, referrals for abnormal laboratory studies occurred significantly more often in the recent cohort of patients. Primary care physicians faced with interpreting abnormal imaging or laboratory results may not feel qualified to advise parents on the significance of the findings. A recent survey of general pediatricians with 5 years or less of experience reported that 51% never or rarely cared for children needing nephrology services and 21% felt additional training in nephrology during residency would have been helpful [12]. Additionally, proximity to subspecialty care would be expected to factor into decision making. In the survey mentioned above, general pediatricians in rural settings were more comfortable managing subspecialty issues on their own as compared to those with local access to subspecialties [12]. In turn, parental expectations for access to pediatric subspecialties may be tempered in geographically remote areas [1].

Another novel finding demonstrated here was a reduction in the frequency of referral for UTIs and VUR. When considered together the proportion of referrals for these indications in our early cohort was 17% which was the same as the 16% reported by Radina et al., during the time period of 2007–2008 [4]. However, in our late cohort (2011–2013) the proportion of referrals for UTIs or VUR dropped in half for each category. In 2011 the American Academy of Pediatrics (AAP) issued guidelines which limited indications for imaging for VUR after UTIs with similar guidelines endorsed in the United Kingdom by the National Institute for Health and Clinical Excellence earlier in 2007 [8, 13]. Thus, our reduction in referrals for VUR may be due in part to a reduction in the frequency of imaging for VUR by community physicians. Additionally, the contribution of bowel and bladder dysfunction to the risk for recurrent UTIs has been increasingly appreciated and emphasized in educational forums for primary care physicians. Enhanced awareness of this connection may have empowered many to feel more comfortable addressing recurrent UTIs as well as various voiding issues on their own [8, 9, 14, 15]. Likewise, the reduction in referrals for urinary tract dilation and hydronephrosis might to some degree reflect increasing experience and evolution of practice in management of antenatal hydronephrosis [16, 17]. A recent multidisciplinary consensus statement on classification of antenatal and postnatal urinary tract dilation reflects a move toward standardization and should be helpful as it becomes more widely adopted [18].

Our study has several limitations. Instead of a full decade between time periods the gap between our study cohorts was approximately nine years. Electronic medical records were not available prior to July 2002 and review of paper records was not feasible due to offsite storage with high risk for incomplete data collection. However, the time span between the two cohorts was considered sufficient given evolving practices for issues such as prenatal hydronephrosis, UTIs and VUR between the study periods. Data were derived from a single general pediatric nephrology practice in a non-academic setting and may not reflect referral patterns in larger centers, or at centers with large catchment areas. However, the small number of nephrologists in our practice is not unusual for pediatric nephrology. The recent Pediatric Nephrology Workforce Survey reported an overall median group size of 4 with 46% of pediatric nephrologists practicing in groups of 3 or less [19]. Also, 27% reported practicing in a non-academic setting [19]. Additionally, use of the primary indication for referral likely resulted in some misclassification. The referral indication as specified by the primary care provider may not describe the actual finding(s) or diagnosis subsequently made by the nephrologist and secondary reasons for referral were not included. Our focus was the primary provider's perception of the issue warranting a pediatric nephrology referral and not the final categorization by the nephrologist. It is possible that the observed decrease in referral for UTIs and VUR might be due to an increase in referrals to urology. Although this possibility cannot be excluded, the number of urology practices in our referral area did not change or enlarge between the two time periods. The reduction in referrals for voiding issues may reflect a change in our practice with more of these children being directed to urology rather than nephrology. Lastly, in rare instances children with known renal disease were referred to our practice after newly relocating to the area, or after pediatric nephrology services at a large nearby military base became unavailable. In such instances these children were considered new patients though in reality reflected a request for ongoing care.

The large proportion of referrals prompted by imaging and laboratory findings noted here supports the need for enhanced communication between providers. A survey of pediatricians conducted by the AAP in 2010 reported that 61% of rural and 46% of non-rural pediatricians perceived inadequate access to pediatric nephrologists

[2]. Traditional access in the form of office consultation will continue to be a challenge as recent surveys by the AAP and the American Society of Pediatric Nephrology indicate that the work force is aging and limited in numbers and location [19]. Investigators from Texas and North Carolina have reported that phone consultations with pediatric subspecialists frequently allowed for continued local management and often obviated the need for an outpatient visit [20, 21]. These studies suggest that improved access to pediatric subspecialists electronically or via telephone could impact on decisions for referral and improve use of limited resources [20].

Conclusion

Changes in indications for referral noted here likely reflect the evolution of clinical practice with regard to increased use of imaging, laboratory testing and updates in UTI/VUR practice guidelines over the two studied time periods of 2002–2004 and 2011–2013. These findings have implications for the education of primary care providers and pediatric nephrologists, particularly with regard to the use and interpretation of imaging studies. Whether increasing utilization of diagnostic studies is impacting referral patterns for other subspecialties is unknown. Further investigation along this line would help determine if our single center findings indicate changes in referrals to Pediatric Nephrology, or are reflective of broad changes in general pediatric practice. Given the ever increasing complexities of diagnostic modalities and the challenges inherent in providing subspecialty services, open communication between primary care providers and pediatric nephrologists is critical to the provision of necessary and timely services.

Abbreviations

OR: odds ratio; UTI: urinary tract infection; VUR: vesicoureteral reflux

Acknowledgments

The authors wish to thank Robin Hamman, RN for her assistance in conducting chart reviews. The authors would like to acknowledge the assistance and help given by Dr. Paul Amoroso and Ms. Anne Reedy from MIRI. We also would like to thank Mary Bridge Children's Foundation and MIRI for making the Open Access choice possible.

Funding

Mary Bridge Children's Foundation and MultiCare Institute for Research & Innovation (MIRI) supported this study through each of their research funding mechanisms.

Authors' contributions

CH conceptualized and designed the study, performed chart reviews, compiled data, prepared manuscript and submitted the final manuscript. SH made a substantial contribution to design of the study, performed chart reviews, performed statistical analyses and participated in preparation and editing of manuscript drafts. JM made a substantial contribution to the analysis and interpretation of results, participated in preparation and editing of manuscript. KY made a substantial contribution to design of the study, performed chart reviews and participated in review of drafts and revisions. All authors have read and approve of the final version of the manuscript.

Competing interests

The authors declare that they have no competing interests.

Author details

[1]Department of Pediatrics, Division of Nephrology, University of Washington, Seattle, WA, USA. [2]MultiCare Institute for Research & Innovation, MultiCare Health System, Tacoma, WA, USA.

References

1. Ray KN, Bogen DL, Bertolet M, Forrest CB, Mehrotra A. Supply and utilization of pediatric subspecialties in the United States. Pediatrics. 2014;133(6):1061–9.
2. Pletcher BA, Rimsza ME, Cull WL, Shipman SA, Shugerman RP, O'Connor KG. Primary care pediatricians' satisfaction with subspecialty care, perceived supply and barriers to care. J Pediatr. 2010;156(6):1011–5.
3. Mayer ML. Are we there yet? Distance to care and relative supply among pediatric medical subspecialties. Pediatrics. 2006;118(6):2313–21.
4. Radina M, Sharma AP, Yarin A, Filler G. Adherence to waiting-time targets for pediatric nephrology clinic referrals. Pediatr Nephrol. 2010;25:311–6.
5. Abbott M, Paulin H, Sidhu D, Naugler C. Laboratory tests interpretation and use of resources. Can Fam Physician. 2014;60(3):e167–72.
6. Alonso-Cerezo MC, Martin JS, Montes MAG, de la Iglesin VM. Appropriate utilization of clinical laboratory tests. Clin Chem Lab Med. 2009;47(12):1461–5.
7. Tompane T, Bush R, Dansky T, Huang JS. Diagnostic imaging studies performed in children over a 9-year period. Pediatrics. 2013;131(1):e45–52.
8. Paintsil E. Update on recent guidelines for the management of urinary tract infections in children: the shifting paradigm. Curr Opin Pediatr. 2013;25(1):88–94.
9. Jackson EC. Urinary tract infections in children: knowledge update and a salute to the future. Pediatr Rev. 2015;36(4):153–64. quiz 165-166
10. Scheinman JI, Foreman JW, Chan JCM. Perspective of a pediatric nephrology program: an 18 year retrospective. Acta Paediatr Sin. 1997;38(5):352–35.
11. Filler G, Payne RP, Orrbine E, Clifford T, Drukker A, McLaine PN. Changing trends in the referral patterns of pediatric nephrology patients. Pediatr Nephrol. 2005;20:603–8.
12. Freed GL, Dunham KM, Switalski KE, Jones MD, McGuinness GA. Recently trained general pediatricians: perspectives on residency training and scope of practice. Pediatrics. 2009;123:S38–43.
13. Roberts KB, Subcommittee on urinary tract infections and steering committee on quality improvement and management. Urinary tract infection: clinical practice guidelines for the diagnosis and management of the initial UTI in febrile infants and children 2-24 months. Pediatrics. 2011;128(3):595–610.
14. Hellerstein S, Linebarger JS. Voiding dysfunction in pediatric patients. Clin Pediatr (Phila). 2003;42:43–9.
15. Vande Walle J, Rittig S, Bauer S, Eggert P, Marschall-Kehrel D, Tekgul S. Practical consensus guidelines for the management of enuresis. Eur J Pediatr. 2012;171:971–83.
16. Cheng AM, Phan V, Geary DF, Rosenblum ND. Outcome of isolated antenatal hydronephrosis. Arch Pediatr Adolesc Med. 2004;158(1):38–40.
17. Becker AM. Postnatal evaluation of infants with an abnormal antenatal renal sonogram. Curr Opin Pediatr. 2009;21(2):207–13.
18. Nguyen HT, Benson CB, Bromley B, et al. Multidisciplinary census on the classification of prenatal and postnatal urinary tract dilation (UTD classification system). J Pediatr Urol. 2014;10(6):982–99.
19. Primack WA, Meyers KE, Kirkwood SJ, Ruch-Ross HS, Radabaugh CL, Greenbaum LA. The US pediatric nephrology workforce: a report commissioned by the American Academy of Pediatrics. Am J Kidney Dis. 2015;66(1):33–9.
20. Lister G. 2011 Joseph W. St Geme Jr lecture: five things I'd like to see changed in American pediatrics, five lessons I've learned. Pediatrics. 2012; 129(5):961–7.
21. Wegner SE, Humble CG, Feaganes J, Stiles AD. Estimated savings from paid telephone consultations between subspecialists and primary care physicians. Pediatrics. 2008;122(6):e1136–40.

18

Folk prescription for treating rhinitis as a rare cause of childhood lead poisoning

Xiao-Lan Ying[1], Morri Markowitz[2] and Chong-Huai Yan[1*]

Abstract

Background: Folk prescriptions continue to be important sources of childhood lead poisoning. Nasal spray folk prescriptions for treating rhinitis has only been reported once previously as a cause of lead poisoning.

Case presentation: We identified three pediatric cases of severe lead poisoning caused by nasal spray folk medicines prescribed for treating rhinitis. The three patients had similar clinical manifestations including: severe abdominal pain, headache, pale appearance and fatigue. Liver function tests were abnormal. Blood lead levels (BLLs) of the three patients were 91 μg/dL, 91 μg/dL, and 105 μg/dL, respectively. After chelation BLLs decreased. The lead content of the three folk remedies as measured by inductively coupled plasma mass spectrometry (ICP-MS) were 14.8, 22.3, and 33.4%. All the symptoms resolved during a course of chelation therapy. There were no severe side effects of treatment.

Conclusions: Nasal spray folk prescriptions for treating rhinitis may contain extremely high bio-accessible lead content and are potential sources of lead poisoning. Clinicians should be alert to this possibility especially in those children presenting with multisystem symptoms.

Keywords: Child, Lead poisoning, Folk medicine, Nasal spray, Rhinitis

Background

Eliminating pediatric lead poisoning remains a world-wide challenge [1, 2]. Since symptoms of lead poisoning are nonspecific, such as abdominal pain, pale appearance, behavioral changes, headaches, fatigue, and irritability [3], the possibility of lead poisoning is easily overlooked. Thus the correct diagnosis can be delayed resulting in progression of toxicity.

The accurate identification of at-risk populations from unusual sources of lead exposure is essential to prevent further toxicity. Some cases of lead poisoning caused by folk medicines have been reported in recent years [4–6]. However, to our knowledge, only one case of lead poisoning due to a nasal spray folk remedy has been reported [7].

Extremely elevated BLLs (BLLs ≥70 μg/dL) now occur rarely in children [8]. We report three cases of severe childhood lead poisoning from folk medications specifically prescribed for treating rhinitis. These cases were complicated by concurrent abnormal liver function which can affect lead poisoning treatment.

Case presentation

Case 1

A 7-year-old boy was referred to our hospital for an elevated BLL (> 60 μg/dL) discovered during routine screening procedures. On admission, a recheck of the BLL, tested by Atomic Absorption Spectrometry (AAS), showed the level to be 91 μg/dL. Thus the diagnosis of lead poisoning was confirmed.

Two months before admission, he started to feel dizzy and developed headaches. Symptoms progressed to poor appetite, mouth-bitterness, repeated vomiting and abdominal pain for more than a month. The abdominal pain was intermittent, without an obvious precipitant and generally lasted for 10 min with spontaneous

* Correspondence: yanchonghuai@xinhuamed.com.cn; yanch@shkeylab-ceh.org
[1]MOE-Shanghai Key Laboratory of Children's Environmental Health, Xinhua Hospital affiliated to Shanghai Jiaotong University School of Medicine, Shanghai 200092, China
Full list of author information is available at the end of the article

resolution. Subsequently, intense joint pain and fatigue occurred causing him to be unable to walk by himself.

Before admission, he had been hospitalized twice elsewhere. At his first presentation 2 months earlier, laboratory examinations found elevated serum liver enzymes: alanine transaminase (ALT) 145 U/L and aspartate aminotransferase (AST) 78 U/L. He also had anemia with a hemoglobin (Hb) level of 96 g/L and red blood cell (RBC) count of 3.67×10^{12}/L). Superficial gastritis and bile reflux were found by endoscopy. An upper abdominal CT angiography showed "a general decrease in liver density; possible superior mesenteric artery syndrome". A descriptive diagnosis of "chronic superficial gastritis, possible superior mesenteric artery syndrome, and abnormal liver function tests" was made. He was treated with omeprazole and sucralfate for 2 weeks which was accompanied by relief of his symptoms. He was discharged from the hospital without an identified etiology.

Ten days after discharge, he was admitted to another hospital for intermittent vomiting and severe abdominal pain. Liver function tests, electroencephalogram and abdominal ultrasonography were normal. An incidental BLL test was performed (this hospital tests lead routinely) and reported as elevated. He was referred to our hospital for further evaluation and treatment.

On admission to our hospital, his examination found a soft, non-tender abdomen without rebound tenderness. Both liver and spleen were impalpable. Neurologic examination was normal. Abnormally increased pigmentation of the gums ("lead line") was observed (Fig. 1). No radiopaque point masses were identified on anteroposterior abdominal radiography. Anteroposterior radiograph of the knees (Fig. 2) showed increased linear radio-density at the distal femoral and proximal tibial and fibular metaphyses. Serum chemistries were normal. The RBC count was 3.68×10^{12}/L (reference range 4.0–5.5×10^{12}/L) and the Hb level was 101 g/L (reference range 120-150 g/L), consistent with anemia.

A more detailed history about sources of lead exposure was taken. He had been using a red-colored folk medicine (Fig. 3), spraying it in the nostrils two to four times a day during the week prior to consulting a doctor. The nasal spray liquid was obtained from a traditional Chinese medicine (TCM) practitioner (Shenzhen, Guangdong, China). Analysis of the liquid revealed a lead concentration of 148,000 mg/kg (14.8%) as measured by ICP-MS.

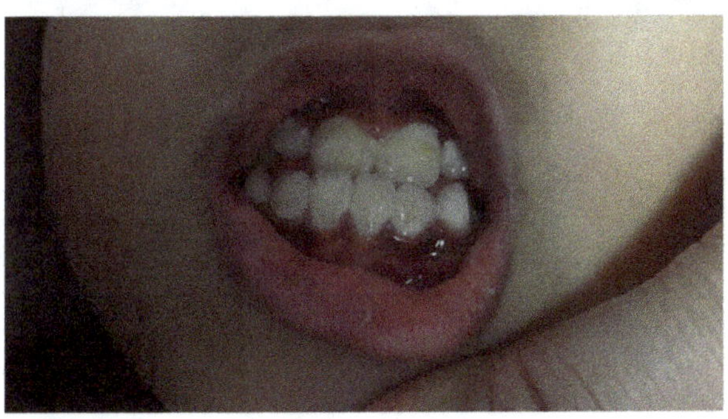

Fig. 1 Gum lead line

Chelation therapy combined orally administered dimercaptosuccinic acid (DMSA) (350 mg/m^2 body surface area, q8h) and intravenous calcium disodium edetate ($CaNa_2EDTA$) (1 g/m^2 body surface area, continuous infusion using a micro-pump over 24 h) for 5 days. Glutathione (600 mg, intravenous drip, once a day) was added as an antioxidant. All the symptoms resolved; and the BLL declined to 21 μg/dL after chelation therapy was completed.

Case 2

An 8-year-old girl with rhinitis had consulted the same TCM practitioner as in case 1 and was prescribed the same nasal spray liquid to be used twice a day for 10 days. She developed severe abdominal colic, vomiting, constipation and felt fatigued. Her venous BLL was 91 μg/dL. The nasal spray contained 223,000 mg/kg (22.3%) lead. Abnormal laboratory test results included: creatine kinase 747 U/L (reference range 30–135 U/L), creatine kinase isoenzyme MB 14.8 ng/mL (reference range 0–6.8 ng/mL); AST 119 U/L (reference range 8–38 U/L), ALT 390 U/L (reference range 0-75 U/L). Radiography of the abdomen revealed shadow of stool and gas as well as points of increased density (Fig. 4).

It could not be determined whether the radiopaque particles seen on the abdominal x-ray contained lead or not. Since chelating agents may increase gut lead absorption, folium sennae was administered as a cathartic to eliminate lead from the intestine prior to initiating chelation. The chelation regimen was identical with case 1. However, after 2 days of therapy the white blood cell count fell to 2.11×10^9/L (normal range: 4.0–10.0×10^9/L). This may be attributed to DMSA, which was withheld subsequently. Chelation continued with an intravenous infusion of $CaNa_2EDTA$ to achieve a BLL of 36 μg/dL at the end of 5 days.

Case 3

A 5-year-old boy had consulted the same TCM practitioner as in Cases 1 and 2 and was prescribed the same medication to be used twice a day for 7 days. Severe abdominal pain and vomiting followed. Prior to transfer to our hospital his initial laboratory data showed markedly elevated liver enzyme levels (ALT 1083 U/L, AST 972 U/L). No abnormality was found on abdominal x-ray. On examination, his liver was palpable 4 cm below the right costal margin. The BLL on admission was 105 μg/dL. The nasal spray contained 33.4% lead.

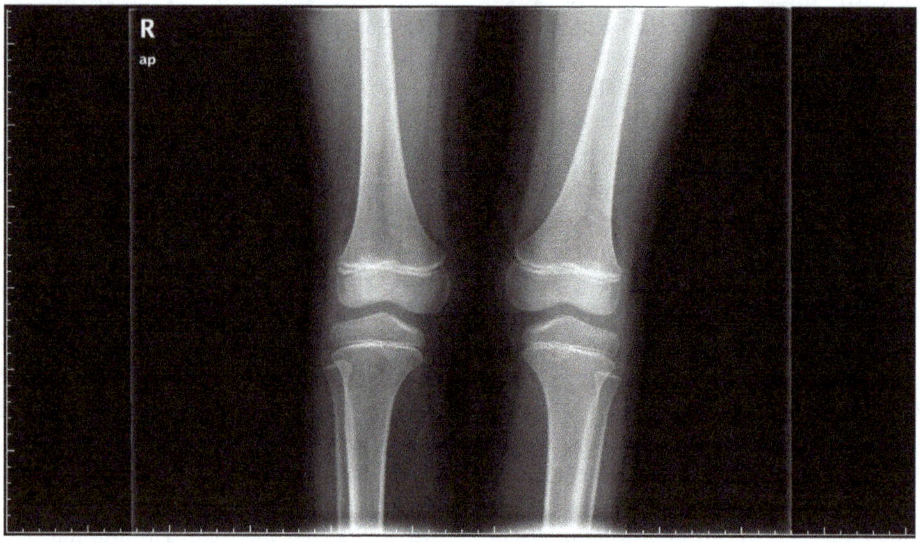

Fig. 2 Anteroposterior radiograph of the knees bilaterally

Chelation therapy was initially withheld because of the severely altered liver enzyme results as both drugs are potentially hepatotoxic. Initially, he received treatment aimed at improving liver function with glutathione and disodium glycyrrhetate (Table 1) and continued to receive these medications during the whole course of treatment. As his liver function tests improved, his BLL went down concomitantly, prior to chelation (Table 1, BLL of Day 1: 105 μg/dL; Day 4: 96 μg/dL; Day 8: 80 μg/dL) at which point chelation treatment was initiated with DMSA and $CaNa_2EDTA$ infusion (same usage as Case 1). The post-chelation lead level for this child was 34 μg/dL. No adverse events happened to all the three children.

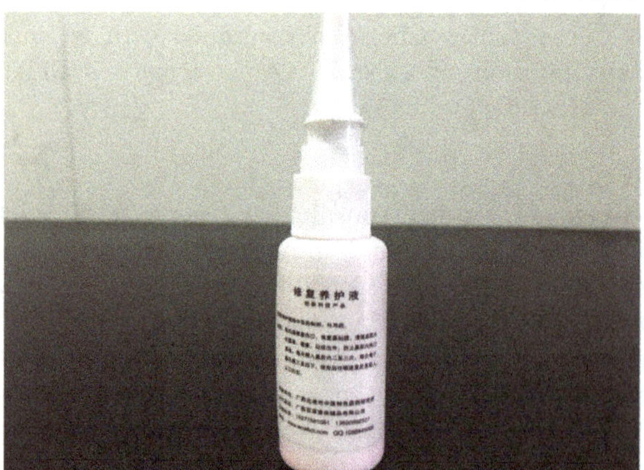

Fig. 3 Folk medicine for treating rhinitis

Discussion

Absorption of lead

Ingestion and inhalation are the two primary modes of lead entry into the body. The former is more common in children due to hand-to-mouth activity, while the latter occurs more frequently in occupationally exposed adults [9]. The percentage of lead absorbed from the gut depends on factors as follows: particle size, gastric pH,

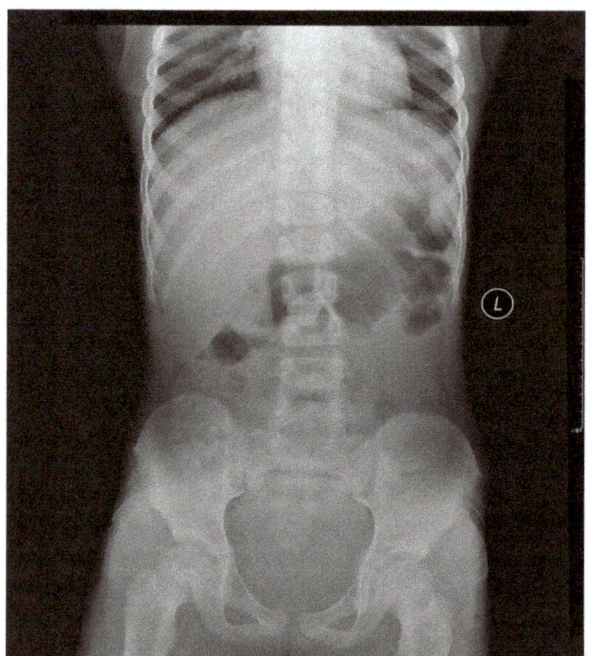

Fig. 4 Radiography of the abdomen

Table 1 Liver function test during therapy

Variable	Reference range	Day1[a]	Day 2	Day 3	Day 4	Day 5	Day 6	Day 7	Day8[b]	Day9	Day10	Day13
ALT (U/L)	0–75	641	521	415	317	254	197	176	117	124	14	67
AST (U/L)	8–38	280	137	102	91	85	75	81	57	93	23	40

[a]Day 1: Start to get liver-protecting treatment in our hospital
[b]Day 8: Start chelation therapy combined with liver-protecting treatment

other material in the gut, and nutritional status of essential elements [10]. Inhalational absorption through the lung depends on particle size.

The three patients had reportedly short-term exposures to nasal spray liquids for treating rhinitis that had extremely high lead concentrations. The short period of exposure is consistent with acute lead poisoning. This folk remedy was sprayed directly into the nostrils. All three children mentioned that they tasted and swallowed the liquid. Thus, the lead was potentially absorbed from multiple sites including the nasal mucosa, the lungs, as well as the gastrointestinal tract.

Diagnosis of lead poisoning

Abdominal pain caused by lead poisoning has been reported [11, 12]. Possibly the delay in diagnosis in our patients was due to a lack of awareness by the physicians of its features in children. This highlights the need to educate clinicians including subspecialists about this disease. Lead poisoning should be in the list of possible diagnoses for children with unexplained multi-systems symptoms, especially of the gastrointestinal and central nervous systems.

These children also had detectable signs of lead poisoning. The line of gingival hyperpigmentation [13] in the first patient has been described in occupationally lead exposed adults [14]. He also had a "lead line" on long bone radiography. The width of the dense metaphysis has been reported to correlate with the length of the period of toxic exposure [15].

Folk remedy as a potential source of lead poisoning

Lead poisoning can be diagnosed through the determination of the lead concentration in whole blood. In children, an elevated BLL indicates the need to identify the sources of exposure that likely lead to ingestion. While typical environmental sources predominate as the cause of lead poisoning, cultural factors are also important. Besides lead-containing paint, various sources of lead were identified for children with BLL ≥ 45 μg/dL in New York City: imported spices, cosmetics, as well as traditional folk medicines [8]. A detailed history about the usage of traditional folk medicine is essential. Laboratory analyses of these medicines will then determine the lead content.

Lead poisoning due to folk remedies for treating skin problems [16], abdominal pain [17], epilepsy [18], or "strengthening eyes" [19] have been reported before. However, a nasal spray folk remedy for treating rhinitis as a potential source of lead poisoning has only been reported in a single adult [7]. As shown in Fig. 3 the container can look completely ordinary for a nasal spray and is clearly not an indicator of safety. Usage of such products in children should prompt clinicians to consider lead screening and public health agencies to educate local communities of the risks of their use.

Historically, the compositions of folk medicines were proprietary and medicine containers did not indicate the constituents. Given the high concentrations that we found it's likely that the Traditional Chinese Healer purposefully added lead to the nasal spray, presumably because he felt it offered a therapeutic benefit. Given the known and potentially lethal toxicity of lead, its medicinal use should be prohibited. These cases highlight the need for governmental oversight of folk medicine content.

Treatment of lead intoxication

Despite intestinal and neurological symptoms the diagnosis of lead poisoning was delayed. Hepatotoxicity was observed in our patients as evidenced by elevated transaminase levels. Both DMSA and $CaNa_2EDTA$ can be hepatotoxic; pretreatment evaluation of liver function is necessary. With DMSA, a transient mild rise of hepatic transaminases is the most common adverse effect reported, generally resolving on discontinuation of treatment without long-term sequelae. Published studies on the frequency of this transaminase increase differ, varying between < 1.5 and 60% of patients [20, 21]. In a multicenter placebo controlled DMSA trial conducted in children with initial BLLs between 20 and 45 μg/dL, no difference in the rate of elevated ALT levels in treated versus untreated children was observed [22].

Although hepatic damage is not a common feature of childhood lead poisoning [23, 24], animal studies have found that chronic lead poisoning caused mild histological and histochemical changes in the liver [25]. The very high liver enzyme levels in case 3 delayed chelation. With the conservative approach taken, liver function recovered quickly and BLLs declined. Spontaneous excretion of lead in patients with acute lead poisoning may have a greater impact on BLLs than those with more chronic lead poisoning since lead has not had time to accumulate in bone.

Conclusions

Although the differential diagnosis of lead poisoning is broad, any child who presents with unexplained GI and CNS symptoms should undergo a BLL test, which will directly support or reject the diagnosis of lead toxicity.

Folk remedies for treating rhinitis can be an unexpected source of lead exposure. It is incumbent on pediatricians to perform a diligent search for unconventional sources of lead when confronted with cases without an apparent etiology.

Abbreviations

AAS: Atomic absorption spectroscopy; ALT: Alanine transaminase; AST: Aspartate Aminotransferas; BLLs: Blood lead levels; $CaNa_2EDTA$: Calcium disodium edetate; DMSA: Dimercaptosuccinic acid; Hb: Hemoglobin; ICP-MS: Inductively coupled plasma mass spectrometry; RBC: Red blood cells; TCM: Traditional Chinese medicine

Acknowledgements

This work was supported by the grant from the National Basic Research Program of China (Technology 973 Program, Grant No. 2012CB525001).

Funding

This work was supported by the National Basic Research Program of China (Technology 973 Program, Grant No. 2012CB525001) in the collection, analysis, and interpretation of data and in writing the manuscript.

Authors' contributions

XY collected the materials of the case, carried out the initial analyses, drafted the initial manuscript, and approved the final manuscript as submitted. MM reviewed and revised the manuscript, and approved the final manuscript as submitted. CY designed the data collection instruments, and coordinated and supervised data collection, critically reviewed the manuscript, and approved the final manuscript as submitted. All authors approved the final manuscript as submitted and agree to be accountable for all aspects of the work.

Competing interests

The authors declare that they have no competing interests.

Author details

[1]MOE-Shanghai Key Laboratory of Children's Environmental Health, Xinhua Hospital affiliated to Shanghai Jiaotong University School of Medicine, Shanghai 200092, China. [2]Division of Environmental Sciences, Children's Hospital at Montefiore, Albert Einstein College of Medicine, Bronx NY10467, USA.

References

1. McClure LF, Niles JK, Kaufman HW. Blood lead levels in young children: US, 2009-2015. J Pediatr. 2016;175:173–81.
2. Falk H. International environmental health for the pediatrician: case study of lead poisoning. Pediatrics. 2003;112(1 Pt 2):259–64.
3. Woolf AD, Goldman R, Bellinger DC. Update on the clinical management of childhood lead poisoning. Pediatr Clin North Am. 2007;54(2):271–94. viii
4. Breeher L, Mikulski MA, Czeczok T, et al. A cluster of lead poisoning among consumers of Ayurvedic medicine. Int J Occup Environ Health. 2015;21(4):303–7.
5. Lin CG, Schaider LA, Brabander DJ, et al. Pediatric lead exposure from imported Indian spices and cultural powders. Pediatrics. 2010;125(4):e828–35.
6. Woolf AD, Hussain J, McCullough L, et al. Infantile lead poisoning from an Asian tongue powder: a case report & subsequent public health inquiry. Clin Toxicol (Phila). 2008;46(9):841–4.
7. Lan F, Lin J, Chen MX. [A case of nonindustrial lead poisoning caused by the nasal spray folk prescription](in Chinese). Strait J Prev Med. 2014; 20(06):93–4.
8. Keller B, Faciano A, Tsega A, et al. Epidemiologic characteristics of children with blood lead levels >/=45 mug/dL. J Pediatr. 2017;180:229–34.
9. Dapul H, Laraque D. Lead poisoning in children. Adv Pediatr Infect Dis. 2014;61(1):313–33.
10. Markowitz M. Lead poisoning. In: Kliegman RM, editor. Nelson textbook of pediatrics [M]. 19th Elsevier Saunders; 2011. p. 2448–53.
11. Shamshirsaz AA, Yankowitz J, Rijhsinghani A, et al. Severe lead poisoning caused by use of health supplements presenting as acute abdominal pain during pregnancy. Obstet Gynecol. 2009;114(2 Pt 2):448–50.
12. Frith D, Yeung K, Thrush S, et al. Lead poisoning–a differential diagnosis for abdominal pain. Lancet. 2005;366(9503):2146.
13. Pearce JM. Burton's line in lead poisoning. Eur Neurol. 2007;57(2):118–9.
14. Nogue S, Culla A. Images in clinical medicine. Burton's line. N Engl J Med. 2006;354(20):e21.
15. Chandrasekar S, Lomasney LM, Derhammer N. Systemic lead toxicity. Orthopedics. 2015;38(10):592. 644–597
16. Mathee A, Naicker N, Teare J. Retrospective investigation of a lead poisoning outbreak from the consumption of an Ayurvedic medicine: Durban, South Africa. Int J Environ Res Public Health. 2015;12(7):7804–13.
17. Cabb EE, Gorospe EC, Rothweiler AM, et al. Toxic remedy: a case of a 3-year-old child with lead colic treated with lead monoxide (greta). Clin Pediatr (Phila). 2008;47(1):77–9.
18. Ying XL, Xu J, Markowitz M, et al. Pediatric lead poisoning from folk prescription for treating epilepsy. Clin Chim Acta. 2016;461:130–4.
19. Jones TF, Moore WL, Craig AS, et al. Hidden threats: lead poisoning from unusual sources. Pediatrics. 1999;104(5 Pt 2):1223–5.
20. Bradberry S, Vale A. Dimercaptosuccinic acid (succimer; DMSA) in inorganic lead poisoning. Clin Toxicol (Phila). 2009;47(7):617–31.
21. Thurtle N, Greig J, Cooney L, et al. Description of 3,180 courses of chelation with dimercaptosuccinic acid in children≤ 5 y with severe lead poisoning in Zamfara, northern Nigeria: a retrospective analysis of programme data. PLoS Med. 2014;11(10):e1001739.
22. Rogan WJ, Bornschein RL, Chisolm JJ, et al. Safety and efficacy of succimer in toddlers with blood lead levels of 20-44 μg/dL. Pediatr Res. 2000;48(5):593–9.
23. Verheij J, Voortman J, van Nieuwkerk CM, et al. Hepatic morphopathologic findings of lead poisoning in a drug addict: a case report. J Gastrointestin Liver Dis. 2009;18(2):225–7.
24. Beattie AD, Mullin PJ, Baxter RH, et al. Acute lead poisoning: an unusual cause of hepatitis. Scott Med J. 1979;24(4):318–21.
25. Jarrar BM, Taib NT. Histological and histochemical alterations in the liver induced by lead chronic toxicity. Saudi J Biol Sci. 2012;19(2):203–10.

19

Xanthine calculi in a patient with Lesch-Nyhan syndrome and factor V Leiden treated with allopurinol

Lisa B. E. Shields[1], Dennis S. Peppas[2] and Eran Rosenberg[2*]

Abstract

Background: Lesch-Nyhan syndrome is a rare inborn error of purine metabolism marked by a complete deficiency of the enzyme hypoxanthine-guanine phosphoribosyltransferase (HPRT). Inherited as an X-linked recessive genetic disorder that primarily affects males, patients with Lesch-Nyhan syndrome exhibit severe neurological impairments, including choreoathetosis, ballismus, cognitive dysfunction, and self-injurious behavior. Uric acid levels are usually abnormally high, leading to kidney and bladder stones which often necessitate urological intervention. Factor V Leiden is an autosomal dominant disorder of blood clotting associated with hypercoagulability, thrombophilia, and renal disease.

Case presentation: We present the first reported case of xanthine calculi in a patient with Lesch-Nyhan syndrome and Factor V Leiden who was treated with allopurinol. A renal ultrasound and CT scan demonstrated bilateral staghorn calculi in the kidneys as well as nephrocalcinosis. Two years earlier the patient underwent cystoscopy with bilateral ureteroscopy and laser lithotripsy, and he was stone free afterwards. The patient subsequently underwent bilateral percutaneous nephrolithotomy (PCNL) and was stone free following the procedure. Patients with endogenous overproduction of uric acid who are being treated with allopurinol have a higher chance of developing xanthine stones.

Conclusions: Pediatricians treating these children should be aware of these rare conditions and promptly manage the potential complications that may require medical or surgical intervention.

Keywords: Pediatrics, Lesch-Nyhan, Kidney stones, Allopurinol, Factor V Leiden

Background

Initially described in 1964, Lesch-Nyhan syndrome is characterized by a triad of hyperuricemia, central nervous system dysfunction, and familial inheritance and has an incidence of 1:100,000 to 1:300,000 [1, 2]. Neurological abnormalities include spasticity, cognitive impairment, impulsivity, hematological disorders such as megaloblastic anemia or microcytic anemia, and compulsive self-injurious behavior, specifically, lip biting or finger chewing [1, 3–5]. Uric acid overproduction often leads to lithiasis and gout [5].

The enzyme hypoxanthine-guanine phosphoribosyltransferase (HPRT) plays an important role in uric acid synthesis and purine metabolism [6]. HPRT-deficient patients have purine overproduction and elevated uric acid levels. A spectrum of diseases results from mutations of the HPRT gene, and the severity of the molecular defect correlates with the clinical phenotype [3, 5, 6]. Partial HPRT deficiency as observed in Kelley-Seegmiller syndrome is manifested by excessive purine synthesis, gout, and no neurological involvement [7, 8]. Inherited as an X-linked recessive disorder generally affecting males, Lesch-Nyhan syndrome represents the most severe phenotype [5].

Factor V Leiden, the most common cause of inherited thrombophilia, is associated with a mutation making it resistant to the action of the natural anticoagulant activated protein C (APC) [9]. APC is unable to prevent Factor V Leiden from producing more fibrin. Heterozygous Factor V Leiden is found in approximately 5% of the

* Correspondence: eran.rosenberg@nortonhealthcare.org
[2]Norton Children's Urology, Norton Healthcare, Louisville, KY 40207, USA
Full list of author information is available at the end of the article

Caucasian population and poses an increased risk of developing deep venous thrombosis, pulmonary embolism, and renal disease [9–13]. Elevated homocysteine levels are associated with an increased risk for atherosclerosis and venous thrombosis as well as microalbuminuria, renal dysfunction, and megaloblastic anemia [14, 15].

We report the first case of xanthine calculi in a patient with Lesch-Nyhan syndrome and Factor V Leiden who was treated with allopurinol and underwent several urological procedures to remove calculi. We discuss the pathophysiology of xanthine stones, the use of allopurinol in patients with HPRT deficiency experiencing uric acid overproduction, the consequences of allopurinol overdosing, the challenges associated with the combined diagnoses of Lesch-Nyhan syndrome and Factor V Leiden, and the myriad medical and surgical managements for urolithiasis associated with Lesch-Nyhan syndrome.

Case presentation

Case report

A 12-year-old boy (height: 51 in.; weight; 44 lbs. 1.5 oz. [20.0 kg]; BMI: 11.93 kg/m^2) with a history of Lesch-Nyhan syndrome presented to our office with a 1 ½ month history of dysuria, hematuria, and pain secondary to nephrolithiasis. He suffered from a non-verbal learning disorder associated with a developmental delay, was wheelchair-dependent, and had undergone extraction of 10 teeth due to biting and grinding his teeth. Due to his self-mutilating behavior, he wore braces on his arms and had surgery of his left thumb as a result of biting himself. Two years prior to presentation, the patient underwent a cystoscopy with bilateral ureteroscopy due to xanthine stones. He was stone free following the procedure. The patient's mother denied a family history of kidney stones, thromboembolism and gout. At the age of 18 months, the boy underwent a test for organic acids in his urine which revealed highly elevated hypoxanthine without an elevation of xanthine and with a slight elevation of uracil. He was diagnosed clinically with Lesch-Nyhan syndrome at that time based on a triad of uric acid overproduction, neurologic dysfunction, and cognitive and behavioral disturbances.

Uric acid crystals were noted intermittently in the patient's diaper which had increased significantly in the preceding days. He had been treated with the medication allopurinol since he was 2 years old. At the time of presentation, the dose of allopurinol was 200 mg administered once per day. He had never experienced gout. The patient was prescribed potassium citrate.

Diagnostic tests

A renal ultrasound demonstrated multiple calculi in both kidneys with the largest measuring 1.8 cm in the right kidney as well as echogenic material in the medullary pyramids bilaterally suggesting nephrocalcinosis (Fig. 1). There were no masses, hydronephrosis, or hydroureter. A urinalysis revealed the following: specific gravity = 1.010; pH = 7.0; leukocyte esterase = 500; trace microscopic hematuria; and negative nitrite. The urine culture was negative. The uric acid level in blood was 2.9 mg/dL (Normal range: 2.5–8.5 mg/dL). Uric acid levels in blood collected in the previous 2 years were all in the normal range, specifically, 5.0 mg/dL, 2.6 mg/dL, and 3.2 mg/dL. There was no evidence of renal failure. The patient underwent six separate urinalyses between the ages of 9 and 12, all of which demonstrated a pH of either 6 or 7.

A CT scan of the abdomen and pelvis demonstrated staghorn calculi in both kidneys, involving all calyces.

Surgery

The patient underwent a right percutaneous nephrolithotomy (PCNL) 2 months after presentation. During the hospital stay, the patient was noted to be anemic and received 5 days of epogen and iron supplementation. He developed a thrombus in the right cephalic vein and was diagnosed with heterozygous Factor V Leiden with elevated homocysteine (16.2 umol/L [Normal range: 6.6–14.8 umol/L]). The methylene tetrahydrofolate reductase (MTHFR) and prothrombin genes were negative. Folic acid was initiated. The Factor V Leiden mutation was detected through a polymerase chain reaction (PCR) test that utilized microarray-based oligonucleotide hybridization and signal amplification to detect the Factor V Leiden mutation.

Seven weeks later, the patient began experiencing aspiration of liquids, gastroesophageal reflux, and markedly delayed gastric emptying, necessitating a laparosc opic Nissen fundoplication with gastrostomy tube and open pyloroplasty. The patient continued to suffer from nephrolithiasis, with visualization of a left renal calculus

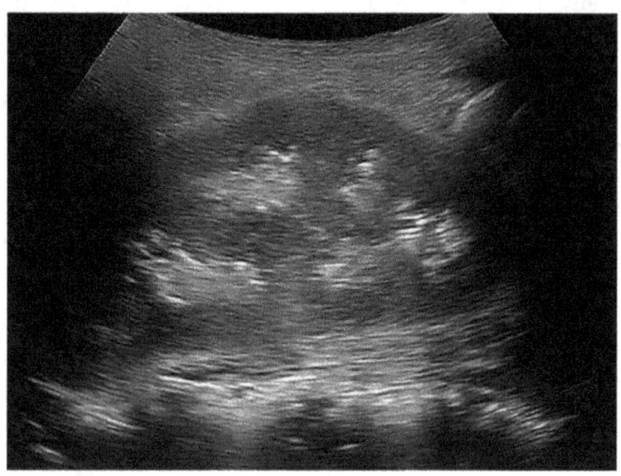

Fig. 1 Renal ultrasound demonstrated multiple calculi and nephrocalcinosis of the kidneys bilaterally

greater than 2 cm. A CT scan demonstrated staghorn calculi in the left kidney (Fig. 2). He underwent a left PCNL and left nephrostomy tube exchange 6 months after the right-sided procedure. A nephrogram revealed evidence of a filling defect in the lower pole calyx which may represent organizing blood clot or residual stone. Renal ultrasounds performed 6 and 9 months later demonstrated extensive bilateral nephrocalcinosis without hydronephrosis or hydroureter. There was no evidence of calculi in the collecting systems.

The calculi that were removed during the ureteroscopies, the ones that the patient had passed while seen as an outpatient, and those that were sent for analysis following the PCNL were all consistent with xanthine calculi.

Discussion

A classic feature of Lesch-Nyhan syndrome is hyperuricemia due to a metabolic deficit caused by a HPRT mutation [16]. The HPRT defect results in the accumulation of hypoxanthine which is oxidized to xanthine by xanthine oxidase and further oxidized to uric acid [5, 17]. Hyperuricemia may lead to hyperuricosuria, uric acid stone formation, and uric acid crystal nephropathy [16]. If the hyperuricemia remains untreated, conditions such as gouty arthritis and fatal uric acid nephropathy may arise [5, 17].

Allopurinol, an inhibitor of xanthine oxidase, stimulates xanthine and hypoxanthine urinary excretion and decreases uric acid production [2, 18]. In contrast with hypoxanthine, the solubility of xanthine in urine is low. While allopurinol is often beneficial in the treatment of the hyperuricemic state associated with Lesch-Nyhan syndrome, there is a risk of developing xanthine stones when the urine is saturated with xanthine [18]. Torres and colleagues performed a 22-year investigation of the use of allopurinol in patients with Lesch-Nyhan syndrome and partial HPRT deficiency [19, 20]. They reported a 47% mean reduction of serum urate concentration, a mean 74% reduction in urinary uric acid-to-creatinine ratio, and increased hypoxanthine and xanthine urinary excretion rates by 5.4 and 9.5 times, respectively [20]. These authors concluded that allopurinol was a safe and efficacious drug for the treatment of uric acid overproduction and did not influence the neurological features associated with Lesch-Nyhan syndrome [19, 20].

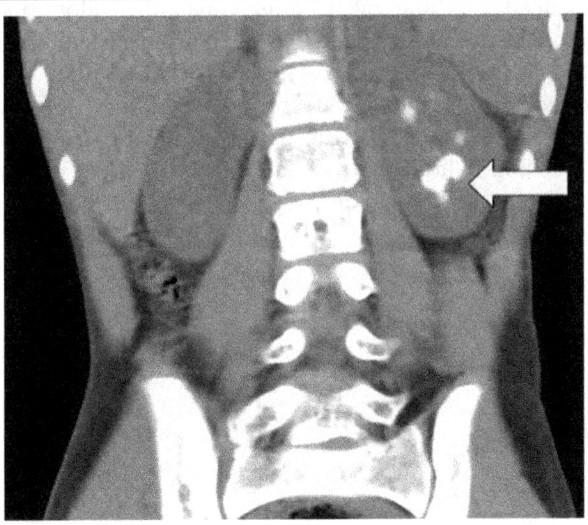

Fig. 2 CT scan of the abdomen and pelvis showed staghorn calculi in the left kidney

Pediatric urinary lithiasis is rarely encountered and, when observed, consists often of calcium oxalate stones [17, 18, 21]. The most common cause of xanthine calculi is primary hereditary xanthinuria which is an autosomal recessive disorder due to a deficiency of the enzyme xanthine oxidase [17, 22]. Individuals with Lesch-Nyhan syndrome are at risk of developing xanthine calculi as a result of treatment with allopurinol [16], however, a paucity of cases have been reported [17–19, 23]. The mechanism of xanthine stone formation may be related to the significant increase of urinary oxypurinol, the metabolite of allopurinol, in response to allopurinol treatment [22]. Patients may present with renal failure secondary to obstructive uropathy and are subsequently diagnosed with Lesch-Nyhan syndrome [16, 24] or may suffer from Lesch-Nyhan syndrome and experience renal failure secondary to uric acid nephropathy or stone obstruction [2, 18].

A fine line exists between lowering serum urate sufficiently to prevent the painful manifestations of gout while not producing excessive xanthine in the urine. Cameron and colleagues stressed the importance of careful monitoring of allopurinol especially in patients with Lesch-Nyhan syndrome as the total urinary oxypurine excretion is sensitive to allopurinol which may result in xanthine and oxypurinol calculi [25]. The allopurinol dose should be closely monitored and reduced to no more than 5 mg/kg per 24 h in children or 100 mg/24 h in adults [25]. The boy presented in our case was treated with an allopurinol dose (10 mg/kg) that was so excessive that his serum urate was at the lower end of normal (5.0 mg/dL, 2.6 mg/dL, and 3.2 mg/dL). Thus, his large urate production was diverted into xanthine and hypoxanthine. Furthermore, Torres and colleagues suggested maintaining the urinary hypoxanthine excretion rate higher than that of xanthine and keeping the serum urate concentration between 5.0 mg/dL and 7.0 mg/dL to prevent xanthine lithiasis associated with allopurinol use in HPRT deficiency [20]. However, the boy in our case had a serum urate level far below this range.

The dangers of excessive allopurinol in this report serves as a significant educational message for physicians. Our report represents a situation of allopurinol overdosing. First, Torres and colleagues' recommendation of keeping the serum urate concentration between 5.0 mg/dL and 7.0 mg/dL was not followed [20]. Secondly, the dose of allopurinol was double the recommended dose of 5 mg/kg [25]. The boy developed xanthine lithiasis as a consequence of these factors, placing him at risk of developing renal failure.

We report the first case in the literature of a patient with Lesch-Nyhan syndrome and Factor V Leiden who was treated with allopurinol and subsequently developed xanthine calculi. Bilateral staghorn calculi were noted, involving all calyces. Nephrocalcinosis was also observed in the medullary pyramids bilaterally. The uric acid levels in the blood remained in the normal range throughout the course of urological follow-up.

Our patient's combined diagnoses of Lesch-Nyhan syndrome and Factor V Leiden created several challenges. The urological course of treating the xanthine calculi was complicated by his Factor V Leiden, with the development of a thrombus in the right cephalic vein. Due to the risk of thrombophilia associated with Factor V Leiden, afflicted individuals are encouraged to remain active and refrain from being immobile for long periods of time. The boy in our report with Lesch-Nyhan syndrome had motor dysfunction and required a wheelchair, preventing him from the recommended walking. Our patient also had anemia and an increased homocysteine level which may be associated with microalbuminuria, megaloblastic anemia, and renal dysfunction. Similarly, patients with Lesch-Nyhan syndrome may experience hematological disorders such as megaloblastic anemia or microcytic anemia in addition to their uric acid overproduction. The renal and hematological risk factors associated with Lesch-Nyhan syndrome, Factor V Leiden, and elevated homocysteine levels may have exacerbated this boy's condition. We believe it is a coincidence that the boy was diagnosed with both heterozygous Lesch-Nyhan syndrome and Factor V Leiden. Lesch-Nyhan syndrome is caused by a deficiency of the enzyme HGPRT due to a mutation in the HPRT gene located on the X chromosome, whereas Factor V Leiden (rs6025) is an autosomal disorder marked by a mutation of human factor V located on chromosome 1q24.2. We have not discerned a genetic correlation between these two conditions.

The first-line treatment of uric acid stones or uric acid crystal nephropathy in individuals with Lesch-Nyhan syndrome consists of medical management (Table 1) [2, 16–18, 22, 23]. It has been suggested that raising the dose of allopurinol may be successful in the decreasing the frequency of stone formation by increasing the hypoxanthine to xanthine ratio [26]. Contrarily, urinary alkalization coupled with reducing the dose of allopurinol may prove more efficacious in preventing xanthine stone formation [17]. If medical management fails or is not tolerated, invasive procedures may be performed (Table 1) [16].

Despite proper medical management consisting of aggressive hydration, an appropriate dose of the allopurinol which was not adjusted during treatment, use of potassium citrate, and routine renal ultrasounds, the patient presented herein underwent numerous urological procedures for calculi, including a cystoscopy with bilateral uteroscopy and laser lithotripsy with bilateral placement of ureteral stents followed by bilateral PCNLs 2 years later. Renal ultrasounds performed 6 and 9 months after the urological interventions showed extensive bilateral nephrocalcinosis without hydronephrosis, hydroureter, or calculi, indicating that the medical and surgical management of the xanthine calculi had proven successful.

Conclusions

Pediatricians should be aware of the rare phenomena of Lesch-Nyhan syndrome and Factor V Leiden and the potential renal disorders inherent in both conditions. To our knowledge, this is the first case involving a single patient who was diagnosed with the genetic diseases Lesch-Nyhan syndrome and Factor V Leiden and experienced xanthine calculi after consuming allopurinol. Prompt medical management of xanthine calculi by a high fluid intake, maintaining an alkaline urine, and monitoring for uric acid nephropathy is warranted. Furthermore, awareness of the consequences of allopurinol overdosing is imperative in the management of patients with Lesch-Nyhan syndrome to decrease the likelihood of renal failure.

Table 1 Treatment of Urolithiasis Associated with Lesch-Nyhan syndrome

Medical Management	Invasive Procedures
■ High fluid intake ■ Maintain alkaline urine with potassium or sodium citrate to prevent uric acid stone formation (urinary pH: 6.5–7.0) ■ Gradually increase allopurinol dose from 2.5 mg/kg doses per day to 10 mg/kg per day and administer 2–3 doses per day ■ Monitor purine metabolites of allopurinol in blood and urine ■ Assess urinary uric acid, xanthine, hypoxanthine, and oxypurinal excretion to determine accurate allopurinol dosage ■ Avoid excess dietary purines, calcium, salts ■ Routine renal ultrasound to monitor for uric acid nephropathy	■ Percutaneous nephrolithotomy ■ Shock wave lithotripsy ■ Ureteroscopy ■ Open surgery

Abbreviations

APC: Activated protein C; HPRT: Hypoxanthine-guanine phosphoribosyltransferase; MTHFR: Methylene tetrahydrofolate reductase; PCNL: Percutaneous nephrolithotomy

Acknowledgments

We acknowledge Norton Healthcare for their continued support.

Authors' contributions

LS made substantial contributions to the conception and design, analyzed and interpreted the data, performed the literature search, and was the major contributor in the writing of the manuscript. DP made substantial contributions to the conception and design and revised the draft critically for important intellectual content. ER made substantial contributions to the conception and design, analyzed and interpreted the data, and revised the draft critically for important intellectual content. All authors read and approved the final manuscript and have agreed to be accountable for all aspects of the work in ensuring that questions related to the accuracy or integrity of any part of the work are appropriately investigated and resolved.

Competing interests

The authors declare that they have no competing interests.

Author details

[1]Norton Neuroscience Institute, Norton Healthcare, Louisville, KY 40202, USA. [2]Norton Children's Urology, Norton Healthcare, Louisville, KY 40207, USA.

References

1. Lesch M. Nyhan WL. A familial disorder of uric acid metabolism and central nervous system function. Am J Med. 1964;36:561–70.
2. Sikora P, Pijanowska M, Majewski M, Bienias B, Borzecka H, Zajczkowska M. Acute renal failure due to bilateral xanthine urolithiasis in a boy with Lesch-Nyhan syndrome. Pediatr Nephrol. 2006;21:1045–7.
3. Jinnah HA, De GL, Harris JC, Nyhan WL, O'Neill JP. The spectrum of inherited mutations causing HPRT deficiency: 75 new cases and a review of 196 previously reported cases. Mutat Res. 2000;463:309–26.
4. Nyhan WL. Lesch-Nyhan disease. J Hist Neurosci. 2005;14:1–10.
5. Torres RJ, Puig JG. Hypoxanthine-guanine phosophoribosyltransferase (HPRT) deficiency: Lesch-Nyhan syndrome. Orphanet J Rare Dis. 2007;2:48.
6. Puig JG, Torres RJ, Mateos FA, et al. The spectrum of hypoxanthine-guanine phosphoribosyltransferase (HPRT) deficiency. Clinical experience based on 22 patients from 18 Spanish families. Medicine (Baltimore). 2001;80:102–12.
7. Kelley WN, Rosenbloom FM, Henderson JF. Seegmiller JE. A specific enzyme defect in gout associated with overproduction of uric acid. Proc Natl Acad Sci U S A. 1967;57:1735–9.
8. Kelley WN, Greene ML, Rosenbloom FM, Henderson JF, Seegmiller JE. Hypoxanthine-guanine phosphoribosyltransferase deficiency in gout. Ann Intern Med. 1969;70:155–206.
9. Ornstein DL, Cushman M. Factor V Leiden. Circulation. 2003;107:e94–7.
10. Irish AB, Green FR, Gray DW, Morris PJ. The factor V Leiden (R506Q) mutation and risk of thrombosis in renal transplant recipients. Transplantation. 1997;64:604–7.
11. Kujovich JL, Factor V. Leiden thrombophilia. Genet Med. 2011;13:1–16.
12. Le Moine A, Chauveau D, Grunfeld JP. Acute renal artery thrombosis associated with factor V Leiden mutation. Nephrol Dial Transplant. 1996;11: 2067–9.
13. Wattanakit K, Cushman M. Chronic kidney disease and venous thromboembolism: epidemiology and mechanisms. Curr Opin Pulm Med. 2009;15:408–12.
14. Jager A, Kostense PJ, Nijpels G, et al. Serum homocysteine levels are associated with the development of (micro) albuminuria: the Hoorn study. Arterioscler Thromb Vasc Biol. 2001;21:74–81.
15. Varga EA, Sturm AC, Misita CP, Moll S. Cardiology patient pages. Homocysteine and MTHFR mutations: relation to thrombosis and coronary artery disease. Circulation. 2005;111:e289–93.
16. Ankem M, Glazier DB, Barone JG. Lesch-Nyhan syndrome presenting as acute renal failure secondary to obstructive uropathy. Urology. 2000;56:1056.
17. Brock WA, Golden J, Kaplan GW. Xanthine calculi in the Lesch-Nyhan syndrome. J Urol. 1983;130:157–9.
18. Pais VM Jr, Lowe G, Lallas CD, Preminger GM, Assimos DG. Xanthine urolithiasis. Urology. 2006;67:1084–11.
19. Torres RJ, Prior C, Puig JG. Efficacy and safety of allopurinol in patients with the Lesch-Nyhan syndrome and partial hypoxanthine-phosphoribosyltransferase deficiency: a follow-up study of 18 Spanish patients. Nucleosides Nucleotides Nucleic Acids. 2006;25:1077–82.
20. Torres RJ, Prior C, Puig JG. Efficacy and safety of allopurinol in patients with hypoxanthine-guanine phosphoribosyltransferase deficiency. Metabolism. 2007;56:1179–86.
21. Cohen TD, Ehreth J, King LR, Preminger GM. Pediatric urolithiasis: medical and surgical management. Urology. 1996;47:292–303.
22. Ogawa A, Watanabe K, Minejima N. Renal xanthine stone in Lesch-Nyhan syndrome treated with allopurinol. Urology. 1985;26:56–8.
23. Kranen S, Keough D, Gordon RB, Emmerson BT. Xanthine-containing calculi during allopurinol therapy. J Urol. 1985;133:658–9.
24. Vargiami E, Printza N, Papadimiditriou E, et al. Nephrocalcinosis and renal failure in Lesch-Nyhan syndrome: report of two familial cases and review of the literature. Urology. 2016;97:194–6.
25. Cameron JS, Moro F, Simmonds HA. Gout, uric acid and purine metabolism in paediatric nephrology. Pediatr Nephrol. 1993;7:105–18.
26. Hiraishi K, Nakamura S, Yamamoto S, Kurokawa K. Prevention of xanthine stone formation by augmented dose of allopurinol in the Lesch-Nyhan syndrome. Br J Urol. 1987;59:362–3.

Generalized arterial calcification of infancy with a novel *ENPP1* mutation

Iole Brunod[1], Barthélémy Tosello[2,3*], Sophie Hassid[1], Catherine Gire[2], Laurent Thomachot[1] and Michel Panuel[3,4]

Abstract

Background: Generalized Arterial Calcification of Infancy (GACI) is a heritable ectopic mineralization disorder resulting in diffuse arterial calcifications and/or stenosis, mostly caused by mutations in the *ENPP1* gene. Here we present a case report of GACI in a male infant with a new familial mutation of the *ENPP1* gene and the clinical outcome after biphosphonates therapy.

Case presentation: The clinical presentation was characterized by a severe early-onset of hypertension refractory to multiple therapy. To investigate this atypical hypertension, a renal Doppler ultra-sonography was performed and diffuse echo-bright arteries were detected; then a low-dose whole-body computed tomography demonstrated extensive arterial calcifications, suggesting GACI. A novel homozygous mutation c.784A > G (p.Ser262Gly) was detected in the *ENPP1* gene. The infant was administered four courses of bisphosphonates: arterial calcifications were found to decrease but severe refractory hypertension was persistent. Although GACI can be a rapidly fatal illness and frequently results in death in infancy, the patient was 24 months of age at the time of writing this report.

Conclusions: Three points of interest: the first one is to remind clinicians of this rare and atypical etiology in neonates with severe hypertension and in fetuses with cardiomyopathy and non-immune hydrops fetalis. The second point is the identification of a novel mutation in the *ENPP1* gene associated with a clinical presentation of GACI. The third point is the fairly favourable outcome of our patient after bisphosphonates therapy, with calcifications regression but not hypertension.

Keywords: *ENPP1*, Generalized arterial calcification of infancy, Arterial calcification, Neonatal hypertension

Background

Generalized Arterial Calcification of Infancy (GACI, OMIM 208000), also known as idiopathic infantile arterial calcification, is a heritable ectopic mineralization disorder resulting in diffuse arterial calcifications [1] mostly caused by mutations in the *ENPP1* gene [2]. GACI is characterized by prenatal or infantile onset of widespread arterial calcifications and/or narrowing of large- and medium-sized arteries [3], without neither gender nor ethnic predilection [4]. Commonly, patients present with variable cardiovascular phenotypes and symptoms with onset in-utero or in the first months of life [4]. GACI is inherited in an autosomal recessive manner. The classic form of GACI is caused by mutations in the *ENPP1* gene (GACI1, OMIM 208000), localized to chromosome 6q22-q23 [5]. To date, therapeutic guidelines are lacking. Being synthetic analogues of inorganic pyrophosphate, the most reported GACI therapy are bisphosphonates: their efficacy is not completely proven as some case reports show inconsistent results and clinical trials are not feasible [3, 6]. Prognosis is poor; most affected individuals die within the first year of life from cardiovascular complications [4].

GACI is a rare disease; data about this condition, especially regarding clinical course and treatment efficacy, is mainly based on clinical series and case reports [4]. This case report of neonatal GACI contributes to enrich the literature with data on a new familial mutation of the *ENPP1* gene and provides details of the specific clinical course after biphosphonates therapy.

* Correspondence: barthelemy.tosello@ap-hm.fr
[2]Department of Neonatology, Hôpital Nord, Assistance Publique des Hôpitaux de Marseille (APHM), Chemin des Bourrely, 13015 Marseille, France
[3]Aix Marseille Univ, CNRS, EFS, ADES, Marseille, France
Full list of author information is available at the end of the article

Case presentation

The male patient was the naturally conceived son of a 34-year-old gravida 2, para 0, miscarriage 1 mother. His healthy parents were consanguineous (first-degree cousins, of Algerian origin), without history of hypertension, calcification or cardiomyopathy. Prenatal concerns included a fetal hypertrophic cardiomyopathy (HCM) associated with a hydrops fetalis and a polyhydramnios, treated by one amnioreduction due to poor maternal tolerance. No other abnormality was noted on the prenatal ultrasound. Furthermore, antenatal investigations of fetal cardiomyopathy were negative or normal (enzyme disorder, maternal viral infection, normal fetal karyotype). Preterm birth was medically indicated because of an abnormal fetal heart rate: the newborn was delivered by urgent caesarean section at 29 weeks' gestation. The newborn was eutrophic (birth weight 1330 g), umbilical cord pH was 7.21; his Apgar scores were 4 at 1 min, 8 at 5 min, 10 at 10 min. Resuscitative and neonatal appropriate care were provided.

At birth, he presented with hydrops fetalis (oedema and mild pericardial effusion); he was not dysmorphic; postnatal echocardiography confirmed the diagnosis of HCM without other heart anomalies and routine x-ray didn't show bone abnormalities. The patient developed severe hypertension a few hours after birth (mean arterial pressure > 70 mmHg, normal range: 35–40 mmHg). This hypertension was refractory to a triple therapy (propranolol, nicardipine, clonidine). To assess this atypical hypertension, extensive blood and urinary tests (for endocrine disease and inborn error of metabolism) were performed, but yielded negative results. A renal artery Doppler ultrasound was performed and detected extensive calcifications of the renal arteries, the abdominal aorta and its major branches. To further elucidate the extent of the calcifications, a low-dose whole-body computed tomography was performed and detected diffuse calcifications of large- and medium-sized arteries (Fig. 1a, b). The brain Magnetic Resonance Imaging was normal at term equivalent age. In view of these findings we retrospectively reviewed the chest x-ray performed at day 1 of life: it is noteworthy that calcifications were already apparent (Fig. 1d). Prenatal ultrasound images were also retrospectively reviewed by several radiologist experts but no arterial calcifications were detected. These singularities were consistent with GACI: the patient's genotype was analysed, and a mutation was found in the *ENPP1* gene.

The treatment consisted of four courses of bisphosphonates administered by intravenous route on day 40 of life, on day 70 of life, on month 21 of life and at 2 years old: each course consisted of 2 or 3 disodium pamidronate infusions (0.50 mg/kg/infusion) delivered over 1 week. At 20 week-follow-up visit, 2 months after the two initial courses of bisphosphonates, the extent of the arterial calcifications was assessed by a whole body computed tomography and an almost complete resolution of the lesions was demonstrated (Fig. 1c). Concurrently, from 2 months-old to one-year-old, the baby developed transiently hypophosphatemia (serum phosphate level of 3.1 mg/dL (1.0 mmol/L); normal infant range = 4.6–7.1 mg/dL and 1.5–2.3 mmol/L) with inappropriate urinary phosphate excretion (fractional excretion of phosphate > 5%). All other relevant markers of phosphate homeostasis were within normal range (serum 1,25-$(OH)_2$-vitamin D level, parathyroid

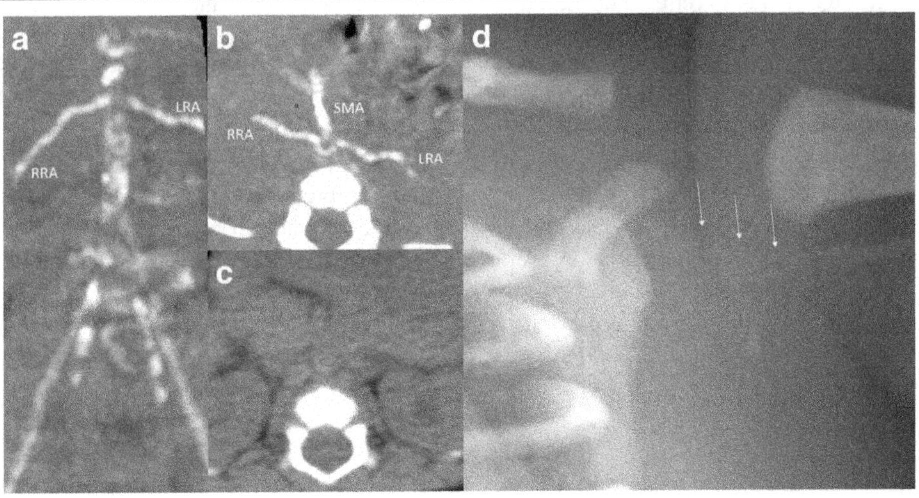

Fig. 1 **a** Abdominal CT-scan frontal view at 1 month of age: huge vascular calcifications of the aorta, the iliac arteries, the renal arteries (RRA: right renal artery, LRA: left renal artery). **b** Abdominal CT-scan axial view at 1 month of age: calcifications of the superior mesenteric artery (SMA), renal arteries (RRA, LRA) and the aorta. **c** Abdominal CT-scan axial view at 5 months of age: the arterial calcifications are no longer visible. **d** Close-up view on the left scapular area of chest X-ray at day 1: subtle calcifications of the left subclavian and left axillary artery (white arrows)

hormone level, serum calcium level, serum alkaline phosphatase level). The infant had no bone deformities. The transient hypophosphatemia was corrected with oral phosphate supplementation and no vitamin D supplementation. Concerning cardiovascular outcome, at 2-year-old follow-up, hypertension was still treated with a triple combination of drugs: blood pressure levels were constantly above 140/80 mmHg. However, hypertrophic cardiomyopathy resolved with this treatment. The patient had normal growth and development. He had neither ocular nor cutaneous manifestations of Pseudoxanthoma Elasticum (PXE).

The investigation of a multi-gene panel was performed by high-throughput next-generation sequencing. Genomic DNA was processed with the TruSight One/Nextera hybrid capture method and coding regions with adjacent intronic regions of the two GACI-associated genes *ENPP1* and *ABCC6* were enriched by PCR (Illumina®). Subsequent analysis was conducted by massive parallel sequencing using the MiSeq Benchtop System (Illumina®). Quality criteria require a minimal coverage of 20× for at least 97% of target regions of the investigated genes: the minimal coverage of 20× achieved for all targeted regions was 98% with an average coverage of 172 sequences per base. For assessment of the variants, the dbSNP, ExAc, HGMD, LOVD and UniProt databases, as well as the prediction programs PredictSNP, PhDSNP, SNAP, SIFT, PolyPhen-1, PolyPhen-2, MutationTaster, SNAP, MAPP and Panther were used. Next-generation sequencing analysis of the patient's *ENPP1* gene revealed a homozygous mutation c.784A > G (p.Ser262Gly). There was no mutation in the *ABCC6* gene. The parents consented to undergo genetic testing. The c.784A > G (p.Ser262Gly) mutation was also present, in the heterozygous state, in the consanguineous parents. The mutation c.784A > G (p.Ser262Gly) has so far not been described in the literature and mutation databases: there are no entries for the variation in the 1000 Genomes project and the Exome Aggregation Consortium, which indicates a very low global minor allele frequency (MAF). The prediction programs PredictSNP, PhDSNP, SNAP, SIFT, PolyPhen-1, PolyPhen-2, MutationTaster and SNAP all classify the variation as pathogenic whereas the prediction programs MAPP and Panther classify the variation as benign.

The combination of cardiovascular findings and extensive calcifications on imaging, together with the *ENPP1* mutation, confirmed the diagnosis of GACI1 in the proband.

Discussion

We report a case of neonatal GACI: clinical presentation was a severe early-onset hypertension, investigations found diffuse calcifications on imaging and a mutation in *ENPP1* gene. The *ENPP1* mutation found in the proband is not yet described in the literature. Even though the clinical presentation, results of investigation and management reported in this publication have been already described, outcome and clinical course after bisphosphonates are of interest. Indeed, biphosphonate is the most reported therapy but guidelines are lacking and results are not consistent, emphasizing the importance of collecting data: here, arterial calcifications were found to decrease (Fig. 1c) but severe refractory hypertension was persistent. Although GACI can be a rapidly fatal illness and frequently results in death in infancy, the patient was 24 months of age at the time of writing this report.

Diagnosis of GACI is made by the combination of clinical, imaging or histopathological findings, together with genetic results. The clinical presentation described in this case report was previously reported in the literature: hypertension was reported in 22% of patients and cardiomegaly in 10% of patients [4]. Cardiovascular phenotype is quite variable in GACI disease, including fetal distress, polyhydramnios, hydrops fetalis, heart failure, hypertension, cardiomegaly, visceral effusion, respiratory distress, cyanosis or reduced peripheral pulse [4]. Some case reports described association with clinical features of PXE such as angioid streaks of the retina and papular skin lesions [2]; PXE is characterized by dystrophic calcification of soft tissues. Patients have normal growth and development [3].

In addition to clinical features, investigations can help establish the diagnosis, especially imaging and histopathological investigations. Vascular calcifications can be revealed as early as during prenatal ultrasound [7]. The preferred imaging modality to assess calcifications extension is whole-body computed tomography [8]. Calcifications can also be detected on routine x-ray films as subtle radiopaque regions. Hence, these findings are easily missed and found by reviewing x-rays, for example the chest x-ray: this pitfall has already been reported [9], and in our case report, has delayed the diagnostic process. Calcifications are also detected, although less frequently, in extravascular sites as periarticular sites [6]. Histopathology, when it is performed, shows diffuse deposition of calcium hydroxyapatite in the internal elastic lamina and diffuse fibrointimal hyperplasia causing patchy luminal narrowing of large- and medium-sized arteries [10].

Our patient's genetic testing revealed a new familial mutation in the *ENPP1* gene: the unaffected and consanguineous parents were heterozygous carriers for the same mutation as their homozygous son, in accordance with the autosomal recessive mode of inheritance of GACI disease. This mutation, c.784A > G (p.Ser262Gly), is not yet described in the literature and mutation databases. To date, biallelic *ENPP1* mutations are detected in about 70% of all cases of GACI [2] with more than 40 different causative mutations [6]. Most of authors in the literature review don't have evidence of genotype-phenotype association [11]. Rutsch et al., in a multicenter genetic study and retrospective observational analysis of 55 subjects affected by GACI, have noted one possible genotype-phenotype correlation: homozygosity for the *ENPP1* pathogenic variant p.Pro305Thr was associated with death in infancy in all 5 cases [6]; otherwise, no clear genotype-phenotype correlation was seen in the other subjects of the study.

The *ENPP1* gene encodes an ectonucleotide pyrophosphatase/phopshodiesterase1 ENPP1, which is a membrane-bound enzyme. The ENPP1 enzyme hydrolyzes extracellular ATP in AMP and inorganic pyrophosphate (PPi) [12]. Under physiologic conditions, PPi is a powerful antimineralization factor: PPi inhibits calcification by binding to nascent hydroxyapatite crystals, thereby preventing further growth of the crystals [13]. ENPP1 is the major generator of extracellular PPi, and so plays a key role in regulating vascular calcification process by controlling the levels of circulating PPi. In GACI1, deleterious mutations affecting ENPP1 enzyme restrict PPi generation, leading to propensity for hydroxyapatite deposition [1]. Less frequently, GACI is linked to a mutation in the ATP-binding cassette subfamily C, member6 (ABCC6) gene (GACI2, OMIM 614473) [2] which encodes an ABCC6 [1]. *ABCC6* gene is affected in the classic form of PXE and so, in the same way as there is an overlap in clinical phenotypes, there is a genotypic overlap between GACI and PXE: some patients with GACI harbor mutations in *ABCC6*, and some patients with clinical manifestations consistent with PXE have mutations in *ENPP1* [2]. These observations have suggested the possibility of shared pathomechanistic pathways for these conditions: GACI and PXE represent likely two ends of a clinical spectrum of ectopic calcification and other organ pathologies rather than two distinct disorders [2]. The protein ABCC6 function is unclear: ABCC6 is a putative transmembrane efflux transporter protein expressed primarily in the basolateral plasma membrane of hepatocytes and in the proximal tubules of the kidney; nevertheless, the molecules transported physiologically by ABCC6 from the intracellular milieu to the extracellular space have not been identified yet [1]. ABCC6 has been shown to influence extracellular ATP levels and therefore has a role in the PPi generating pathway. Also, it has been shown that ABCC6 deficiency leads to low extracellular PPi levels [14, 15].

Our patient encountered transient hypophosphatemia: several cases of GACI reported association with hypophosphatemia, and even hypophosphatemic rickets [16]. Hypophosphatemia was found to be associated with a milder phenotype and with a better prognosis [6]. The physiopathology is not well understood. It is hypothesized that hypophosphatemia in GACI might reflect a physiologic compensation mechanism rather than a primary defect. However, a phenotype of autosomal-recessive hypophosphatemic rickets without any arterial calcification was encountered in patients with mutations in the ENPP1 gene, suggesting a different pathway involved in the generation of hypophosphatemic rickets [1].

Due to lack of guidelines, biphosphonates therapy was administered to our patient, as it is the most reported GACI therapy: arterial calcifications were found to decrease (Fig. 1c) but severe refractory hypertension and hypertrophic cardiomyopathy were persistent. Data from literature are not consistent: in a non-randomized, comparative, retrospective study on few patients (n = 43), infants treated with bisphosphonates showed a significantly increased survival [6]. However, both spontaneous resolution of calcifications and fatal outcome despite early therapy have been reported [9, 17]. Hence, it is difficult to determine if bisphosphonates therapy is truly protective or if resolution of calcifications reflects the natural history of the disease. Our patient's outcome after treatment is consistent with other reports in that resolution of calcifications didn't correlate with resolution of all cardiovascular findings: it may be a consequence of the persistence of arterial stenosis due to persistent vascular remodelling and damage [6]. A better understanding of this rare disease is provided thanks to animal models (such as tiptoe-walking (ttw/ttw) mouse, ages with stiffened joints (asj/asj) mouse and Enpp1 knock-out mouse). New therapeutic strategies are emerging from encouraging animal studies. A recombinant enzyme therapy with subcutaneous administration of an ENPP1-Fc fusion protein was shown to prevent the mortality, vascular calcifications and sequelae in the asj/asj mouse model [18]. Another preclinical work, using *Enpp1*^{asj} mice as a model of GACI, demonstrated the dual beneficial effects of bisphosphonates treatment by preventing ectopic mineralization while correcting decreased bone mineralization [19].

Another point to note in this case is the rather favourable outcome: at 2-year-old, the infant presented with severe hypertension but a disappearance of hypertrophic cardiomyopathy. Prognosis in GACI is likely to be poor, most affected individuals die within the first year of life from cardiovascular complications: the mortality rate during the first 6 months of life varies among studies between 85% [10] and 55% for the most recent study [6]. Nevertheless, there are reports in the literature of long-term survival, with several in their 20s [20].

Conclusion

We report a case of neonatal GACI with three points of interest: the first one is to remind clinicians of this rare and atypical etiology in neonates with severe hypertension and in fetuses with cardiomyopathy and non-immune hydrops fetalis. The second point is the identification of a novel mutation in the *ENPP1* gene associated with a clinical presentation of GACI. The third point is the fairly favourable outcome of our patient after bisphosphonates therapy, with calcifications regression but not hypertension. A better understanding of this rare disease could lead to a better comprehension of more common diseases also associated with calcification impairment (such as chronic kidney disease).

Abbreviations

ABCC6: ATP-binding cassette subfamily C, member6; asj/asj: ages with stiffened joints mouse; GACI: Generalized Arterial Calcification of Infancy; HCM: hypertrophic cardiomyopathy; PPi: inorganic pyrophosphate; PXE: Pseudoxanthoma Elasticum; ttw/ttw: tiptoe-walking mouse

Acknowledgements

The authors acknowledge our patient and his family for their participation.

Authors' contributions

IB contributed to conception and design of the manuscript, clinical management of the patient, and drafted the manuscript. IB, BT, and LT contributed to acquisition, analysis and interpretation of data, and drafting of the manuscript. SH, CG and MP contributed to critical revision of the manuscript for important intellectual content. All authors read and approved the final version of the manuscript.

Consent for publication

This report was approved by the Ethics Committee of the Aix-Marseille University. Written informed consent was obtained from the patient's parents for publication of this case report and any accompanying images.

Competing interests

The authors declare that they have no competing interests.

Author details

[1]Pediatric and Neonatal Intensive Care Unit, Hôpital Nord, Assistance Publique-Hôpitaux de Marseille, Chemin des Bourrely, 13015 Marseille, France. [2]Department of Neonatology, Hôpital Nord, Assistance Publique des Hôpitaux de Marseille (APHM), Chemin des Bourrely, 13015 Marseille, France. [3]Aix Marseille Univ, CNRS, EFS, ADES, Marseille, France. [4]Department of Medical Imaging, Assistance Publique-Hôpitaux de Marseille, Hôpital Nord, Chemin des Bourrely, 13015 Marseille, France.

References

1. Nitschke Y, Rutsch F. Inherited arterial calcifications syndromes: etiologies and treatment concepts. Curr Osteoporos Rep. 2017;15:255–70.
2. Nitschke F, Baujat G, Botschen U, Wittkampf T, Du Moulin M, Stella J, et al. Generalized arterial calcification of infancy and pseudoxanthoma elasticum can be caused by mutations in either ENPP1 or ABCC6. Am J Hum Genet. 2012;90:25–39.
3. Ferreira C, Ziegler S, Gahl W. Generalized arterial calcification of infancy. In: GeneReviews®; 1993. https://www.ncbi.nlm.nih.gov/pubmed/25392903. Accessed 13 Nov 2014.
4. Chong CR, Hutchins GM. Idiopathic infantile arterial calcification: the spectrum of clinical presentations. Pediatr Dev Pathol. 2008;11:405–15.
5. Ruf N, Uhlenberg B, Terkeltaub R, Nurnberg P, Rutsch F. The mutational spectrum of ENPP1 as arising after the analysis of 23 unrelated patients with generalized arterial calcification of infancy (GACI). Hum Mutat. 2005;25:98.
6. Rutsch F, Böyer P, Nitschke Y, Ruf N, Lorenz-Depierieux B, et al. Hypophosphatemia, hyperphosphaturia, and bisphosphonate treatment are associated with survival beyond infancy in generalized arterial calcification of infancy. Circulation. 2008;1:133–40.
7. Spear R, Mack LA, Benedetti TJ, Cole RE. Idiopathic infantile calcification: in utero diagnosis. J Ultrasound Med. 1990;9:473–6.
8. Greenberg SB, Gibson J. New findings in idiopathic arterial calcification of infancy detected by MDCT. AJR Am J Roentgenol. 2005;185:530–2.
9. Stuart G, Wren C, Bain H. Idiopathic infantile arterial calcification in two siblings: failure of treatment with diphosphonate. Br Heart J. 1990;64:156–9.
10. Moran JJ. Idiopathic arterial calcification of infancy: a clinicopathologic study. Pathol Annu. 1975;10:393–417.
11. Cheng KS, Chen MR, Ruf N, Lin SP, Rutsch F. Generalized arterial calcification of infancy: different clinical courses in two affected siblings. Am J Med Genet A. 2005;136:210–3.
12. Stefan C, Jansen S, Bollen M. NPP-type ectophosphodiesterases: unity in diversity. Trends Biochem Sci. 2005;30:542–50.
13. Fleisch H, Russell RG, Straumann F. Effect of pyrophosphate on hydroxyapatite and its implications. Nature. 1996;212:901–3.
14. Jansen RS, Küçükosmanoglu A, de Haas M, Sapthu S, Otero JA, Hegman IE, et al. ABCC6 prevents ectopic mineralization seen in pseudoxanthoma elasticum by inducing cellular nucleotide release. Proc Natl Acad Sci U S A. 2013;110(50):20206–11.
15. Jansen RS, Duijst S, Mahakena S, Sommer D, Szeri F, Váradi A, et al. ABCC6-mediated ATP secretion by the liver is the main source of the mineralization inhibitor inorganic pyrophosphate in the systemic circulation-brief report. Arterioscler Thromb Vasc Biol. 2014;34(9):1985–9.
16. Lorenz-Depiereux B, Schnabel D, Tiosano D, Häusler G, Strom TM. Loss-of-function ENPP1 mutations cause both generalized arterial calcification of infancy and autosomal-recessive hypophosphatemic rickets. Am J Hum Genet. 2010;90:25–39.
17. Sholler GF, Yu JS, Bale PM, Hawker RF, Celermajer IM, Kozlowski K. Generalized arterial calcification of infancy: three case reports, including spontaneous regression with long term survival. J Ped. 1984;105:257–60.
18. Albright RA, Stabach P, Cao W, Kavanagh D, Mullen I, et al. ENPP1-FC prevents mortality and vascular calcifications in rodent model of generalized arterial calcification of infancy. Nat Commun. 2015;6:10006.
19. Li Q, Kingman J, Sundberg JP, Levine MA, Uitto J. Dual effects of bisphosphonates on ectopic skin and vascular soft tissue mineralization versus bone microarchitecture in a mouse model of generalized arterial calcification of infancy. J Invest Dermatol. 2016;136:275–83.
20. Ciana G, Trappan A, Bembi B, Benettoni A, Mao G, Zennaro F, et al. Generalized arterial calcification of infancy: two siblings with prolonged survival. Eur J Pediatr. 2006;4:258–63.

21

Long-term effects of the *SLC2A9* G844A and *SLC22A12* C246T variants on serum uric acid concentrations in children

Hye Ah Lee[1,2], Bo Hyun Park[1], Eun Ae Park[3], Su Jin Cho[3], Hae Soon Kim[3] and Hyesook Park[1*]

Abstract

Background: We evaluated the effects of two single-nucleotide polymorphisms on UA concentrations in the first decade of life using repeated-measures data.

Methods: We included all subjects who were followed-up at least once and for whom we had both UA and genotypic data (i.e., 375, 204, 307, and 363 patients aged 3, 5, 7, and 9 years, respectively). All participated in the Ewha Birth and Growth Cohort study. We used a mixed model analysis to estimate the longitudinal association of serum UA concentration due to the rs3825017 (*SLC22A12* c. 246C > T) and rs16890979 (*SLC2A9* c. 844G > A) genotypes.

Results: Overall, the tracking coefficient of UA concentrations in children 3 to 9 years of age was 0.31, and was higher in boys than in girls (0.34 vs. 0.29, respectively). Regarding individual variance, serum UA concentrations decreased as age increased ($\beta = -0.07$, $p < 0.05$), but there were no significant differences by sex. The effects of rs3825017 on UA concentration were significant in boys, but not in girls. Boys with the T allele of rs3825017 had higher concentrations than their counterparts regardless of the time of follow-up. The rs16890979 genotypes were not significantly associated with serum UA concentration in either sex.

Conclusion: This study showed that rs3825017 in the *SLC22A12* gene was associated with UA concentration in childhood.

Keywords: Children, Longitudinal study, Urate transporter 1, Uric acid

Background

Uric acid (UA) is the major endpoint of purine metabolism in humans [1, 2]. Serum UA concentration is modulated by urate excretion and reabsorption, which mainly occurs in the kidneys [1, 2]. An abnormally high serum concentration of UA is a predictor of vascular disease, gout, and renal disease [1], and is also associated with pediatric hypertension [3]. In addition, a longitudinal cohort study of the Bogalusa Heart Study reported that UA concentration in childhood is a significant predictor of blood pressure later in life [4].

It has been suggested that genetic variants markedly contribute to UA concentrations [5], with an estimated heritability of ~70% [6]. Genome-wide association (GWA) studies of common variants identified more than 30 genetic loci associated with the UA concentrations, mostly in urate transporters, such as the genes encoding solute carrier family 2 facilitated glucose transporter member 9 (also known as *SLC2A9* encoding GLUT9), solute carrier family 22 (organic anion/cation transporter) member 12 (also known as *SLC22A12* encoding URAT1), and the ATP-binding cassette transporter subfamily G member 2 (*ABCG2*) [2, 5]. The importance of URAT1 and GLUT9 for regulating blood urate levels was confirmed, and mutations in *SLC22A12* and *SLC2A9* have been reported to be responsible for hypouricemia [7]. *ABCG2* is also known to be a major cause of gout and hyperuricemia that acts by decreasing urate excretion [8]. Among these candidate genes, the missense single-nucleotide polymorphisms (SNPs) rs3733591 (c. 881G > A) and rs16890979 (c. 844G > A) in the *SLC2A9* gene had significant effects on gout in an Asian population [9]. Both polymorphisms protected against the

* Correspondence: hpark@ewha.ac.kr
[1]Department of Preventive Medicine, College of Medicine, Ewha Womans University, 1071, Anyangcheon-ro, Yangcheon-ku, Seoul 158-710, Korea
Full list of author information is available at the end of the article

development of gout, and rs16890979 showed a stronger association than rs3733591 [9]. The protective effect of common variant p.V12 M (rs2231137) in *ABCG2* on gout was also reported in a meta-analysis (odds ratio = 0.73, $p < 0.0001$) [10], but the functional characterization of this variant did not show altered urate transport activity [11]. As variants in *SLC22A12* related to hypouricemia, c.774G > A and c.269G > A were identified in Japanese [12] and Korean [13] subjects, and c.1245_1253del and c.1400C > T were found in the Roma population [14]. In addition, a recent study of Korean men reported five tagging SNPs of URAT1, of which rs3825017 (c. 246C > T) showed a strong association with hyperuricemia despite the small sample size [15]. Except for genetic effects, birth weight [16], dietary intake [1, 17], and body mass index (BMI) [18] are also correlated with UA concentrations.

Evidence from GWA and epidemiology studies has suggested a number of candidate genes and a recent study from the Viva La Familia Study also reported genetic variants in *SLC2A9* associated with UA concentrations in children [19]. Studies evaluating the effects of gene variants in the context of controlling UA concentrations are important, but insufficient research has been conducted in children. On reviewing the literature and considering the possibility of genotype analysis, we assessed the effects of two SNPs (rs3825017 genotype of *SLC22A12* and rs16890979 genotype of *SLC2A9*) of UA-related genes on the UA concentration in childhood using repeated-measures UA data derived from the Ewha Birth & Growth Cohort study to determine whether genetic variants influence the UA concentrations during the first 10 years of life. Because there is little data on how the UA concentration is maintained over time, we also estimated the tracking coefficient of the UA concentrations during childhood.

Methods

Study subjects

This study was conducted as part of the ongoing Ewha Birth & Growth Cohort study, a single-hospital-based prospective cohort that was established in 2001–2006. The cohort was started to investigate the risk and preventive factors that may be associated with growth and disease susceptibility via longitudinal observations. The study enrolled 940 subjects at 24–28 weeks pregnancy who visited Ewha Womans University Mokdong Hospital, Seoul, Korea for prenatal care. We conducted follow-up when their offspring reached the ages of 3, 5, and 7 years and annually thereafter. By 2016, the follow-up of children aged 9 years had been completed. The methodology of the cohort study has been reported elsewhere [20, 21]. In this study, two SNPs were genotyped in the subjects who were followed up at least once. There were 471, 400, 364, and 400 cohort members who were followed up at the ages of 3, 5, 7, and 9 years, respectively. Of these, we included subjects who had both UA and genotype data (i.e., 375, 204, 307, and 363 at ages 3, 5, 7, and 9 years, respectively). This study was composed of 620 children because many children attended multiple follow-up visits. Written informed consent for participation in the study was obtained from the parents or guardians of all of the study participants at the time of follow-up. The study protocol was approved by the Institutional Review Board of Ewha Womans University Hospital (approval No. EUMC 2015–04-048). All processes were performed in accordance with relevant guidelines and regulations.

Uric acid measurements

When visiting a hospital to participate in the follow-up program, we collected a blood sample from an antecubital vein in a vacutainer tube containing ethylenediaminetetraacetic acid (EDTA). All blood sample were obtained after fasting at least 8 h. Serum UA concentrations were measured using the uricase-peroxidase coupled reaction method on a Hitachi Auto-analyzer 7600 (Hitachi, Fukuoka, Japan) in the Clinical Biochemistry Department of the Seegene Medical Foundation, Seoul, Korea. UA measurements during follow-up were performed in the same way.

Genotyping the two SNPs

The genotypes of rs3825017 in *SLC22A12* and rs16890979 in *SLC2A9* were screened using the TaqMan fluorogenic 5′ nuclease assay (ABI, Foster City, CA, USA). The final volume of the polymerase chain reaction (PCR) was 5 μL, and each reaction contained 10 ng genomic DNA, 2.5 μL TaqMan Universal PCR Master Mix, and 0.13 μL 20× Assay Mix. The thermal cycle conditions were as follows: 50 °C for 2 min to activate the uracil N-glycosylase and to prevent carry-over contamination, 95 °C for 10 min to activate the DNA polymerase, followed by 45 cycles at 95 °C for 15 s and 60 °C for 1 min. All of the PCR reactions were performed using 384-well plates on a Dual 384-Well GeneAmp PCR System 9700 (ABI). The endpoint fluorescent readings were performed on an ABI PRISM 7900 HT Sequence Detection System (ABI). Duplicate samples and negative controls were included to ensure the accuracy of genotyping, which was performed at DNA Link Inc. in Seoul, Korea. The distribution of the two SNPs in the study subjects satisfied Hardy–Weinberg equilibrium.

Covariates

As covariates, we considered BMI and birth weight, based on previous studies [16, 18]. Maternal education level was used as a measure of socioeconomic status because it changes little over time (graduated from high school or some college or higher). Anthropometric data were collected by trained researchers when the subjects visited the hospital to participate in the follow-up program. Height and weight were measured to the nearest 0.1 cm and 0.1 kg, respectively, while wearing light clothing and no shoes using a stadiometer and calibrated scale. BMI was calculated as weight (kg)/height^2 (m^2). BMI at each follow-up point was considered a covariate. Birth weight was obtained from the hospital birth records.

Statistical analysis

Numerical variables are presented as the mean and standard deviation and categorical variables were presented as the number of subjects and percent. Using repeated-measures data for UA concentrations in subjects aged 3, 5, 7, and 9 years, we estimated the intra-class correlation (ICC) as the tracking coefficient through mixed model analysis [22]. There was no critical tracking value. We interpreted < 0.3 as weak, 0.3–0.6 as moderate, and > 0.6 as strong, based on a previous study [23]. The average difference in UA concentration by sex was evaluated using Student's *t*-test. The average UA concentration according to genotype was analyzed using a generalized linear model.

To investigate the long-lasting effects of genetic variants on UA concentration, we used mixed model analysis with a random intercept model. Analyses were conducted using a variance component structure based on lower Akaike information criterion (AIC) values for model selection. The genetic variant used a dominant model (CC vs. CT + TT genotypes) to ensure that the groups had sufficient subjects. Maternal education level and birth weight were treated as time-independent covariates. The BMI at each follow-up visit was considered a time-dependent covariate. To assess the effect modifier, we also included the interaction between sex and genotype as a dominant model.

All of the statistical tests were conducted using SAS 9.4 (SAS Institute, Cary, NC, USA) with two-sided tests, and a p value < 0.05 was considered statistically significant. For the interaction, P values < 0.1 were considered to be significant, based on a previous report [24].

Results

Two SNPs were examined in 620 children. The rs3825017 allele frequencies of CC, CT, and TT were 61.1%, 34.9%, and 4.0%, respectively. The rs16890979 allele frequencies of GG, GA, and AA were 99.0%, 1.0%, and 0.0%, respectively (Table 1). The genetic polymorphism distribution did not differ by sex ($p > 0.05$, χ^2 test) and there was no sex difference in UA concentration with follow-up time ($P > 0.05$). Overall, the tracking coefficient of UA concentration from 3 to 9 years of age was 0.31, and was higher in boys than in girls (0.34 vs. 0.29, respectively). While the tracking coefficient of UA concentration from 5 to 9 years of age was higher (total = 0.37, boys = 0.39, girls = 0.34), these values can interpreted as showing moderate stability.

Table 2 shows the average UA concentration for genetic models of the two polymorphisms. There was a limited ability to assess the effects of rs16890979 on UA concentration because the minor allele frequency was very low. Thus, its result was not presented in the table. The effects of rs3825017 on UA concentration were significant in boys, but not in girls. Boys with the T allele of rs3825017 had higher concentrations than their counterparts at baseline (Table 2). In boys, carriers with one or two T alleles (i.e., CT or TT) had a higher mean UA concentration than non-carriers regardless of the time of follow-up, even after adjusting for birth weight, maternal education level, time, and BMI at each follow-up point. In girls, no effects of rs3825017 on UA concentration were apparent (Fig. 1).

The longitudinal effects of rs3825017 genotype on individual UA concentration are presented in Table 3. The random intercept model showed that UA concentration at baseline varied among the children. When estimating changes in UA concentration with age, we found that concentration decreased by 4.39 μmol/L with every 2-year increase in age ($P < 0.001$). Individual UA concentrations changed at the same rate with age in the children, indicating that there were no significant effects of a random slope in time. The rs3825017 genotypes had significant effects on the changes in UA concentration in the first decade of life in boys only (Table 3). The effect of BMI on the UA concentrations was not significant in either sex. Maternal education level as a measure of socioeconomic status and birth weight had no effect on UA concentration. After adjusting for the interaction between genotypes and sex, the difference in sex was significant (P for interaction = 0.08). The longitudinal effects of rs16890979 were not assessed due to the very low frequency of the minor allele.

Discussion

This study used a longitudinal approach to examine the relationship between two candidate SNPs and UA concentration in a general pediatric population. The rs3825017 genotype of *SLC22A12* had a notable effect on UA concentration in the first 10 years of life in boys. Although there was no sex difference in UA concentration, the genetic effects of rs3825017 on concentration differed by sex ($P_{\text{genotype} \times \text{sex}} = 0.08$) during childhood. The tracking coefficient of UA from 3 to 9 years of age showed moderate stability.

Both *SLC22A12*, which encodes urate transporter 1 (URAT1), and *SLC2A9*, which encodes glucose transporter 9 (GLUT9), are involved in modulating urate reabsorption in the renal tubules. A meta-analysis of GWA studies identified multiple candidate loci related to UA level in European (*SLC2A9*, *ABCG2*, *SLC17A1*, *SLC22A11*, *SLC22A12*, *SLC16A9*, *GCKR*, *LRRC16A*, and *PDZK1*) and East Asian (*SLC2A9*, *ABCG2*, *SLC22A12*,

Table 1 Distribution of *SLC2A9* G844A and *SLC22A12* C246T variants and characteristics of the study subjects

	Unit: *n* (%) or mean (standard deviation)		
	Total	Boys	Girls
Genetic variants			
rs3825017 polymorphism			
CC	377 (61.1%)	197 (62.5%)	180 (59.6%)
CT	215 (34.9%)	107 (34.0%)	108 (35.8%)
TT	25 (4.0%)	11 (3.5%)	14 (4.6%)
rs16890979 polymorphism			
GG	614 (99.0%)	312 (98.7%)	302 (99.3%)
GA	6 (1.0%)	4 (1.3%)	2 (0.7%)
Serum uric acid concentration (μmol/L) at each FU age			
UA at 3 years of age	223.44 (46.44)	225.38 (43.98)	221.52 (48.78)
UA at 5 years of age	235.94 (42.55)	234.60 (41.55)	237.28 (43.69)
UA at 7 years of age	223.97 (55.64)	219.92 (57.03)	227.94 (54.12)
UA at 9 years of age	211.59 (48.85)	214.19 (52.04)	208.97 (45.41)
Covariates			
Birth weight (kg)	3.09 (0.59)	3.15 (0.59)	3.03 (0.58)
BMI (kg/m^2) at 3 years of age	15.47 (1.31)	15.49 (1.33)	15.45 (1.29)
BMI (kg/m^2) at 5 years of age	15.71 (1.67)	15.94 (1.78)	15.47 (1.53)
BMI (kg/m^2) at 7 years of age	15.95 (2.10)	16.19 (2.18)	15.72 (2.01)
BMI (kg/m^2) at 9 years of age	17.50 (2.58)	17.88 (2.75)	17.14 (2.35)
Maternal education level			
Graduated from high school	132 (22.2%)	64 (21.2%)	68 (23.3%)
Some college or higher	462 (77.8%)	238 (78.8%)	224 (76.7%)

UA uric acid, *FU* follow-up, *BMI* body mass index

and *MAF*) populations [2, 25]. Mutations in *SLC22A12* or *SLC2A9* were initially reported in Japanese patients with renal hypouricemia, although patients from various ethnic groups have subsequently been identified [7]. A study of children in the Viva La Familia Study also recently showed that the serum UA concentration was associated strongly with genetic variants in *SLC2A9* through GWA analysis [19]. Of genetic variants, the Hereditary and Phenotype Intervention (HAPI) Heart Study found that rs16890979 in *SLC2A9* was associated

Table 2 Baseline differences in the uric acid concentrations (μmol/L) for each genetic model[a]

	Total				Boys				Girls			
	n	Mean	S.D.	*p*	*n*	Mean	S.D.	*p*	*n*	Mean	S.D.	*p*
Dominant model for rs3825017												
CC	222	221.58	47.98	0.37	112	219.17	45.44	0.02	110	224.02	50.52	0.40
CT + TT	151	226.02	44.40		73	234.66	40.44		78	217.94	46.64	
Recessive model for rs3825017												
CC + CT	355	223.19	46.79	0.73	178	224.02	43.97	0.05	177	222.36	49.57	0.33
TT	18	227.02	42.81		7	257.46	36.13		11	207.64	35.63	
Codominant model for rs3825017												
CC	222	221.58	47.98	0.66	112	219.17	45.44	0.02	110	224.02	50.52	0.53
CT	133	225.89	44.77		66	232.24	40.36		67	219.63	48.21	
TT	18	227.02	42.81		7	257.46	36.13		11	207.64	35.63	

S.D standard deviation

[a] For the baseline differences, the results were obtained using the uric acid concentrations at 3 years of age

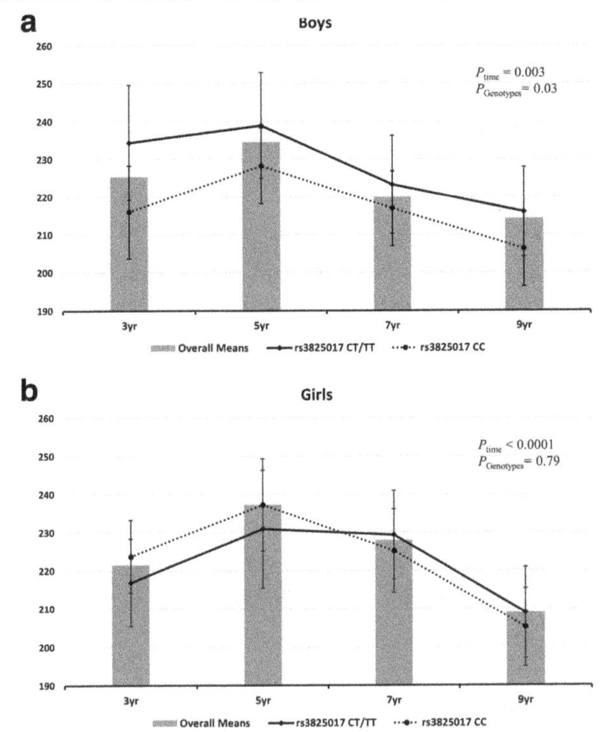

Fig. 1 The average uric acid concentrations (μmol/L) with the dominant model of rs3825017 genotypes from 3 to 9 years of age, by sex. **a** Boys, **b** Girls The least-squared mean by genotypes (as a dominant model) at each follow-up age were obtained from a mixed model under a random intercept model with variance components structure. It was estimated while controlling for time, birth weight, maternal education level, and body mass index at each time point. Genetic variants and time were applied as categorical values to obtain the mean values for the genetic variant at each time point. The box indicates the average UA concentration, and the vertical lines show the standard error

with UA concentrations and it accounted for 4.3% of the variance [26]. This association was also reported in studies of the Framingham and Rotterdam cohorts [5] and a Czech population [27], but there was a discrepancy in the direction of association. This might involve additional factors, such as diet, lifestyle, and different linkage disequilibrium structures [8, 27]. Although two meta-analyses reported that the dominant model of rs16890979 was associated with gout in an Asian population [9, 28], our study had limited statistical strength due to the low minor allele frequency; the minor allele frequency of rs16890979 was less than 0.02 in the populations of China and Japan, was greater than 0.29 in a European population [29], 0.23 in the Framingham Heart Study, and was 0.21 in the Rotterdam Study [5]. In addition, *SLC2A9* rs16890979 showed possible associations with gout [9] and hyperuricemia [30]. However, functional characterization of *SLC2A9* rs16890979 in an experimental validation study revealed no significant difference in the expression of GLUT9 [30]. Functional studies are likely to be important in determining the causality of disease-related SNPs.

In our study, rs3825017 in *SLC22A12* affected UA concentration in boys, but not in girls. Three other studies have examined rs3825017 [12, 15, 31]. In line with our study, one study of Korean men found an association with hyperuricemia (odds ratio = 2.29, 95% confidence interval 1.78 to 2.93), while studies from Japanese and Chinese population found no significant effect. The latter studies did not assess sex differences, which needs further study. Regarding to *SLC2A9*, several studies have suggested sex differences by genotype including rs16890979; the effects were seen more clearly in women than in men [2, 32]. The sex difference can be explained by sex hormones. Because estrogen is uricosuric [33], the differences with the rs3825017 genotype are expected to be more distinct around puberty. A recent GWA study of gout and its subtypes revealed that *HIST1H2BF-HIST1H4E*, *NIPAL1*, and *FAM35A* were novel risk loci [8]. However, detailed knowledge of the functional pathways of these genes affecting UA concentrations remains limited and further studies are required.

Although the pathological mechanism of UA is unclear, Mazzali et al. reported that rats with induced mild hyperuricemia develop mild hypertension and slightly reduced renal function [34]. In addition, injury was seen in the afferent arterioles of the renal microvasculature in the hyperuricemic rat [35, 36]. These experimental studies also suggested that these

Table 3 Longitudinal effects of rs3825017 genotypes on individual serum uric acid concentrations

	Total			Boys			Girls		
	β	S.E.	*p*	*β*	S.E.	*p*	*β*	S.E.	*p*
Sex	0.48	3.37	0.89	–			–		
FU time	−4.39	1.18	< 0.001	−4.51	1.71	< 0.01	−4.06	1.65	0.01
Dominant model for rs3825017	5.13	3.44	0.14	11.98	4.94	0.02	−0.88	4.77	0.85
BMI	1.47	0.76	0.05	1.90	1.02	0.06	0.92	1.16	0.43
Birth weight	−1.50	2.92	0.61	2.57	4.08	0.53	−4.79	4.20	0.25
Maternal education	5.46	4.02	0.17	8.95	5.76	0.12	3.09	5.61	0.58

FU follow-up, *BMI* body mass index
The rs3825017 genotypes for the dominant model (CC and CT + TT)
The coefficients (*β*) were obtained from a mixed model under random intercept model with variance components structure

changes could be prevented by maintaining UA concentration in the normal range [1, 34, 35].

Even in children, UA had an independent effect on higher blood pressure after controlling for adiposity factors, renal function, and pubertal status [18]. A cohort study with an average 12-year follow-up also reported that the UA concentration in childhood and changes in concentration were significant predictors of blood pressure in later life [4]. Feig et al. suggested that serum UA concentration is directly correlated with blood pressure, and that hyperuricemia showed a stronger association in childhood primary hypertension than in secondary or white-coat hypertension [3]. Therefore, control of UA levels may be important to prevent disease. In our study, the tracking coefficient of UA during the 6-year follow-up period beginning at 3 years of age showed moderate stability (ICC = 0.31). The tracking coefficient of UA from 5 to 9 years of age was slightly higher (ICC = 0.37). The UA concentration in blood can vary with age, sex, and pubertal status [4, 19]. Unlike previous studies, we found no differences in UA concentration with sex, and the average UA concentration decreased with increasing age during the first decade of life. Our study examined younger subjects than those used in previous studies [4, 18, 37], and there are few prospective studies of UA using repeated measures. Thus, it is difficult to explain the difference.

To the best of our knowledge, this is the first study to assess the persistent effects of genetic variants on the UA concentration during childhood. Compared with non-carriers, boys with carriers of at least one rs3825017 T allele exhibited elevated UA concentrations. Our results support those of an earlier study conducted in Korean males [15]. Additionally, BMI was positively associated with the UA concentration during childhood, with borderline significance in boys but not in girls.

This study had several weaknesses. First, we assessed the effect of one tag SNP; other genetic variants near URAT1 may also be important. In addition, residual confounding by unmeasured factors may affect UA concentration. Conversely, our results are less likely to be influenced by unhealthy factors such as alcohol consumption and comorbidities compared to adult studies and case-control studies, because this study examined a general pediatric population. We assumed that the genetic variants were dichotomized by a dominant effect of the risk allele due to the low frequency of homozygous carriers of the risk allele. It is necessary to confirm this in a large-scale study and in studies of different ethnic groups. To verify the statistical power, we calculated the required sample size for linear mixed model with random intercept. As a result, 41 subjects per group were required to evaluate the significance of a difference in the UA concentration between the two groups (non-carriers vs carriers of at least one rs3825017 T allele), assuming that the power was 80% with $\alpha = 0.05$, four repeated measurements, and mean difference − 11.3. Thus, we found that the statistical power of our study was adequate. Finally, there is a limit to generalizing our findings because the evidence is still insufficient.

Conclusions

In summary, we estimated the stability of UA concentration over 6 years beginning in early childhood, and observed moderate stability. A single measurement of UA during childhood may have a limited ability to predict disease in later life. Through a longitudinal approach, we also found that rs3825017 genotype had a notable effect on UA concentration in boys during childhood. Our study considered only two SNPs (rs3825017 in *SLC22A12* and rs16890979 in *SLC2A9*). Therefore, further studies with extended follow-up periods are required to consider other major genetic loci associated with UA concentrations, such as glucokinase regulatory protein (*GCKR*) and *ABCG2* [2].

Abbreviations

ABCG: ATP-binding cassette transporter; AIC: Akaike information criterion; BMI: Body mass index; EDTA: Ethylenediaminetetraacetic acid; *GCKR*: Glucokinase regulatory protein; GLUT9: Glucose transporter 9; GWA: Genome-wide association; ICC: Intra-class correlation; PCR: Polymerase chain reaction; *SLC22A12*: Solute carrier family 22 (organic anion/cation transporter) member 12; *SLC2A9*: Solute carrier family 2 facilitated glucose transporter member 9; SNP: Single-nucleotide polymorphism; UA: Uric acid; URAT1: Urate transporter 1

Funding

This research was supported by the Basic Science Research Program through the National Research Foundation of Korea (NRF), funded by the Ministry of Science, ICT& Future Planning (NRF-2014R1A1A3051023).

Authors' contributions

Conceptualization, EAP, SJC, HSK, and HP; formal analysis, HAL; data curation, HAL, BHP, EAP, SJC, HSK, and HP; writing the original draft, HAL; reviewing and editing the manuscript, BHP, EAP, SJC, HSK and HP; supervision, HP; approval of the final manuscript, all authors.

Competing interests

The authors declare that they have no competing interests.

Author details

[1]Department of Preventive Medicine, College of Medicine, Ewha Womans University, 1071, Anyangcheon-ro, Yangcheon-ku, Seoul 158-710, Korea. [2]Clinical Trial Center, Mokdong Hospital, Ewha Womans University, Seoul, Korea. [3]Department of Pediatrics, College of Medicine, Ewha Womans University, Seoul, Korea.

References

1. Kutzing MK, Firestein BL. Altered uric acid levels and disease states. J Pharmacol Exp Ther. 2008;324(1):1–7.

2. Kolz M, Johnson T, Sanna S, Teumer A, Vitart V, Perola M, et al. Meta-analysis of 28,141 individuals identifies common variants within five new loci that influence uric acid concentrations. PLoS Genet. 2009;5(6):e1000504.
3. Feig DI, Johnson RJ. The role of uric acid in pediatric hypertension. J Ren Nutr. 2007;17(1):79–83.
4. Alper AB Jr, Chen W, Yau L, Srinivasan SR, Berenson GS, Hamm LL. Childhood uric acid predicts adult blood pressure: the Bogalusa heart study. Hypertension. 2005;45(1):34–8.
5. Dehghan A, Köttgen A, Yang Q, Hwang SJ, Kao WL, Rivadeneira F, et al. Association of three genetic loci with uric acid concentration and risk of gout: a genome-wide association study. Lancet. 2008;372(9654):1953–61.
6. Whitfield JB, Martin NG. Inheritance and alcohol as factors influencing plasma uric acid levels. Acta Genet Med Gemellol. 1983;32:117–26.
7. Claverie-Martin F, Trujillo-Suarez J, Gonzalez-Acosta H, Aparicio C, Justa Roldan ML, Stiburkova B, Ichida K, Martín-Gomez MA, Herrero Goñi M, Carrasco Hidalgo-Barquero M, Iñigo V, Enriquez R, Cordoba-Lanus E, Garcia-Nieto VM, RenalTube Group. URAT1 and GLUT9 mutations in Spanish patients with renal hypouricemia. Clin Chim Acta. 2018;481:83–9. https://doi.org/10.1016/j.cca.2018.02.030.
8. Nakayama A, Nakaoka H, Yamamoto K, Sakiyama M, Shaukat A, Toyoda Y, et al. GWAS of clinically defined gout and subtypes identifies multiple susceptibility loci that include urate transporter genes. Ann Rheum Dis. 2017;76(5):869–77. https://doi.org/10.1136/annrheumdis-2016-209632.
9. Chen Y, Ying Y, Shi S, Li L, Huang Y, Ye H, Gong O, Huang H, Ji H, Huang T, Duan S. A systematic review and meta-analysis of 4 candidate polymorphisms with the risk of gout. Int J Clin Exp Med. 2016;9(8):16025–33.
10. Stiburkova B, Pavelcova K, Zavada J, Petru L, Simek P, Cepek P, Pavlikova M, Matsuo H, Merriman TR, Pavelka K. Functional non-synonymous variants of ABCG2 and gout risk. Rheumatology (Oxford). 2017;56(11):1982–92.
11. Higashino T, Takada T, Nakaoka H, Toyoda Y, Stiburkova B, Miyata H, et al. Multiple common and rare variants of ABCG2 cause gout. RMD Open. 2017; 3(2):e000464.
12. Iwai N, Mino Y, Hosoyamada M, Tago N, Kokubo Y, Endou H. A high prevalence of renal hypouricemia caused by inactive SLC22A12 in Japanese. Kidney Int. 2004;66(3):935–44.
13. Lee JH, Choi HJ, Lee BH, Kang HK, Chin HJ, Yoon HJ, Ha IS, Kim S, Choi Y, Cheong HI. Prevalence of hypouricaemia and SLC22A12 mutations in healthy Korean subjects. Nephrology (Carlton). 2008;13(8):661–6. https://doi.org/10.1111/j.1440-1797.2008.01029.x.
14. Gabrikova D, Bernasovska J, Sokolova J, Stiburkova B. High frequency of SLC22A12 variants causing renal hypouricemia 1 in the Czech and Slovak Roma population; simple and rapid detection method by allele-specific polymerase chain reaction. Urolithiasis. 2015;43(5):441–5. https://doi.org/10.1007/s00240-015-0790-4.
15. Cho SK, Kim S, Chung JY, Jee SH. Discovery of URAT1 SNPs and association between serum uric acid levels and URAT1. BMJ Open. 2015;5(11):e009360.
16. Franco MC, Christofalo DM, Sawaya AL, Ajzen SA, Sesso R. Effects of low birth weight in 8- to 13-year-old children: implications in endothelial function and uric acidlevels. Hypertension. 2006;48(1):45–50.
17. Lin WT, Huang HL, Huang MC, Chan TF, Ciou SY, Lee CY, et al. Effects on uric acid, body mass index and blood pressure in adolescents of consuming beverages sweetened with high-fructose corn syrup. Int J Obes (Lond). 2013;37(4):532–9.
18. Viazzi F, Antolini L, Giussani M, Brambilla P, Galbiati S, Mastriani S, et al. Serum uric acid and blood pressure in children at cardiovascular risk. Pediatrics. 2013;132(1):e93–9.
19. Voruganti VS, Laston S, Haack K, Mehta NR, Cole SA, Butte NF, et al. Serum uric acid concentrations and SLC2A9 genetic variation in Hispanic children: the viva La Familia study. Am J Clin Nutr. 2015;101(4):725–32.
20. Lee HA, Park EA, Cho SJ, Kim HS, Kim YJ, Lee H, et al. Mendelian randomization analysis of the effect of maternal homocysteine during pregnancy, as represented by maternal MTHFR C677T genotype, on birth weight. J Epidemiol. 2013;23(5):371–5.
21. Lee HA, Kim YJ, Lee H, Gwak HS, Hong YS, Kim Q, et al. The preventive effect of breast-feeding for longer than 6 months on early pubertal development among children aged 7-9 years in Korea. Public Health Nutr. 2015;18(18):3300–7.
22. Twisk JWR. Applied longitudinal data analysis for epidemiology: a practical guide. Cambridge: Cambridge University Press; 2003. p. 225–7.
23. Pearson N, Salmon J, Campbell K, Crawford D, Timperio A. Tracking of children's body-mass index, television viewing and dietary intake over five-years. Prev Med. 2011;53(4–5):268–70.
24. Prado EL, Maleta K, Ashorn P, Ashorn U, Vosti SA, Sadalaki J, Dewey KG. Effects of maternal and child lipid-based nutrient supplements on infant development: a randomized trial in Malawi. Am J Clin Nutr. 2016;103:784–93.
25. Okada Y, Sim X, Go MJ, Wu JY, Gu D, Takeuchi F, et al. Meta-analysis identifies multiple loci associated with kidney function-related traits in east Asian populations. Nat Genet. 2012;44(8):904–9.
26. Parsa A, Brown E, Weir MR, Fink JC, Shuldiner AR, Mitchell BD, et al. Genotype-based changes in serum uric acid affect blood pressure. Kidney Int. 2012;81(5):502–7.
27. Stibůrková B, Pavlíková M, Sokolová J, Kožich V. Metabolic syndrome, alcohol consumption and genetic factors are associated with serum uric acid concentration. PLoS One. 2014;9(5):e97646. https://doi.org/10.1371/journal.pone.0097646. eCollection 2014.
28. Meng Q, Yue J, Shang M, Shan Q, Qi J, Mao Z, et al. Correlation of GLUT9 polymorphisms with gout risk. Medicine (Baltimore). 2015;94(44):e1742.
29. Yang B, Mo Z, Wu C, Yang H, Yang X, He Y, et al. A genome-wide association study identifies common variants influencing serum uric acid concentrations in a Chinese population. BMC Med Genomics. 2014;7:10.
30. Hurba O, Mancikova A, Krylov V, Pavlikova M, Pavelka K, Stibůrková B. Complex analysis of urate transporters *SLC2A9, SLC22A12* and functional characterization of non-synonymous allelic variants of GLUT9 in the Czech population: no evidence of effect on hyperuricemia and gout. PLoS One. 2014;9(9):e107902.
31. Li C, Han L, Levin AM, Song H, Yan S, Wang Y, et al. Multiple single nucleotide polymorphisms in the human urate transporter 1 (hURAT1) gene are associated with hyperuricaemia in Han Chinese. J Med Genet. 2010; 47(3):204–10.
32. McArdle PF, Parsa A, Chang YC, Weir MR, O'Connell JR, Mitchell BD, et al. A common non-synonymous variant in GLUT9 is a determinant of serum uric acid levels in old order Amish. Arthritis Rheum. 2008;58(9):2874–81.
33. Adamopoulos D, Vlassopoulos C, Seitanides B, Contoyiannis P, Vassilopoulos P. The relationship of sex steroids to uric acid levels in plasma and urine. Acta Endocrinol. 1977;85(1):198–208.
34. Mazzali M, Kanellis J, Han L, Feng L, Xia Y-Y, Chen Q, et al. Hyperuricemia induces a primary arteriolpathy in rats by a blood pressure-independent mechanism. Am J Physiol Renal Physiol. 2002;6:F991–7.
35. Sánchez-Lozada LG, Tapia E, Avila-Casado C, Soto V, Franco M, Santamaría J, et al. Mild hyperuricemia induces glomerular hypertension in normal rats. Am J Physiol Renal Physiol. 2002;283(5):F1105–10.
36. Watanabe S, Kang DH, Feng L, Nakagawa T, Kanellis J, Lan H, et al. Uric acid, hominoid evolution, and the pathogenesis of salt-sensitivity. Hypertension. 2002;40(3):355–60.
37. Feig DI, Johnson RJ. Hyperuricemia in childhood primary hypertension. Hypertension. 2003;42(3):247–52.

22

Type 1 tympanoplasty in pediatric patients

Deniz Baklaci*, Ismail Guler, Ihsan Kuzucu, Rauf Oguzhan Kum and Muge Ozcan

Abstract

Background: The aim of this study was to investigate the success of type 1 tympanoplasty in pediatric patients with chronic otitis media, and to evaluate the prognostic factors that may influence its success.

Materials and methods: Medical records of 102 children aged between 8 and 18 years (46 female, 56 male) who underwent type 1 tympanoplasty for chronic tympanic membrane perforation between January 2010 and July 2017 were reviewed. Age, gender, condition of contralateral ear (unilateral, bilateral), type (central, marginal) and location of perforation (anterior, posterior, inferior), graft material (fascia, cartilage), pre- and post-operative hearing levels, mean air-bone gap (ABG), surgical approach (postauricular, endaural) and length of follow up were recorded.

Results: Anatomical and functional success (ABG < 20 dBHL) rates were 86.3% (88 patients) and 74.5% (76 patients) after a mean follow-up of 32 ± 16.55 months, respectively. The mean hearing improvement was 10.77 ± 10.45 dBHL. The graft success rates were significantly higher in tragal cartilage group (95.1%) than in temporalis fascia group (80.3%) ($p = 0.033$). Graft success was negatively affected by contralateral perforation ($p = 0.003$). All patients with bilateral perforations and graft failure were in temporalis fascia group. Age, type and location of perforation and surgical approach did not influence graft success ($p > 0.05$).

Conclusion: Our results showed that type 1 tympanoplasty can be performed effectively in pediatric population regardless of age, location and type of perforation and surgical approach. Bilateral perforations are prone to reperforation, and should be treated with cartilage graft.

Keywords: Type 1 tympanoplasty, Children, Prognostic factors, Graft success, Hearing

Background

Tympanoplasty was popularized by Zollner and Wullstein [1] in the middle of 1950s. Today, the success rate of tympanoplasty still remains a considerable interest. There has been a particular attention to the outcomes of tympanoplasty in the pediatric age group since 1960s [2, 3]. In the literature, a success rate of tympanoplasties in children ranging from 35 to 94% [4, 5]. Numerous factors have been proposed for the reason of poorer tympanoplasty outcomes in children than in adults: higher frequency of upper respiratory infection and otitis media, poorer eustachian tube function and presence of hypertrophic adenoid tissue, and immaturity of the immune system [6–10]. Therefore, some authors do not propose tympanoplasty in pediatric age [10, 11]. They advocate that eustachian tube dysfunction results in inadequate ventilation to the middle ear, leading to the tympanic membrane (TM) perforation [7–10]. These results mitigating against delaying tympanoplasty in pediatric patients allows for the spontaneous closure of TM perforations. Another problem in pediatric tympanoplasty is thata narrow external auditory canal may complicate the surgery in some patients while postoperative dressings and care may be compelling and unpleasant, especially in uncooperative children.

Nevertheless, studies showed that tympanoplasty success rates in pediatric population were similar to adults [6, 12, 13]. The philosophy of performing tympanoplasty on the pediatric population is based on facts that cannot be disregarded. The presence of hearing loss in childhood has negative effects on the development of speech, language and learning skills. It has been showed that children with hearing loss have some difficulties with reaching their full academic potential [14]. Since

* Correspondence: doktorent@gmail.com
Numune Training and Research Hospital, Department of Otolaryngology, 931st Avenue 945st Street No:5/3 Çankaya, Ankara, Turkey

children have an excellent cochlear reserve, they are more likely to benefit from tympanoplasty in terms of hearing improvement. On the other hand, the risk for a long-standing perforation isthat the squamous epithelium may enter the middle ear through the perforation and this may result in cholesteatoma formation in the middle ear cavity [15]. Therefore, closure of TM perforation prevents cholesteatoma formation and ossicular damage in the long-term. A successful tympanoplasty provides children a safe, non-draining and care-free ear and also the ability to participate in water activities and other social activities without restriction.

There are various factors that may affect the surgical success of tympanoplasty in children, such as age, the size and location of perforation, previous otological operations (ventilation tube, myringotomy, tympanoplasty), condition of the operated and contralateral ear (dry vs draining), presence of adenoid hypertrophy, function of the eustachian tube, choice of graft material, surgical technique and surgeon's experience [8–10, 16]. However, there is still a lack of certainty on which factors contribute to a successful closure due to inconsistencies in demographic and surgical parameters have been evaluated in the literature.

In this study, we aimed to investigate the surgical and functional outcomes of type 1 tympanoplasty in pediatric population and determine the factors influencing the success of tympanoplasty.

Methods

Medical records of 147 pediatric patients who underwent primary tympanoplasty in our clinic between January 2010 and July 2017 were reviewed. The casespresenting with wet ear, cholesteatoma, tympanosclerosis, ossicular chain erosion, combined with mastoidectomy or ossiculoplasty, and patients younger than 8 years old and older than 18 at the time of the surgery and whose first follow-ups were less than 12 months,were excluded from the study.

The study was approved by the local ethics committee (no: E-18-1907), and conducted in accordance with the ethical principles described by the Declaration of Helsinki. Prior written informed consent was obtained from the parents or guardians of the children who served as participants, and of participants 16 years or older, and assent form participants under 16 years of age.

For each patient we analyzed age, gender, condition of contralateral ear (unilateral/bilateral), type (central/marginal) and location of the perforation (anterior/posterior/inferior), graft material (temporal fascia/tragal cartilage), preoperative and postoperative hearing levels, surgical approach (postauricular/endaural), and length of follow-up. Patients were divided into two groups by age: ≤12 years and 13–18 years, as those that are thirteen years old and older are considered adolescents, while those twelve years old and younger are considered children [17].

Type of perforation was described as marginal in cases which the anulus was involved, otherwise it was described as central. Location of perforation categorized into three groups regarding its relation to handle of malleus: anterior, posterior and inferior.

The nasal cavity and nasopharynx were examined by nasal endoscopy. The patients with allergic rhinitis were treated with nasal steroids and antihistaminic drugs for at least two months, and the operation was performed following the evaluation of allergic rhinitis symptoms and nasal cavity examination after treatment. The patients with adenoid vejetation were treated with adenoidectomy, and the operation was performed after three months from adenoidectomy surgery.

All the children were operated witha microscope (Möller-Wedel Optical®; Hamburg, Germany) under general anesthesia. All tympanoplastieswere performed using the underlay technique with temporalis fascia or tragal cartilage through postauricular or endaural incision.

All the children underwent detailed preoperative and postoperative 6th month pure-tone audiometry (PTA) measurements at 0.5, 1, 2 and 4 kHz frequencies using an Interacoustic AC-40 (Middelfart, Denmark) clinical audiometer. Preoperative and postoperative air and bone conduction thresholds were measured for four frequencies. The air–bone gap (ABG) was calculated as the average difference between the air conduction and the bone conduction at 0.5, 1, 2, and 4 kHz. A successful functional result wasdefined as a postoperative ABG of 20 dB (dB) or less [18].

The postoperative follow-up controls take place generally at hospital at the 1st, 3rd, 6th, and 12th months, and annually there after. The surgical performance is measured by otoscopic and microscopic examinations 12 months after the surgery.

Statistical data analysis was performed using SPSS 21 (SPSS Inc., IBM company, Chicago). Data was expressed as mean ± standard deviation (S.D) and as proportion (%). Chi-square test was used for comprising of categorical data. Wilcoxon and Mann-Whitney U tests were used for non-parametric variables whereas independent and paired sample t test were used for parametric variables. The multivariate logistic regression analysis was used to identify independent predictors of functional success. A p value < 0.05 was accepted as statistically significant.

Results

A total of 102 patients (46 female, 56 male) with 102 operated ears (66 left, 36 right) who met the criteria mentioned above were included in this study. The mean length of follow-up was 32 ± 16.55 months (range 12 to 66 months).

The prognostic factors regarding age, statue of contralateral ear, location and type of perforation, graft material and surgical approach are given in Table 1.

The mean age was 14 ± 2.10, ranging from 8 to 18 years old. There were 28 patients (27.4%) in the younger group and 74 patients (78.6%) in the older group. The mean ages were 11.21 ± 1.01 for 12 years old and younger and 14.92 ± 1.37 for 13 years old and older. Graft success rates were 85.5% (24 ears) for 12 years old and younger and 86.5% (64 ears) for 13 years old and older. There was no statistically significant difference in the graft success rates between age groups ($p = 1.000$). The distribution of tympanoplasty outcomes by age was given in Fig. 1.

The overall anatomical success rate of tympanoplasty was 86.3% (88 ears) at the last visit. During the follow-up period, recurrent perforation occurred in 13.7% of patients (14 ears) (Table 2).73 patients (71.6%) had unilateral perforation, 29 patients (28.4%) had bilateral perforation. Graft success rates were 93.2% (68 ears) in patients with unilateral perforations and 69.0% (20 ears) in patients with bilateral perforations, and the difference was statistically significant ($p = 0.003$).

Of the 102 ears, 45 ears (44.1%) perforations were anterior, 45 (44.1%)were posterior, and 12 (11.8%) were inferior. Graft success rates were 86.7% (39 ears) in anterior perforations, 86.7% (39 ears) in posterior perforations, and 83.3% (10 ears) in inferior perforations. There was no statistically significant difference in the graft success rates between the location of perforations ($p = 0.952$).

Table 1 Comparison of prognostic factors for surgical outcomes

	n	Graft success (*n*, %)	*p*
Younger group	28	24 (85.5)	
(≤12 ages)			N.S.*
Older group	74	64 (86.5)	
(13–17 ages)			
Unilateral perforation	73	68 (93.2)	0.003
Bilateral perforation	29	20 (69)	
Location of perforation			
Anterior	45	39 (86.7)	
Posterior	45	39 (86.7)	N.S.*
İnferior	12	10 (83.3)	
Type of perforation			
Central	77	68 (88.3)	N.S.*
Marjinal	25	20 (80)	
Graft material			
Fascia	61	49 (80.3)	0.033
Cartilage	41	39 (95.1)	
Approach			
Postauricular	78	67 (85.9)	N.S.*
Endaural	24	21 (87.5)	

N.S., *$p > 0.05$

Seventy seven ears (75.5%) were with a central perforation and 25 ears (24.5%) were marginal perforation. Graft success rate of central perforations was 88.3% (68 ears) and marginal perforations was 80.0% (20 ears). There was no statistically significant difference in the graft success rates between the type of perforations ($p = 0.294$).

Temporal fascia was used in 61 ears (59.8%) and tragal cartilage was used in 41 ears (40.2%). Graft success rate of fascia group was 80.3% (49 ears) and cartilage group was 95.1% (39 ears), and the difference was statistically significant ($p = 0.033$).

Seventy eight ears (76.5%) were operated via postauricular approach, 24 ears (23.5%) were operated via endaural. Graft success rate of postauricular group was 85.9% (67 ears) and endaural group was 87.5% (21 ears). There was no statistically significant difference in the graft success rates between the type of surgical approach ($p = 0.573$).

The mean preoperative and postoperative bone conduction thresholds were12.51 ± 8.18 dB and 9.74 ± 8.60 dB, respectively, and the difference was statistically significant ($p < 0.001$). The mean preoperative and postoperative air conduction thresholds were 39.36 ± 14.10 dB and 25.79 ± 15.57 dB, respectively, and the difference was statistically significant ($p < 0.001$). The mean preoperative and postoperative ABG were 26.85 ± 9.47 dB and 16.08 ± 10.46 dB, respectively, and the difference was statistically significant ($p < 0.001$) (Table 3). The mean hearing improvement was 10.77 ± 10.45 dB. The postoperative ABG was less than 20 dB in 76 patients, and the functional success rate was 74.5% (Table 2).

Discussion

Success of pediatric tympanoplasty has been a topic of discussion for many years. In the literature, there are numerous studies that investigated it with quite variable results [4, 5, 10, 12]. The disparity of outcomes in pediatric tympanoplasty is attributed to different definition of success and heterogenity of the patients included. In the present study, the success rate of pediatric tympanoplasty was 86.3%, and this result is consistent with rates based on the literature. Factors such as age, location and type of perforation, surgical approach have no statistically significant effect on tympanoplasty outcomes. Status of contralateral ear and graft material influence the outcomes of tympanoplasty.

The timing of pediatric tympanoplasty is controversial. Improvement of eustachian tube function continues with

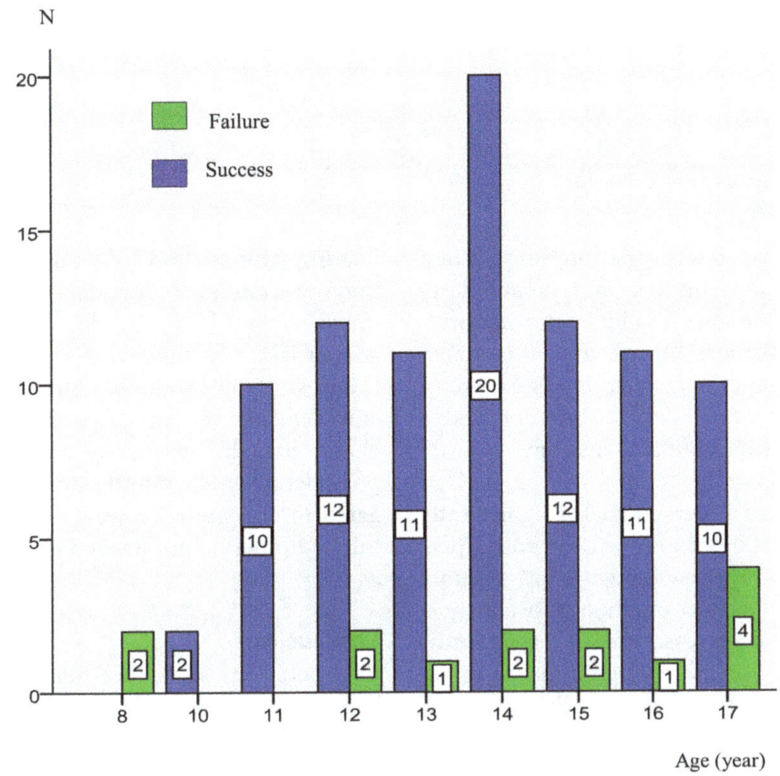

Fig. 1 Tympanoplasty outcomes by age. Shows the distribution of graft take results of patients according to age

aging children [19]. The reasons for the failure of the tympanoplasty results in early ages are thought to be inadequate function of the eustachian tube, weak immune system and recurrent upper respiratory tract infections [6, 8, 20]. There have been various suggestions by different authors regarding the age of the child before the surgery. Some recommended waiting until the ages of 6 [5], 7 [21] or 8 [9] for the operation while others observed more favorable results in children aged 9 [22], 10 [10] or 12 [8]. On the contrary, some authors declared that there was no correlation between age and surgical success [12, 22]. In a study [23], which included the surgical outcomes of tympanoplasty in 52 patients aged between 13 and 17 years old, the success rate was 80.8% similar to those found in adults. In our study, we compared two pediatric age groups (age 8–12 and age 13–18) in terms of tympanoplasty outcome, and found that tympanoplasty outcomes were favorable and similar in both groups ($p > 0.05$). Although a small number of patients were in the younger group, this is the first study to compare the success of tympanoplasty between adolescent and childhood groups.

Table 2 The anatomical and functional success

	n	%
Anatomical success	88	86.3
Functional success (< 20 dBHL ABG)	76	74.5

ABG air-bone gap

Eustachian tube function is an important factor affecting the success of surgery [9, 17]. The status of contralateral ear can be a guide about eustachian tube dysfunction. Some authors [12] showed that the success rates of bilateral perforations decreased by half of unilateral perforations, and they proposed that high graft failures would be a result of severe eustachian dysfunction. In the present study, we used the status of contralateral ear as a predictor of eustachian tube function. There were five graft failures in unilateral group, and nine graft failures in bilateral group. Our results showed that the patients with unilateral perforation had higher graft success (93.2%) than patients with bilateral perforations (69%) ($p = 0.003$). Furthermore, we found that in all bilateral perforations that postoperative graft failure occurred, the temporal fascia had been used as graft material. We may state that when contemplating tympanoplasty in children with bilateral perforations, tragal cartilage should be considered firstly.

Location and type of perforation have been shownto be prognostic factors influencing surgical outcomes of tympanoplasty. The repair of anterior perforations might be technically difficult especially when the anterior canal is prominent, and blocks accessing the perforation. Some

Table 3 Comparison of pre- and post-operative mean air-bone thresholds and ABG

	Pre-operative (dB ± S.D.)	Post-operative (dB ± S.D.)	p
Air conduction	39.36 ± 14.10	25.79 ± 15.57	< 0.001
Bone conduction	12.51 ± 8.1	9.74 ± 8.60	< 0.001
ABG	26.85 ± 9.47	16.08 ± 10.46	< 0.001

dB decibel, *ABG* air-bone gap, *S.D.* Standard deviation, $p < 0.05$

authors [24] proposed that anterior perforations have a tendency to slow and poor healing in tympanoplasty while others [25] found the lowest failure rates in anterior perforations. Some authors [9], on the other hand, did not find any correlation between the location of perforation and graft success. We also did not find a significant correlation between surgical outcome and site of perforation ($p > 0.05$).

Graft success rates were observed to be significantly lower in marginal perforations compared to central perforationsin some studies [5] even though some authors [26] did not find a significant correlation between type of perforation and surgical success. In the present study, even though graft failure was more common in marginal perforations, we did not find any statistically significant relationship between type of perforation and surgical outcome ($p > 0.05$). Marginal perforations have a tendency tolead to cholesteatoma development, which results in ossicular chain erosion and hearing loss, hence it may be stated that a successful tympanoplasty in pediatric patients may prevent the complications associated with a long-term marginal perforation.

Temporalis fascia and tragal cartilage grafts have been most commonly usedin tympanoplasty for many years. Tragal cartilage is strong, thick and easy to place compared to temporal fascia. In a study by Ozbek et al. [27] a higher success rate was observed in the use of tragal cartilage compared to temporal fascia in type 1 pediatric tympanoplasty. In concordance with their results, we found a significantly higher rateof graft success in cartilage group (95.1%) ($p = 0.033$).

In our clinic, postauricular and endaural approaches were performed mostly. Halim et al. [28] compared the success rates of postauricular and endaural approach, and foundno statistically significant difference between two approaches. In this study, 76.5% of operations were performed via the postauricular approach while the rest were performed via the endaural approach. We did not find any correlation between success rate and surgical approach and the findings shows that both two techniques can be performed safely in pediatric patients.

Tympanoplasty is performed to achieve an intact tympanic membrane and hearing improvement. In our study, postoperative ABG significantly decreased compared to preoperative ABG ($p < 0.001$, $p < 0.001$, respectively). Previous studies reported a postoperative mean hearing gain up to 12 dB and a functional success rate ranging from 50 to 88% depending on the definition for improvement [4–6, 10, 12, 25, 27]. Our results were concordant with the literature.

Our study has some limitations. This is a retrospective study and the records of patients obtained from medical charts may be inaccurate or missing. Moreover, only postoperative 6th month hearing results were investigated in our study. However, Future studies with longer follow-up period are needed to support our results.

Conclusion

In conclusion, we believe that type 1 tympanoplasty can be performed effectively in pediatric population regardless of age, location and type of perforation and surgical approach. Early tympanoplasty has an excellent potential for restoring hearing function and may prevent future complications and deterioration associated with long-term perforations. Bilateral perforations are prone to reperforation, and should be treated with cartilage graft.

Abbrevations

ABG: Air-Bone gap; dB: Decibel; N.S: Non-significant; PTA: Pure Tone Audiometry; S.D.: Standard deviation; TM: Tympanic membrane

Acknowledgements

Not applicable.

Funding

The author(s) received no specific funding for this work.

Authors' contributions

DB: Conception, design, writer, IG: Data collection, design, IK: Literature review, design, ROK: Analysis and interpretation, MO: Supervision, critical review. All authors read and approved the final manuscript.

Ethics approval and consent to participate

The study was approved by the ethics committee of Ankara Numune Training and Research Hospital (no: E-18-1907), and conducted in accordance with the ethical principles described by the Declaration of Helsinki. An informed consent was obtained from all participating subjects prior to surgery.

Prior written informed consent was obtained from the parents or guardians of the children who served as participants, and of participants 16 years or older, and assent form participants under 16 years of age.

Competing interests

The authors declare that they have no competing interests.

References

1. Wullstein H. Theory and practice of tympanoplasty. Laryngoscope. 1956; 66(8):1076–93.
2. Gans H. Tympanoplasty in children. Arch Otolaryngol. 1963;77:350.
3. Pyman C. Signposts to successful tympanoplasty, With special reference to children. J Otolaryngol Soc Aust. 1964;1:233–47.
4. Lau T, Tos M. Tympanoplasty in children. An analysis of late results. Am J Otol. 1986;7(1):55–9.
5. Kessler A, Potsic WP, Marsh RR. Type 1 tympanoplasty in children. Arch Otolaryngol Head Neck Surg. 1994;120(5):487–90.
6. Bluestone CD, Cantekin EI, Douglas GS. Eustachian tube function related to the results of tympanoplasty in children. Laryngoscope. 1979;89(3):450-8.
7. Berger G. Myringoplasty in children. J Laryngol Otol. 1974;88:1223–36.
8. Raine C, Singh S. Tympanoplasty in children: a review of 472 cases. Ann Otol Rhinol Laryngol. 1980;89:331–4.
9. Koch WM, Friedman EM, McGill TJ, Healy GB. Tympanoplasty in children: the Boston Children's Hospital experience. Arch Otolaryngol Head Neck Surg. 1990;116(1):35–40.
10. Shih L, de Tar T, Crabtree JA. Myringoplasty in children. Otolaryngol Head Neck Surg. 1991;105(1):74–7.
11. Lancaster J, Makura Z, Porter G, McCormick M. Paediatric tympanoplasty. J Laryngol Otol. 1999;113(7):628–32.
12. Caylan R, Titiz A, Falcioni M, De Donato G, Russo A, Taibah A, et al. Myringoplasty in children: factors influencing surgical outcome. Otolaryngol Head Neck Surg. 1998;118(5):709–13.
13. Collins WO, Telischi FF, Balkany TJ, Buchman CA. Pediatric tympanoplasty: effect of contralateral ear status on outcomes. Arch Otolaryngol Head Neck Surg. 2003;129(6):646–51.
14. Rapin I. Conductive hearing loss effects on children's language and scholastic skills: a review of the literature. Ann Otol Rhinol Laryngol. 1979;88(5_suppl):3–12.
15. Schuknecht HF. Cholesteatoma. Pathology of the Ear. 2nd ed. Philadelphia: Lea & Febiger; 1993. p. 204–206.
16. Manning SC, Cantekin EI, Kenna MA, Bluestone CD. Prognostic value of eustachian tube function in pediatric tympanoplasty. Laryngoscope. 1987;97(9):1012–6.
17. Panel SA. Referral to pediatric surgical specialists. Pediatrics. 2014;133(2):350–6.
18. Balkany TA, Gates GA, Goldenberg RA, Meyerhoff WL, House JW, SURG OHN. Committee on hearing and equilibrium guidelines for the evaluation of results of treatment of conductive hearing loss. Otolaryngol Head Neck Surg. 1995;113(3):186–7.
19. Bylander A, Tjernström Ö. Changes in Eustachian tube function with age in children with Normal ears: a Longiudinal study. Acta Otolaryngol. 1983;96(5–6):467–77.
20. Glasscock ME. Symposium: contraindications to tympanoplasty: II. An exercise in clinical judgment. Laryngoscope. 1976;86(1):70–6.
21. MacDonald RR, Lusk RP, Muntz HR. Fasciaform myringoplasty in children. Arch Otolaryngol Head Neck Surg. 1994;120(2):138–43.
22. Carr MM, Poje CP, Nagy ML, Pizzuto MP, Brodsky LS. Success rates in paediatric tympanoplasty. J Otolaryngol Head Neck Surg. 2001;30(4):199.
23. Rodrigues J, Sousa AC, Gomes A, Gomes P, Mexedo A, Fonseca R. Type I Tympanoplasty in adolescence: prognostic factors and surgical outcomes. Small. 2017;25(16):30.8.
24. Kumar S, Acharya A, Hadjihannas E, Panagamuwa C, McDermott AL. Pediatric myringoplasty: definition of "success" and factors affecting outcome. Otol Neurotol. 2010;31(9):1417–20.
25. Castro O, Pérez-Carro AM, Ibarra I, Hamdan M, Meléndez JM, Araujo A, et al. Myringoplasties in children: our results. Acta Otorrinolaringol (English Edition). 2013;64(2):87–91.
26. Rozendorn N, Wolf M, Yakirevich A, Shapira Y, Carmel E. Myringoplasty in children. Int J Pediatr Otorhinolaryngol. 2016;90:245–50.
27. Ozbek C, Çiftçi O, Tuna EEU, Yazkan Ö, Ozdem C. A comparison of cartilage palisades and fascia in type 1 tympanoplasty in children: anatomic and functional results. Otol Neurotol. 2008;29(5):679–83.
28. Halim A, Borgstein J. Pediatric myringoplasty: postaural versus transmeatal approach. Int J Pediatr Otorhinolaryngol. 2009;73(11):1580–3.

23

Splenic embolization for a giant splenic hemangioma in a child

Woosun Choi[1] and Young Bae Choi[2*]

Abstract

Background: Splenic hemangioma is the most common benign tumor of the spleen. However, it remains a rare medical condition in children. Although the natural course of splenic hemangioma is slow growth, treatment for large splenic hemangiomas has been recommended due to the risk of spontaneous rupture causing life-threating hemorrhage. However, the optimal treatment for splenic hemangioma in children is unclear.

Case presentation: An 11-year-old girl had an enhancing mass, 61 × 54 × 65 mm in size and numerous daughter nodules throughout the entire spleen on a contrast-enhanced computed tomography scan of the abdomen and angiography. The patient was treated by complete embolization at the distal level of splenic artery, which resulted in total splenic infarction. Treatment-related complications were thrombocytosis and postembolization syndrome, including abdominal pain and, intermittent fever below 39 °C. There were no other serious complications, including bleeding.

Conclusion: Splenic embolization may be a safe and less invasive intervention for children with a large splenic hemangioma. Further studies are needed to confirm the effectiveness of our approach.

Keywords: Splenic hemangioma, Embolization, Child

Background

While splenic hemangioma is the most common benign tumor of the spleen, it is nevertheless a rare medical condition. Less than 100 cases of splenic hemangioma have been reported, with fewer 20 being pediatric cases [1–3]. Splenic hemangiomas are most commonly found incidentally since patients are seldom symptomatic. Although the natural course of splenic hemangioma is slow growth, treatment for large splenic hemangiomas exceeding 4 cm in size has been recommended due to the risk of spontaneous rupture causing life-threating hemorrhage [4]. However, the optimal treatment approach to splenic hemangioma including surgery or other interventions in children has been unclear. We present a pediatric case in which a giant splenic hemangioma treated with splenic embolization.

Case presentation

An 11-year-old girl was admitted to our hospital due to abdominal pain and diarrhea of 1 week's duration. She had no medical history of abdominal trauma or surgery. In addition, she had no travel history and there were no pets at her home. Initial assessment of vital signs showed a blood pressure of 116/70 mmHg, a heart rate of 86 beats per minute, body temperature of 36 °C, respiratory rate of 20 breaths/min, and oxygen saturation of 99%, all of which were within normal range for her age. On physical examination, she had tenderness in the right lower quadrant of the abdomen without rebound tenderness. The spleen and liver were not palpable. Laboratory examinations yielded normal results with a leukocyte count of 6,050 cells/μL, hemoglobin concentration of 13.7 g/dL, platelet count of 318,000 platelets/μL, prothrombin time of 12.3 s, and activated partial thromboplastin time of 30.6 s. Initially, she was diagnosed with acute gastroenteritis, and a contrast-enhanced computed tomography (CT) scan of the abdomen was performed to rule out acute appendicitis. A CT scan of the abdomen revealed an enhancing mass, 61 × 54 × 65 mm in size and several subcentimeter enhancing nodules in the spleen, suggesting possible hemangioma, as well as diffuse edematous wall thickening in the colon (Fig. 1). She was diagnosed with acute colitis and a giant splenic hemangioma that was found incidentally, and treated with intravenous hydration and

* Correspondence: zero-ship@hanmail.net
[2]Department of Pediatrics, Chungbuk National University Hospital, Cheongju, Republic of Korea
Full list of author information is available at the end of the article

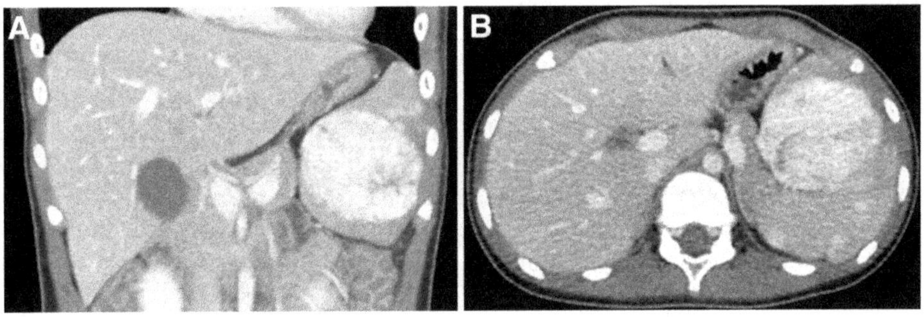

Fig. 1 a and **b** Computed tomography scans shows a giant enhancing mass 61 × 54 × 65 mm in size and several subcentimeter enhancing nodules in the spleen, suggesting possible hemangiomas

medication for acute colitis. After the symptoms of acute colitis resolved, she received vaccinations for encapsulated bacteria including *Haemophilus influenzae* type b, *Streptococcus pneumoniae*, and *Neisseria meningitidis*.

Two weeks after completion of the vaccinations, the patient underwent splenic embolization at the interventional center by a clinically experienced interventional radiologist. The procedure was performed with the patient under general anesthesia and the electrocardiogram, blood pressure, and oxygen saturation with pulse oximetry were continuously monitored during the procedure.

The right common femoral artery was accessed under sonographic guide via the Seldinger technique and a 5-F arterial sheath was placed. A 5-Fr angiographic catheter (Yashiro Glidecath; Terumo, Tokyo, Japan) was used for access and to perform angiography of the celiac trunk and splenic artery. On celiac angiography, a giant hemangioma and multiple daughter nodules were identified in the spleen. Before performing the angiography, we had initially planned selectively embolize of the main mass and the large daughter nodules (Fig. 2a). However, numerous daughter nodules throughout the entire spleen were observed on angiography, and complete splenic artery embolization was performed. For splenic artery embolization, a 1.9-Fr microcatheter (Tellus; Asahi Intecc; Aichi, Japan) was inserted through the angiographic catheter and advanced through the distal splenic artery at the level of the hilum. Polyvinyl alcohol (Contour SE; Boston Scientific, Fremont, CA, USA) particles were initially used for splenic artery embolization and N-butyl cyanoacrylate (Histoacryl; Braun, Sempach, Switzerland) was additionally used for more complete embolization. We occluded the splenic artery at the distal level. Following embolization, angiography demonstrated complete occlusion of the splenic artery (Fig. 2b). There were no acute complications after splenic embolization including bleeding.

At 4 h post-embolization, she developed mild abdominal pain, which was managed with alternating acetaminophen and ketorolac. At 12 h post-embolization, she developed intermittent fever below 39 °C, which was managed with acetaminophen. Blood and urine cultures were subsequently performed. On day 5 post-splenic embolization, hematologic studies showed thrombocytosis, with a platelet count of 502,000/μL. On day 6, a contrast-enhanced CT scan of the abdomen revealed

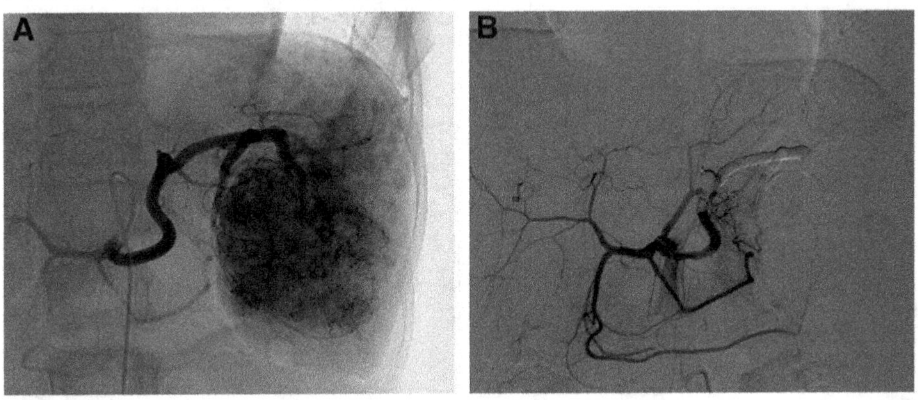

Fig. 2 a Angiography of the splenic artery shows a giant hemangioma and multiple daughter nodules in the spleen. Numerous more daughter nodules were observed throughout the entire spleen on angiography. **b** Post embolization celiac angiography shows complete occlusion of the splenic artery at the distal level

total infarction of the spleen. There were no complications observed, including splenic abscess or bleeding (Fig. 3). On day 7, culture studies showed an absence of bacteria. The abdominal pain and fever had subsided, and the patient was discharged. During outpatient follow-up, the platelet counts peaked at 950,000/μL on day 20 post-splenic embolization and returned to normal 2 months after splenic embolization. No other complications related to the embolization, including pulmonary complications, severe infection, or portal vein thrombosis, occurred during 6 months of follow-up. The patient was prescribed daily prophylaxis with oral amoxicillin for 1 year post-embolization due to her functional asplenia.

Discussion and conclusion

Splenic hemangioma is a rare disease, with an incidence between 0.03 and 14% in autopsy series, most commonly detected in middle-aged adults [4–6]. As hemangiomas are slow-growing benign tumors consisting of numerous blood vessels, small (< 4 cm) asymptomatic splenic hemangiomas have been managed with observation [6]. However, a previous study reported that spontaneous rupture occurs in 25% of patients and large splenic hemangiomas (≥4 cm) had a higher risk of spontaneous rupture [6]. Therefore, splenectomy has been recommended for large splenic hemangiomas due to the risk of life-threatening bleeding.

Splenic embolization was first introduced for hypersplenism treatment by Maddison in 1973 [7]. Compared with splenectomy, splenic embolization had several advantages such as less invasiveness, shorter hospital stays, decreased blood loss, and fewer operative and postoperative complications [7]. Therefore, the indications for splenic embolization included abdominal trauma, hypersplenism, and splenic neoplasm, and have been extended further as the technique continued to improve [8]. In previously reported pediatric cases, most splenic hemangiomas were treated with partial or total splenectomy, and splenic embolization was infrequently performed [1, 2, 9]. In our case, there were no significant complications and only mild abdominal pain and intermittent fever occurred over the 7 days after splenic embolization. This was attributed to postembolization syndrome, which has been reported to be a common complication of splenic embolization and generally resolves without sequelae [7, 10].

Thrombocytosis has been observed 12 to 24 h after splenic embolization and the peak count is reached in 1 or 2 weeks [11]. The degree of thrombocytosis is positively correlated with the degree of spleen infarction and the decreased portal vein flow and increased platelet counts may result in portal vein thrombosis [7, 11]. In our case, the platelet counts reached a peak of 950,000/μL, and there were no thrombotic complications.

As most patients with splenic hemangioma are asymptomatic, an incidental abdominal mass is the most common clinical finding in children with splenic hemangioma. Some patients may have early satiety or abdominal pain due to a mass effect. In our case, although the patient had abdominal pain and diarrhea, it was associated with acute colitis rather than the large splenic hemangioma. There have been reports of heart failure, portal hypertension and gastrointestinal bleeding, thrombocytopenia, anemia, and consumptive coagulopathies such as Kasabach-Merritt syndrome associated with large splenic hemangiomas [1, 2, 4, 6]. The treatment of splenic hemangioma in children has been mostly partial or total splenectomy [1, 2], while Islam et al. reported that the use of oral prednisolone that had an effective antiangiogenic effect in a large splenic hemangioma in an infant [3]. Recently, propranolol has been used for primary therapy of infantile hemangioma; however, to our knowledge, there have been no reports of propranolol for splenic hemangiomas [12]. Further studies may be needed to determine the effectiveness propranolol for splenic hemangioma.

Although splenic embolization may have serious complications such as splenic abscess, splenic rupture,

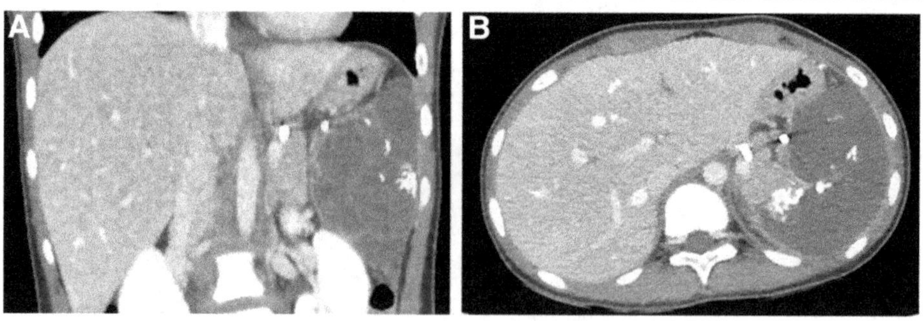

Fig. 3 **a** and **b** Computed tomography on day 6 after embolization shows total infarction of the spleen. Embolic material at the distal splenic artery is also seen on the scans

pancreatitis, and sepsis, it is a less invasive intervention and carries a reduced risk of bleeding compared with splenectomy. As our study was a case report, we cannot provide definite conclusion on the effectiveness of splenic embolization for large splenic hemangiomas. Therefore, further studies are needed to confirm the effectiveness of our approach.

Abbreviation

CT: Computed tomography

Acknowledgements

We thank gratefully professor Kwi-Won Park for helping to take care of the patient.

Author contributions

WC and YBC cared for the patient, drafted the manuscripts and carried out the literature research. Both authors read and approved the final manuscript.

Funding

This work was supported by the research grant of the Chungbuk National University Hospital in 2018.

Competing interests

The authors declare that they have no competing interests.

Author details

[1]Department of Radiology, Chung-Ang University Hospital, Seoul, Republic of Korea. [2]Department of Pediatrics, Chungbuk National University Hospital, Cheongju, Republic of Korea.

References

1. Sencer S, Coulter-Knoff A, Day D, Foker J, Thompson T, Burke B. Splenic hemangioma with thrombocytopenia in a newborn. Pediatrics. 1987;79: 960–6.
2. Panuel M, Ternier F, Michel G, Scheiner C, Bourliere B, Faure F, et al. Splenic hemangioma--report of three pediatric cases with pathologic correlation. Pediatr Radiol. 1992;22:213–6.
3. Islam S, Newman EA, Strouse PJ, Geiger JD. Antiangiogenic therapy for a large splenic hemangioma. Pediatr Surg Int. 2005;21:1007–10.
4. Husni EA. The clinical course of splenic hemangioma with emphasis on spontaneous rupture. Arch Surg. 1961;83:681–8.
5. Coffin CM, Dehner LP. Vascular tumors in children and adolescents: a clinicopathologic study of 228 tumors in 222 patients. Pathol Annu. 1993; 28(Pt 1):97–120.
6. Willcox TM, Speer RW, Schlinkert RT, Sarr MG. Hemangioma of the spleen: presentation, diagnosis, and management. J Gastrointest Surg. 2000;4:611–3.
7. Guan YS, Hu Y. Clinical application of partial splenic embolization. ScientificWorldJournal. 2014;2014:961345.
8. Madoff DC, Denys A, Wallace MJ, Murthy R, Gupta S, Pillsbury EP, et al. Splenic arterial interventions: anatomy, indications, technical considerations, and potential complications. Radiographics. 2005;25(1):S191–211.
9. Raabe EH, Keefer JR, Mitchell SE, Hong K, DiFazio M, Strouse JJ. Subtotal splenic embolization is a safe and effective treatment for isolated splenic vascular tumors associated with consumptive coagulopathy. J Pediatr Hematol Oncol. 2011;33:383–6.
10. Piffaretti G, Tozzi M, Lomazzi C, Rivolta N, Riva F, Caronno R, et al. Splenic artery aneurysms: postembolization syndrome and surgical complications. Am J Surg. 2007;193:166–70.
11. Nio M, Hayashi Y, Sano N, Ishii T, Sasaki H, Ohi R. Long-term efficacy of partial splenic embolization in children. J Pediatr Surg. 2003;38:1760–2.
12. Grzesik P, Wu JK. Current perspectives on the optimal management of infantile hemangioma. Pediatric Health Med Ther. 2017;8:107–16.

24

High rate of antibiotic resistance among pneumococci carried by healthy children in the eastern part of the Democratic Republic of the Congo

Archippe M. Birindwa[1,2,3,5*], Matilda Emgård[1], Rickard Nordén[1], Ebba Samuelsson[1], Shadi Geravandi[1], Lucia Gonzales-Siles[1], Balthazar Muhigirwa[2], Théophile Kashosi[3], Eric Munguakonkwa[2], Jeanière T. Manegabe[2], Didace Cibicabene[2], Lambert Morisho[2], Benjamin Mwambanyi[2], Jacques Mirindi[2], Nadine Kabeza[2], Magnus Lindh[1], Rune Andersson[1,4] and Susann Skovbjerg[1]

Abstract

Background: Pneumococcal conjugate vaccines have been introduced in the infant immunisation programmes in many countries to reduce the rate of fatal pneumococcal infections. In the Democratic Republic of the Congo (DR Congo) a 13-valent vaccine (PCV13) was introduced in 2013. Data on the burden of circulating pneumococci among children after this introduction are lacking. In this study, we aimed to determine the risk factors related to pneumococcal carriage in healthy Congolese children after the vaccine introduction and to assess the antibiotic resistance rates and serotype distribution among the isolated pneumococci.

Methods: In 2014 and 2015, 794 healthy children aged one to 60 months attending health centres in the eastern part of DR Congo for immunisation or growth monitoring were included in the study. Data on socio-demographic and medical factors were collected by interviews with the children's caregivers. Nasopharyngeal swabs were obtained from all the children for bacterial culture, and isolated pneumococci were further tested for antimicrobial resistance using disc diffusion tests and, when indicated, minimal inhibitory concentration (MIC) determination, and for serotype/serogroup by molecular testing.

Results: The pneumococcal detection rate was 21%, being higher among children who had not received PCV13 vaccination, lived in rural areas, had an enclosed kitchen, were malnourished or presented with fever (p value < 0.05). The predominant serotypes were 19F, 11, 6A/B/C/D and 10A. More than 50% of the pneumococcal isolates belonged to a serotype/serogroup not included in PCV13.

Eighty per cent of the isolates were not susceptible to benzylpenicillin and non-susceptibility to ampicillin and ceftriaxone was also high (42 and 37% respectively). Almost all the isolates (94%) were resistant to trimethoprim-sulphamethoxazole, while 43% of the strains were resistant to ≥3 antibiotics.

(Continued on next page)

* Correspondence: birindwaarchippe@gmail.com; archippe.muhandule.birindwa@gu.se
[1]Department of Infectious Diseases, Institute of Biomedicine, University of Gothenburg, Gothenburg, Sweden
[2]Panzi Hospital, Bukavu, Democratic Republic of the Congo
Full list of author information is available at the end of the article

(Continued from previous page)

Conclusions: Our study shows alarmingly high levels of reduced susceptibility to commonly used antibiotics in pneumococci carried by healthy Congolese children. This highlights the importance of local antibiotic resistance surveillance and indicates the needs for the more appropriate use of antibiotics in the area. The results further indicate that improved living conditions are needed to reduce the pneumococcal burden, in addition to PCV13 vaccination.

Keywords: *Streptococcus pneumoniae*, Antibiotic resistance, DR Congo, Nasopharyngeal carriage, Children, PCV13

Background

Streptococcus pneumoniae, or the pneumococcus, is a leading bacterial cause of death in young children worldwide, mainly due to pneumonia [1, 2]. The bacterium is also an important pathogen in other community-acquired respiratory infections, including acute *otitis media*, and in invasive infections, such as meningitis and sepsis.

Pneumococcal infections are estimated to cause 11% of all deaths in children less than 5 years of age worldwide, with a disproportionate number of these deaths in low- and middle income countries [3]. In sub-Saharan Africa, where most of the under-five deaths occur, the leading cause of death is pneumonia and children under the age of 2 years are the most affected [3, 4].

The Democratic Republic of the Congo (DR Congo) is one of the countries with the highest mortality due to childhood pneumonia; in 2015, pneumonia was the leading cause of death under 5 years of age, killing 46,000 Congolese children [5, 6].

Many risk factors, including malnutrition, lack of pneumococcal immunisation, parental smoking and crowded living conditions, [7, 8], as well as exposure to smoke due to the household use of solid fuels has been associated with an increased risk of pneumonia in children [9, 10]. Women and children living in severe poverty have the greatest exposure to household air pollution [11]. In DR Congo, open fires are commonly used in rural villages, while charcoal stoves and electricity are more often used in the cities.

To lower the burden of severe pneumococcal infections among children, pneumococcal conjugate vaccines, covering up to 13 of 98 known pneumococcal serotypes [12], have been introduced in the infant vaccination programmes in many countries. The 13-valent conjugate pneumococcal vaccine (PCV13), containing the serotypes 1, 3, 4, 5, 6A, 6B, 7F, 9 V, 14, 18C, 19A, 19F and 23F, was introduced in DR Congo in 2013. A recent study from Kenya showed that the prevalence of vaccine serotypes was reduced by two-thirds in children younger than 5 years of age after the introduction of PCV10, suggesting that the conjugate vaccines will have substantial effects in reducing invasive pneumococcal disease in Africa [13]. However, in many countries, pneumococcal disease caused by non-vaccine serotypes has increased after the start of vaccination [14] and, in the Gambia, an increase in non-typeable serotypes was noted after the introduction of PCV13; the clinical significance of this finding is not known [15].

There are some reports on the carriage rate and serotype distribution of pneumococci in healthy sub-Saharan children before and after PCV13 vaccination [13, 16, 17], but there are no available data on the child population in DR Congo, either before or after the introduction of PCV13.

According to recommendations revised by the World Health Organisation (WHO) in 2014, oral amoxicillin is the drug of choice for children with pneumonia, while parenteral ampicillin (or penicillin) together with gentamicin should be used in severe cases. Ceftriaxone is recommended as the second-line treatment in children with severe pneumonia who have failed with the first-line treatment. There might, however, be a delay of several years before these recommendations are implemented in local treatment guidelines. Since December 2016, the national policy in DR Congo recommends amoxicillin rather than trimethoprim-sulphamethoxazole (TMP-SMX) for the treatment of pneumonia at community level. As in many other low-income countries, the prescription of antibiotics is, however, not restricted solely to physicians, and children may be treated by people other than educated health workers [18]. Children hospitalised in the South-Kivu province, in eastern DR Congo, due to pneumonia are currently treated with ceftriaxone or ampicillin, together with gentamicin, according to local guidelines, while a combination of ceftriaxone and cloxacillin is used after 48 h without clinical improvement [19].

Resistance to antibiotics is a worldwide concern and the proportion of pneumococci that are not susceptible to penicillin even exceeds 50% in some countries [20]. Before the introduction of the conjugate vaccine, more than two thirds of the pneumococci detected in healthy children in Dar Es Salaam, Tanzania, were non-susceptible to penicillin [21], while the rate was 45% in Gambia [22]. A Peruvian study showed no changes in antibiotic resistance in colonising pneumococci after the introduction of the vaccine, suggesting significant antibiotic resistance in non–PCV7 strains [23], while other studies from South Africa

[24], the United States of America [25] and Canada [26] have shown a decrease in the antibiotic resistance of invasive pneumococci.

Here, we report on the first study of nasopharyngeal carriage and predisposing conditions for pneumococcal colonisation in healthy Congolese children after the introduction of PCV13. The profiles of the circulating pneumococcal serotypes/serogroups and the antibiotic susceptibility of the carried pneumococci were also assessed.

Methods

Study population

From January 2014 to June 2015, 794 healthy children aged one to 60 months attending one of seven health centres in the South-Kivu province in the eastern part of DR Congo for immunisation or growth monitoring were included in the study. The health centres were located in the city of Bukavu ($n = 3$), in the suburban area ($n = 1$), or in the surrounding rural area (n = 3) (Additional file 1).

Written questionnaires about immunisation status and demographic factors were completed by trained final-year medical students or nurses in the presence of a paediatrician and a basic physical examination of the children was performed to monitor current signs of a respiratory tract infection. When available, the immunisation card was checked to confirm the vaccination status of the child. For the 284 healthy children enrolled in 2015, another questionnaire containing questions about socio-economic conditions and previous illness was added. The weight and height were measured and standardised for age using the Emergency Nutrition Assessment (ENA) software 2011 [27].

Signed informed consent was obtained from the parent or guardian of each included child. The study was approved by the Ethics Committees at the Université Catholique de Bukavu, DR Congo, and at the University of Gothenburg, Sweden.

Specimen collection

A nasopharyngeal specimen was obtained from all participating children using an Eswab (Copan Diagnostics Inc., Murrieta, CA). A single trained investigator at each centre obtained the sample following a standardised procedure. The head of the child was tipped backwards and gently immobilised. The bent swab was inserted into the nostril and then passed into the nasopharynx to a distance equal to that from the nose to the tip of the ear and kept in that position for 5 s. The samples were shipped to the Clinical Laboratory at Panzi Hospital within two to 6 h for subsequent pneumococcal culture.

Culture and antibiotic susceptibility testing of pneumococci

The samples were cultured for *Streptococcus pneumoniae* on 5% human blood agar plates (Oxoid Columbia Blood Agar Base – Thermo Fisher Scientific, Waltham, MA), incubated overnight at 34–36 °C in closed jars (Oxoid Limited, Thermo Fisher Scientific, Hampshire, UK) supplied with CO_2 paper sachets (BD GasPak™ EZ CO_2 Container System, Becton, Dickinson and Company, Franklin Lakes, New Jersey) and CO_2 indicators (BD CO_2 Indicator 0.5 mL, Becton, Dickinson and Company).

Suspected pneumococci were identified by a positive optochin test (diameter ≥ 14 mm) and were further tested for antibiotic susceptibility using a disc diffusion test against oxacillin (1 μg) (screening for beta-lactam resistance), trimethoprim-sulphamethoxazole (TMP-SMX) (1.25/23.75 μg), norfloxacin (10 μg) (screening for fluoroquinolone resistance, i.e. levofloxacin and moxifloxacin), tetracycline (30 μg), erythromycin (15 μg) and clindamycin (2 μg) (all from Oxoid Limited), using breakpoints according to the European Committee on Antimicrobial Susceptibility Testing, 2017 [28]. The bacteria and antibiotic discs were applied to Muller Hinton agar plates (Oxoid Limited) supplied with 5% sheep blood (Thermo Fisher Scientific) and 20 mg/L β-Nicotinamide adenine dinucleotide (NAD) (AppliChem GmbH, Darmstadt, Germany) that were incubated over night at 34–36 °C in a CO_2 environment as described above. Pneumococcal isolates with reduced sensitivity to oxacillin (diameter < 20 mm) were further tested using minimal inhibitory concentration (MIC) determination against penicillin G, ampicillin and ceftriaxone (all 0.016–256 μg/mL, bioMérieux, Marcy l'Etoile, France). Pneumococci with an MIC of > 0.06 mg/L were defined as having reduced susceptibility to benzylpenicillin. Multi-drug resistant (MDR) isolates were defined as those that were non-susceptible (intermediate or resistant) to at least one drug from three or more different classes of antimicrobial agents, including the beta-lactams (the penicillins benzylpenicillin and ampicillin and the cephalosporin ceftriaxone) [29]. Apart from the beta-lactams, all drugs tested belong to different classes, namely fluoroquinolones (norfloxacin), lincosamides (clindamycin), macrolides (erythromycin), folate pathway inhibitors (trimethoprim-sulphamethoxazole) and tetracyclines (tetracycline) [29]. The isolates were frozen (– 20 °C) in STGG storage medium [30] before being transported to Gothenburg, Sweden, for further analyses.

Reproducibility of the antibiotic susceptibility results

Out of the 163 pneumococcal strains isolated at the Clinical Laboratory at Panzi Hospital in Bukavu, 151 isolates were transported frozen in STGG medium to Gothenburg. Of these, 32 isolates could be re-cultured after storage and transport, and were tested for antibiotic susceptibility at the Department of Infectious Diseases, University of Gothenburg, Sweden, as well (Fig. 1). When the results were compared with those obtained at the laboratory in Bukavu for the same isolates, the diameter zones for all the tested antibiotic discs varied by 6 mm or less in at least 75% of the cases (Table 1). The resulting interpretation into Sensitive (S), Intermediate (I) or Resistant (R) was similar in both groups (Table 1).

The distributions of MIC values were also compared between the analyses performed in Bukavu and Gothenburg, respectively (Additional file 2). There was an even distribution of MIC values between the two sites for all of penicillin G, ampicillin and ceftriaxone. When interpreting the MIC values for penicillin G, all the isolates were categorised in the same SIR category. For ampicillin, one isolate was differently categorised into sensitive and intermediate, respectively, and the same was true in two cases for ceftriaxone. We also compared the MIC distributions between 2014 and 2015 for all the isolates tested in Bukavu and found an even distribution of the MIC values between the 2 years for ampicillin (Additional file 3). We concluded that the reproducibility was satisfactory for both the disc diffusion tests and the MIC determinations performed in Bukavu and all the results shown in the results section are therefore from the antibiotic susceptibility tests performed in Bukavu.

Nucleic acid extraction and multiplex real-time PCR

The pneumococcal isolates were further analysed by molecular methods in Gothenburg for confirmation of species identification, and for determination of serotypes/serogroups. For those isolates that could be re-cultured after storage and transport ($n = 32$), one colony of each isolate was suspended in 1 mL of PBS prior to the extraction of nucleic acids. For unculturable isolates, 100 μL of STGG storage medium containing non-viable bacteria was diluted in 900 μL of phosphate buffered saline (PBS). DNA was extracted from 200 μL of the suspended isolates or diluted non-viable isolates using a MagNA Pure LC instrument (Roche Diagnostics, Mannheim, Germany) and the Total Nucleic acid Isolation kit (Roche Diagnostic). The extracted nucleic acids were eluted in 100 μL elution buffer. The samples were stored at – 20 °C until further analysis.

A multiplex real-time PCR, able to detect 40 different serotypes, was used according to a protocol published by Centers for Disease Control and Prevention (CDC) using previously published primers with slight modifications (preprint available at https://www.biorxiv.org/content/early/2018/09/12/415422).

The multiplex real-time PCR assays were performed using the Quant Studio 6 Flex with a 384-well system (Applied Biosystems, Carlsbad, CA). Each reaction consisted of a 20 μL reaction volume, including 4 μL of template nucleic acid, along with 1 μM of each of the forward and reverse primers, 0.85 μM of the probe,

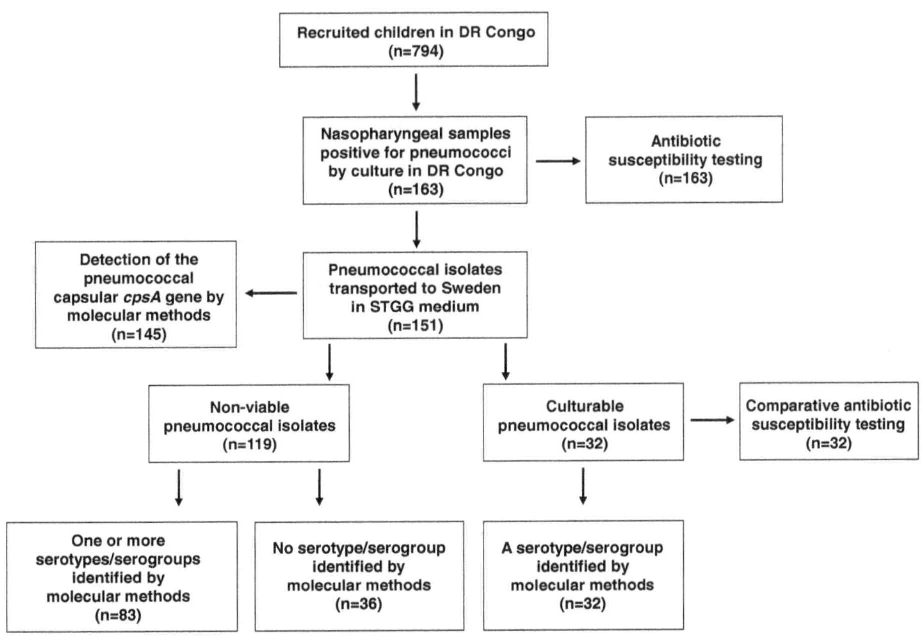

Fig. 1 A flowchart showing the analyses performed in Bukavu, DR Congo, and in Gothenburg, Sweden, respectively, and the number of isolates included in each analysis

Table 1 Comparison of disc diffusion tests on pneumococcal isolates performed in Bukavu and in Gothenburg, respectively ($n = 32$)

	Oxacillin[a] N (%)	TMP-SMX[b] N (%)	Erythromycin N (%)	Clindamycin N (%)	Norfloxacin[c] N (%)	Tetracycline N (%)
Difference in disc diffusion test (mm)						
≤ 3	23 (73)	29 (91)	22 (69)	23 (73)	25 (79)	14 (44)
4–6	5 (15)	1 (3)	3 (11)	3 (11)	5 (15)	10 (31)
> 6	4 (12)	2 (6)	7 (32)	6 (18)	2 (6)	8 (25)
Difference in SIR[d] interpretation[e]	0	0	0	0	0	0

[a] Screening disc for beta-lactam resistance
[b] *TMP-SMX* Trimethoprim-sulphamethoxazole
[c] Screening disc for fluoroquionolone resistance, i.e. levofloxacin and moxifloxacin
[d] *SIR* Sensitive, Intermediate, Resistant
[e] Breakpoints used according to EUCAST 2017

10 µl of 2X Universal Master Mix for DNA targets (Applied Biosystems) [31] and RNAase free water. The Tecan Freedom EVO PCR setup workstation (Tecan Group Ltd., Männedorf, Switzerland) was used to prepare the PCR reactions in a 384-well plate. The PCR reaction conditions were as follows: one initial cycle at 46 °C for 2 min, followed by denaturation at 95 °C for 10 min and 45 amplification cycles of 95 °C for 15 s and 58 °C for 1 min. Each multiplex performance was evaluated using an internal control (*CpsA*) to verify the presence of pneumococcal DNA in the sample, as well as two pUC57 plasmids containing each PCR target amplicon for all serotype systems.

Sequetyping

For eight out of the 32 pneumococcal isolates that could be re-cultured after storage and transport to Gothenburg, Sweden, and in which the multiplex PCR serotyping method was inconclusive, the serotypes/serogroups were determined using a modified Sequetyping protocol (https://www.biorxiv.org/content/early/2018/09/12/415422). Briefly, two PCR reactions were set up to amplified the whole cpsB gene. The PCR products were sent to GATC Biotech (Cologne, Germany) for purification and sequencing using the four PCR primers. The 1006 bp sequence product was matched to a reference database for determination of the serotype.

Data management and statistical analysis

Descriptive analysis was performed using the SPSS package (version 24.0) for logistic regression to analyse the relationship between carriage and socio-demographic or medical factors. Prevalence rates and the 95% CI were calculated. Potential variables associated with pneumococcal carriage were assessed by odds ratios (OR) with 95% CI and tested by univariate analysis with the Pearson chi-square or Fisher's exact test ($n < 5$). Associations with $p < 0.05$ were re-analysed by multivariate analysis. A p-value of < 0.05 was considered significant. Malnutrition was defined as the weight for age or weight for height as a Z score ≤ -2 standard deviations, determined by ENA for smart software 2011.

Results

Characteristics of the included children

From seven health care centres located in the city of Bukavu, in the suburban area or in the surrounding rural area, 794 children (age range one to 60 months, median 9.0 months) were included in the study and sampled from the nasopharynx. The background health data and living conditions of the children are shown in Additional file 1.

Socio-demographic risk factors for pneumococcal carriage

Overall, 163 (20.5%) of the children were culture positive for *S. pneumoniae* in the nasopharynx. The detection rate was associated with age but not with sex. Children aged 24–60 months had a more than three times higher rate of pneumococcal carriage that children below 6 months of age (p-value < 0.0001) (Table 2).

A higher frequency of pneumococcal carriage was observed in children living in the rural area as compared with the urban sites (28% versus 13%) and among children who lived in a house with an enclosed kitchen, i.e. with an open fire located inside the house, directly connected to the living room and/or the bedrooms, and these associations remained significant in multivariate analysis (Table 2). The type of stove and fuel for cooking did not correlate with carriage. Nor were there any associations between pneumococcal carriage and the number of rooms, having siblings, parents smoking tobacco, type of building material in the walls or the roof of the house, or having an animal in the household (Additional file 4).

Medical risk factors

Immunisation with PCV13 was strongly associated with lower rates of pneumococcal carriage, which was observed in only 3% of children who had received two or three doses of PCV13 as compared with approximately 30% of the unvaccinated children ($p < 0.0001$) (Table 2). Malnourished children, children with current fever and those who had had recent antibiotic treatment were

Table 2 Socio-demographic and medical factors related to nasopharyngeal carriage of pneumococci in children living in eastern DR Congo

Socio-demographic factors:	N carrier/N (%)	Univariate analysis		Multivariate analysis	
		OR (95% CI)	*p*-value	OR (95% CI)	*p*-value
Age in months					
< 6	29/302 (9.6)	1.00			
6–12	46/184 (25)	1.41 (0.85–2.36)	0.170	0.14 (0.08–0.26)	0.750
> 12–24	32/125 (26)	2.12 (1.25–3.62)	0.005	0.77 (0.44–1.36)	0.381
> 24–60	56/183 (31)	3.45 (2.19–5.44)	< 0.0001	0.90 (0.48–1.68)	< 0.0001
Sex, male	91/402 (23)	1.30 (0.92–1.84)	0.13	1.17 (0.78–1.77)	0.437
Living in rural area	98/355 (28)	2.51 (1.67–3.77)	< 0.0001	0.57 (0.33–0.97)	0.039
No of people sleeping in the same room as the child					
< 3	3/31 (9.7)	1.00			
≥ 3	74/253 (29)		0.018	1.27 (0.45–3.55)	0.644
Enclosed kitchen[a] (*N* = 77)	43/77 (56)	6.47 (3.62–11.56)	< 0.0001	10.18 (4.93–21.02)	< 0.0001
Medical factors					
Undernutrition[b] (*N* = 286)	83/286 (29)	2.18 (1.54–3.10)	< 0.0001	0.48 (0.32–0.73)	0.001
Current fever[c] (*N* = 22)	14/22 (64)	5.52 (2.21–13.78)	< 0.0001	7.96 (2.38–26.58)	0.001
Previous hospitalisation (*N* = 74)	27/74 (36)	1.83 (1.04–3.25)	0.035	1.61 (0.72–3.59)	0.244
Antibiotics last month (*N* = 55)	23/55 (42)	2.32 (1.25–4.31)	0.006	2.42 (1.07–5.45)	0.033
Neonatal problems[d] (*n* = 284)	22/51 (43.1)	2.45 (1.30–4.61)	0.004	1.27 (0.53–3.02)	0.580
PCV13 immunisation					
2 or 3 doses (*n* = 646[e])	9/283 (3.2)	1.00			
1 dose (*n* = 773)	46/159 (29)	12.39 (5.87–26.16)	< 0.0001	30.12 (14.36–63)	< 0.0001
0 dose (n = 773)	108/331 (33)	13.47 (6.68–27.17)	< 0.0001	20.57 (9.41–44.96)	< 0.0001

[a]Enclosed kitchen = Kitchen with an open fire located inside the house directly connected to the living room and/or the bedrooms
[b]Undernutrition = weight for age or weight for height as a Z score ≤ −2 standard deviations, determined by ENA for smart software 2011
[c]Fever = 37.5–39.0 °C
[d]Neonatal problems = neonatal hospitalisation, neonatal asphyxia or neonatal resuscitation
[e]645 = the number of children that were supposed to be given ≥2 doses of PCV13 when they were older than 10 weeks or two and a half months

more commonly colonised with pneumococci than children without these factors ($p < 0.05$). In contrast, neonatal problems, asthma, a recent history of malaria or gastroenteritis, or immunisation against measles, tuberculosis or *Hemophilus influenzae* type B were not associated with carriage, nor were symptoms of upper respiratory airway infection, such as a runny nose or cough (Table 2 and Additional file 5).

Taken together, age, living in a household with an enclosed kitchen, living in a rural area, undernutrition, current fever and antibiotic treatment during the last month were significantly associated with a higher, and vaccination with PCV13 with a lower, frequency of pneumococcal detection (Table 2).

Antimicrobial susceptibility of S. pneumoniae isolates

The antimicrobial susceptibility pattern was determined at the Clinical Laboratory, Panzi Hospital, Bukavu, for the 163 pneumococcal strains that were isolated from the children (Fig. 2). Using disc diffusion tests, 145 (89%) of the isolates were shown to be non-susceptible to oxacillin and they were therefore regarded as resistant to phenoxymethylpenicillin. These 145 strains were further tested by MIC determination against penicillin G and 101 (62%) strains were categorised as intermediate (MIC 0.06–2 mg/L), while 30 (18%) were resistant (MIC > 2 mg/L). Taken together, 131/163 (80%) of the strains showed reduced susceptibility to benzylpenicillin, as confirmed by MIC determination (Fig. 2). Sixty-eight isolates (42%) had reduced susceptibility to ampicillin, of which 18 were resistant (MIC > 2 mg/L), and 61 isolates (37%) had reduced susceptibility to ceftriaxone (Fig. 2). High rates of non-susceptibility were also found for tetracycline and as many as 94% of the isolates were resistant to trimethoprim-sulphamethoxazole (TMP-SMX), also known as co-trimoxazole (Fig. 2). Notably, 70 (43%) of the pneumococci were multidrug resistant (non-susceptible to ≥3 classes of antimicrobial agents, including the beta-lactams).

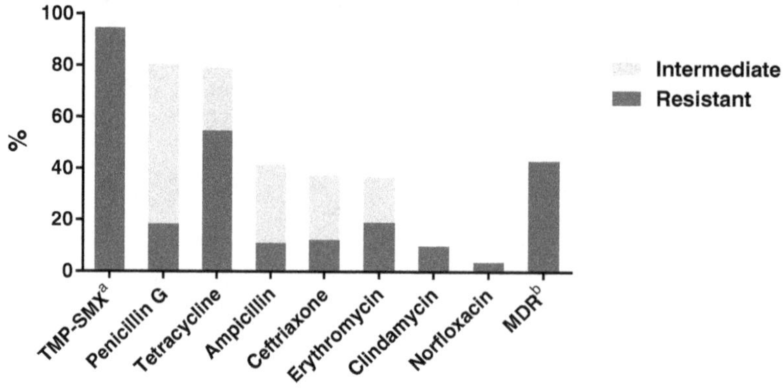

Fig. 2 The antimicrobial susceptibility pattern was determined in Bukavu, DR Congo for 163 pneumococcal strains isolated from healthy Congolese children. Disc diffusion tests were performed to detect reduced susceptibility to oxacillin, trimethoprim-sulfamethoxazole (TMP-SMX), tetracycline, erythromycin, clindamycin or norfloxacin (screening for fluoroquinolone resistance, i.e. levofloxacin and moxifloxacin). For oxacillin non-susceptible isolates, the minimal inhibitory concentration (MIC) was determined for penicillin G, ampicillin and ceftriaxone. [a]TMP-SMX = trimethoprim-sulfamethoxazole, [b]MDR = multi-drug resistant, i.e. non-susceptible to ≥3 classes of antibiotics including the beta-lactams

Serotype distribution

The serotypes or serogroups of the isolated pneumococci were determined by multiplex real-time PCR or by the modified Sequetyping protocol, both performed in Gothenburg, Sweden. Among the 32 living isolates the most common serotype was 19F ($n = 11$), followed by 11A/D ($n = 5$) and 35B/35C (n = 5). The pneumococcal capsular *cpsA* gene was detected in all viable isolates, confirming their species identification.

The serotypes/serogroups of the pneumococci that could not be re-cultured were determined by multiplex PCR after isolation of genomic material from the non-viable isolates in the STGG storage medium ($n = 119$). In 62/119 cases (52%), one serotype/serogroup could be identified, whereas in 21 cases more than one serotype/serogroup was detected. Of these, two serotypes/groups were determined in 17 cases, three serotypes/groups in three cases, while one tube contained four serotypes/groups. In 36/119 cases (30%), no serotype or group could be determined by multiplex real-time PCR. The combined results for all 141serotypes/serogroups that were identified in the viable and non-viable pneumococcal isolates are shown in Fig. 3.

Hence, out of the 141 identified serotypes/serogroups, 76 (54%) belonged to a serotype/serogroup included in

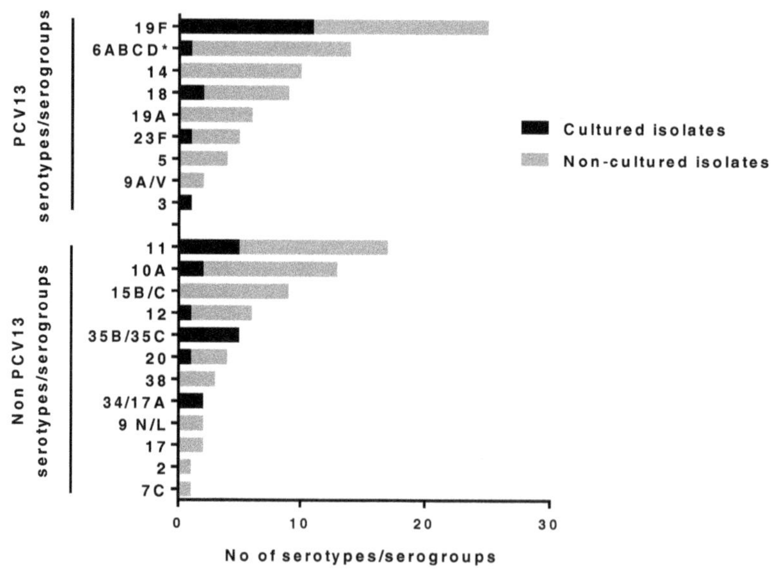

Fig. 3 The combined results of the 141 serotypes/serogroups identified by multiplex PCR or Sequetyping in the cultured, living pneumococcal isolates ($n = 32$) and by multiplex PCR in the non-viable pneumococcal isolates stored in tubes containing bacteria and STGG medium ($n = 83$). In 21 of these tubes containing non-viable bacteria, two or more serotypes/serogroups could be detected (two serotypes/serogroups in 17 cases; three serotypes/groups in three cases and four serotypes/groups in one case). * One culturable isolate could be determined by Sequetyping as 6B

PCV13. However, these 76 included 13 pneumococcal strains that could not be distinguished between 6A, 6B, 6C and 6D, of which only 6A and 6B are included in PCV13. Two further strains could not be separated between 9A and 9 V, of which only 9 V is included. Sixty-five (46%) of the identified serotypes/serogroups could, however, be categorised as non-PCV13-containing types/groups. Thus, the proportion of identified serotypes/serogroups belonging to PCV13 was similar to those not belonging to the vaccine. In the nine children who had received two or three doses of PCV13, vaccine serotypes/groups ($n = 9$) were as commonly detected as were serotypes/groups not included in the vaccine ($n = 7$). There was no significant difference in the distribution of penicillin non-susceptibility between strains whose serotypes/serogroups are included in the PCV13 compared to strains with non-vaccine serotypes/groups (Additional file 6).

In 113/119 non-viable isolates, the pneumococcal capsule gene, *CpsA*, could be detected in the STGG medium.

In the 36 samples, in which no serotype/serogroup could be identified using the multiplex real-time PCR method, the capsule gene, *CpsA*, was detected in 34 cases, verifying the presence of pneumococcal genomic material in the samples, and excluding a complete pneumococcal degradation during transport and storage.

Discussion

This is the first study to report the prevalence, serotype distribution and antimicrobial susceptibility of *Streptococcus pneumoniae* carried by healthy children in DR Congo.

By using culture for pneumococcal detection, we found that the prevalence of nasopharyngeal carriage was 21%. Generally higher levels of carriage have been reported from several other African countries, but there is also a great deal of variation between different regions [21, 32–35].

Differences in carriage rates can be due to geographical and regional variations, or to methodological differences. Limitations of the culture procedures in the present study include use of human blood in the agar plates. The pneumococci were initially identified in Bukavu, DR Congo, using the optochin test, which is not recommended as single test for *S. pneumoniae* identification [36]. However, molecular methods performed in Sweden confirmed the species identification in all but two isolates, either by detection of the pneumococcal capsular gene *CpsA*, or by serotype/serogroup determination. The low rate of positive culture in Sweden after storage and transport could be due to activation of the pneumococcal enzyme autolysin, LytA, which causes the bacterium to lyse and die. If activation of the autolysin also had an impact on the initial cultures performed in Bukavu can only be speculated upon. Apart from potential methodological limitations, our relatively low detection rate could indeed reflect an early effect of the newly introduced pneumococcal conjugate vaccine. To our knowledge, only a few studies have determined the carrier rate of pneumococci among sub-Saharan children after the introduction of the pneumococcal conjugate vaccine [13, 16].

Our study showed that living in a rural area was associated with a higher rate of pneumococcal carriage than in an urban area, in agreement with other studies showing the socio-economic and geographical disparity of pneumococcal carriage [37, 38]. We also found a strong association between pneumococcal carriage and living in a house with an enclosed kitchen, i.e. with an open fire located inside the house, similar to what has been reported before [39]. Many studies have shown that an increased risk of pneumonia and other lower respiratory infections correlates with household air pollution and poverty, but few have studied the association with pneumococcal carriage. Hussey et al. have reported that air pollution alters pneumococcal biofilms, antibiotic tolerance and colonisation [40]. Here, we also confirm the relationship between malnutrition and pneumococcal carriage, as described before [37, 41, 42].

We found an increased prevalence of pneumococci with age, in agreement with the results from Niger [33], while other studies in Africa showed the contrary [38, 43, 44]. One explanation of this could be that the sampling started a few months after the introduction of a PCV13 vaccine programme in DR Congo. Since the children are given vaccine doses when they are six, ten and 14 weeks old, without a catch-up programme, most of the under 2 year olds were vaccinated, while most of the children older than 2 years of age were not. The majority of the children under 6 months of age had already received three doses of PCV13.

Although the vaccination status could not be confirmed by checking the immunisation child cards in all cases, but instead relied on self-reports of the caretakers, we found that PCV13 immunisation was highly protective against pneumococcal carriage. Only 3% of the children that had received two or three doses of PCV13 carried pneumococci, compared with approximately 30% in those that were unvaccinated or had only been given one dose. Among the 141 serotypes/serogroups that were identified, approximately half belonged to a serotype/serogroup included in PCV13, which is similar to other studies [38, 44–47]. Since 24% of the isolates could not be identified to serotype/serogroup and the fact that the multiplex PCR was developed mainly to cover PCV-containing serotypes, it is possible that the number of non-vaccine serotypes/serogroups could be even higher. In Kenya, the prevalence of vaccine serotypes was reduced from 34 to 13% after the introduction of PCV10 [13]. The predominant serotype circulating in the eastern part of DR Congo was found to be the vaccine-type 19F, corroborating the results from Mozambique [48] and Ghana [22]. We detected equally numbers of vaccine- and non-vaccine-serotypes/groups in the nine children who had received two or more doses of PCV13. The distribution of penicillin non-susceptible strains was also similar between the identified vaccine- and non-vaccine serotypes/groups, indicating a limited effect of PCV13 on the carriage of antibiotic resistant strains in the area shortly after introduction of the vaccine.

The relatively high prevalence of serotype 11A/D and 35B/35C, which are not included in the PCV13 vaccine, among the living isolates was unexpected and has not been reported in other African studies [21, 38, 49]. As there are no studies of pneumococcal carriage in DR Congo prior to the introduction of PCV13, no evaluation of serotype replacement can be performed.

In some of the samples containing non-viable pneumococci, we unexpectedly detected more than one serotype/serogroup, although the STGG medium was supposed to contain only one pure cultured pneumococcal isolate. This might reflect the difficulties to visually separate different pneumococcal strains according to their colony morphology on the agar plate, and also confirms other observations that children often carry more than one pneumococcal strain in nasopharynx [50, 51].

We found an association between antibiotic treatment within 1 month prior to sampling and pneumococcal carriage among the children, similar to a study from Iran [39], but contrary to the results from Kenya [52] and Niger [33]. This finding indicates the carriage of pneumococci resistant to antibiotics used in the area and we were in fact able to show alarmingly high resistance rates to the antibiotics commonly used in the eastern part of DR Congo. Amoxicillin (or intravenous ampicillin in severe cases) is recommended by the WHO as the first-line treatment for pneumonia. We found that 42% of the isolated pneumococci had reduced susceptibility to ampicillin, while the rate of non-susceptibility to benzylpenicillin was 80%. High rates of pneumococcal non-susceptibility to ampicillin and/or penicillin have been reported in other sub-Saharan countries [53, 54], but lower rates have also been observed [21, 22, 33]. There is some reported high resistance to TMP-SMX, as we found in this study (94%) [44, 55]. One of the rare post-PCV studies in sub-Saharan Africa reported a limited impact on antibiotic resistance [56]. TMP-SMX or co-trimoxazole and penicillin are the two most available and accessible antibiotics in DR Congo [57]. Self-medication is fairly common in the country, due to inadequate access to formal health care and the wide availability of antibiotics without prescription [57].

Due to the absence of a national antibiotic use policy in DR Congo, non-governmental organisations have introduced their guidelines on empirical antibiotic treatment recommendations, without having enough data on local antibiotic resistance rates. Until recently, co-trimoxazole was recommended as empirical treatment for acute lower respiratory infections in DR Congo, instead of amoxicillin, as recommended by the WHO, and the use of this antibiotic is still widespread in the country. In addition, in many cases, HIV-positive children are likely to be administered TMP-SMX as prophylaxis for *Pneumocystis jirovecii* infections, which might contribute to the development of TMP-SMX-resistant pneumococci.

In DR Congo, the cephalosporin ceftriaxone is the most commonly used antimicrobial drug for severe pneumococcal infections like meningitis. Here, we demonstrate a higher level of resistance (37%), compared with previous studies from Botswana [58] and Tanzania [21].

Moreover, many isolated pneumococcal strains also had reduced susceptibility to erythromycin, tetracycline and clindamycin. Notably, a large proportion of pneumococcal isolates (43%) were multi-drug resistant, i.e. non-susceptible to ≥3 classes of antimicrobial agents, in contrast to the situation in other countries close to DR Congo [21, 44, 53].

The high level of antimicrobial resistance found in our study can be explained by the absence of regulation for the use of antibiotics and no national guidelines for the management of frequent diseases in DR Congo. Moreover, there is an urgent need for microbiological competence and knowledge, as well as well-equipped laboratories, capable of clinical diagnostics and antibiotic resistance surveillance.

Conclusions

To conclude, this study was performed on healthy children below 5 years of age in the eastern part of DR Congo after the introduction of PCV13. Living in rural areas, having an enclosed kitchen with an open fire and undernutrition correlated with higher pneumococcal carriage and PCV13 vaccination with a lower carriage rate. Moreover, it highlights an alarmingly high level of reduced susceptibility to commonly used antibiotics, especially ampicillin and ceftriaxone, among the isolated pneumococcal strains. This underlines the need for new antibiotic treatment guidelines, as well as necessitating local and national antibiotic resistance surveillance programmes.

Additional files

Additional file 1: Socio-demographic factors of the children as reported by the parents

Additional file 2: Susceptibility testing of Penicillin G, Ampicillin and Ceftriaxone performed in Bukavu, D.R. Congo and in Gothenburg, Sweden. To compare the antibiotic susceptibility tests performed in Bukavu, DR Congo, with those performed in Gothenburg, Sweden, the minimal inhibitory concentration (MIC) was determined for penicillin G, ampicillin and ceftriaxone in 32 pneumococcal isolates at both sites.

Additional file 3: The distribution of MIC values for penicillin G, ampicillin and ceftriaxone, respectively, obtained in Bukavu during 2014 and 2015.

Additional file 4: Socio-demographic factors of the children in relation to nasopharyngeal pneumococcal carriage.

Additional file 5: Medical factors of the children in relation to pneumococcal carriage.

Additional file 6: Distribution of penicillin non-susceptibility (intermediate or resistant) among pneumococcal isolates in which a serotype/serogroup included in the PCV13 was detected, and among isolates in which a serotype/group not included in the vaccine was determined

Abbreviations

CARe: Center for Antibiotic Resistance ResearchGothenburg; CDC: Centers for Disease Control and Prevention; CI: Confidence interval; DR Congo: Democratic Republic of the Congo; ENA: Emergency Nutrition Assessment; EUCAST: European committee on antimicrobial susceptibility testing; HIV: Human immunodeficiency virus; MIC: Minimum inhibitory concentration; MSF: Médecins Sans Frontières; OR: Odds ratio; PCV: Pneumococcal conjugate vaccine; PCV10: 10 valent pneumococcal conjugate vaccine; PCV13: 13 valent pneumococcal conjugate vaccine; PCV7: 7-valent pneumococcal conjugate vaccine; TMP-SMX: Trimethoprim-sulphamethoxazole; WHO: World Health Organisation

Acknowledgements

Acknowledgments to the Gothenburg University Research Fund for starting up research in global health.

Our sincere appreciation is also due to all the staff at Panzi Hospital, Kaziba Hospital, the Malkiya Wa Amani health centre, the Muhanzi health centre, the Kadutu BDOM health centre, the Muku health centre and the Nyantende health centre for their co-operation and collaboration in this study.

We thank the staff at the Clinical Laboratory, Microbiology Department, at Panzi Hospital, especially Maombi Chibashimba Ezekiel and Mugisho Muhandule David, for assisting Balthazar and Erick in performing excellent lab work.

Funding

This study was supported by the Sahlgrenska Academy, University of Gothenburg. The funding body had no role in the design of the study, the collection, analysis, interpretation of data, nor in writing of the manuscript.

Authors' contributions

SS, RA and RN designed and supervised the study. AMB, JM1, DC, LM, BM2, JM2 and NK obtained consent from the parents/guardians to participate, acquired information for the questionnaires and collected the samples. Further, AMB, BM1, TK, EM assisted by local lab-technicians performed the lab-work in DR Congo and ME, LG, ES, AMB and SG performed the lab-work in Sweden. AMB analysed the data with close communication with SS, RA and RN under the orientation of statistician at Goteborg University. AMB was mainly responsible for writing the manuscript which was critically revised by SS, RA, RN, and ML. All authors read and approved of the final manuscript.

Competing interests

The authors declare that they have no competing interests.

Author details

[1]Department of Infectious Diseases, Institute of Biomedicine, University of Gothenburg, Gothenburg, Sweden. [2]Panzi Hospital, Bukavu, Democratic Republic of the Congo. [3]Université Evangélique en Afrique, Bukavu, Democratic Republic of the Congo. [4]CARe – Center for Antibiotic Resistance Research, Gothenburg University, Gothenburg, Sweden. [5]Hôpital Général de Référence de Panzi, BP: 266 Bukavu, DR, Congo.

References

1. Zar HJ, Ferkol TW. The global burden of respiratory disease-impact on child health. Pediatr Pulmonol. 2014;49(5):430–4.
2. Rudan I, Boschi-Pinto C, Biloglav Z, Mulholland K, Campbell H. Epidemiology and etiology of childhood pneumonia. Bull World Health Organ. 2008;86(5): 408–16.
3. Hea W. Global, regional, national, and selected subnational levels of stillbirths, neonatal, infant, and under-5 mortality, 1980–2015: a systematic analysis for the Global Burden of Disease Study 2015. Lancet. 2017;388(Issue 10053):1725–74.
4. Lea L. Global, regional, and national causes of under-5 mortality in 2000–15: an updated systematic analysis with implications for the sustainable development goals. Lancet. 2016;388(Issue 10063):3027–35.
5. Amouzou A, Velez L, Tarekegn H, Young M. One is too many: ending child deaths from pneumonia and diarrhoea; 2016.
6. Troeger C, Forouzanfar M, Rao PC, Khalil I, Brown A, Swartz S, Fullman N, Mosser J, Thompson RL, Reiner RC Jr. Estimates of the global, regional, and national morbidity, mortality, and aetiologies of lower respiratory tract infections in 195 countries: a systematic analysis for the global burden of disease study 2015. Lancet Infect Dis. 2017;17(11):1133–61.
7. Ram PK, Dutt D, Silk BJ, Doshi S, Rudra CB, Abedin J, Goswami D, Fry AM, Brooks WA, Luby SP, et al. Household air quality risk factors associated with childhood pneumonia in urban Dhaka, Bangladesh. Am J Trop Med Hyg. 2014;90(5):968–75.
8. Shibata T, Wilson JL, Watson LM, LeDuc A, Meng C, Ansariadi LAR, Manyullei S, Maidin A. Childhood acute respiratory infections and household environment in an eastern Indonesian urban setting. Int J Environ Res Public Health. 2014;11(12):12190–203.
9. Karki S, Fitzpatrick AL, Shrestha S. Risk factors for pneumonia in children under 5 years in a teaching Hospital in Nepal. Kathmandu Univ Med J (KUMJ). 2014;12(48):247–52.
10. Panosian Dunavan C. From cookstoves to oxygen concentrators: a few important tools can help tackle global respiratory disparities. Am J Respir Crit Care Med. 2012;186(9):811–2.
11. SBea G. Respiratory risks from household air pollution in low and middle income countries. Lancet Respir Med. 2014;2(10):823–60.
12. Geno KA, Saad JS, Nahm MH. Discovery of novel pneumococcal serotype 35D, a natural WciG-deficient variant of serotype 35B. J Clin Microbiol. 2017; 55(5):1416–25.
13. Hammitt LL, Akech DO, Morpeth SC, Karani A, Kihuha N, Nyongesa S, Bwanaali T, Mumbo E, Kamau T, Sharif SK, et al. Population effect of 10-valent pneumococcal conjugate vaccine on nasopharyngeal carriage of Streptococcus pneumoniae and non-typeable Haemophilus influenzae in Kilifi, Kenya: findings from cross-sectional carriage studies. Lancet Glob Health. 2014;2(7):e397–405.
14. DMea W. Serotype replacement in disease after pneumococcal vaccination. Lancet. 2011;378(9807):1962–73.
15. Roca A, Bojang A, Bottomley C, Gladstone RA, Adetifa JU, Egere U, Burr S, Antonio M, Bentley S, Kampmann B. Effect on nasopharyngeal pneumococcal carriage of replacing PCV7 with PCV13 in the expanded Programme of immunization in the Gambia. Vaccine. 2015;33(51):7144–51.
16. Klugman KP. Herd protection induced by pneumococcal conjugate vaccine. Lancet Glob Health. 2014;2(7):e365–6.
17. Roca A, Hill PC, Townend J, Egere U, Antonio M, Bojang A, Akisanya A, Litchfield T, Nsekpong DE, Oluwalana C, et al. Effects of community-wide vaccination with PCV-7 on pneumococcal nasopharyngeal carriage in the Gambia: a cluster-randomized trial. PLoS Med. 2011;8(10):e1001107.
18. Van Boeckel TP, Gandra S, Ashok A, Caudron Q, Grenfell BT, Levin SA, Laxminarayan R. Global antibiotic consumption 2000 to 2010: an analysis of national pharmaceutical sales data. Lancet Infect Dis. 2014;14(8):742–50.
19. Grouzard V, Rigal J, Sutton M. Clinical guidelines: Diagnosis and treatment manual for curative programmes in hospitals and dispensaries: guidance for prescribing. 7th revised ed. Medecins Sans Frontieres. 2007. ISBN 978-2-37585-029-9. http://www.refbooks.msf.org/.
20. World Health Organization. Antimicrobial resistance: global report on

surveillance. World Health Organization; 2014. www.who.int/drugresistance/documents/surveillancereport/en/.

21. Moyo SJ, Steinbakk M, Aboud S, Mkopi N, Kasubi M, Blomberg B, Manji K, Lyamuya EF, Maselle SY, Langeland N. Penicillin resistance and serotype distribution of Streptococcus pneumoniae in nasopharyngeal carrier children under 5 years of age in Dar Es Salaam, Tanzania. J Med Microbiol. 2012;61(7):952–9.
22. Dayie NT, Arhin RE, Newman MJ, Dalsgaard A, Bisgaard M, Frimodt-Moller N, Slotved HC. Penicillin resistance and serotype distribution of Streptococcus pneumoniae in Ghanaian children less than six years of age. BMC Infect Dis. 2013;13:490.
23. Hanke CR, Grijalva CG, Chochua S, Pletz MW, Hornberg C, Edwards KM, Griffin MR, Verastegui H, Gil AI, Lanata CF, et al. Bacterial density, serotype distribution and antibiotic resistance of pneumococcal strains from the nasopharynx of Peruvian children before and after pneumococcal conjugate vaccine 7. Pediatr Infect Dis J. 2016;35(4):432–9.
24. Klugman KP, Madhi SA, Huebner RE, Kohberger R, Mbelle N, Pierce N. A trial of a 9-valent pneumococcal conjugate vaccine in children with and those without HIV infection. N Engl J Med. 2003;349(14):1341–8.
25. Tomczyk S, Lynfield R, Schaffner W, Reingold A, Miller L, Petit S, Holtzman C, Zansky SM, Thomas A, Baumbach J. Prevention of antibiotic-nonsusceptible invasive pneumococcal disease with the 13-valent pneumococcal conjugate vaccine. Clin Infect Dis. 2016;62(9):1119–25.
26. Tyrrell GJ, Lovgren M, Chui N, Minion J, Garg S, Kellner JD, Marrie TJ. Serotypes and antimicrobial susceptibilities of invasive Streptococcus pneumoniae pre-and post-seven valent pneumococcal conjugate vaccine introduction in Alberta, Canada, 2000–2006. Vaccine. 2009;27(27):3553–60.
27. ENA 2011(july 9: *smartmethodologyorg//smart-emergency-nutrition-assessment/e.*
28. http://www.eucast.org/clinical_breakpoints/: *wwweucastorg/clinical_breakpoints/* Accessed 29 Sept 2017.
29. Neves FP, Cardoso NT, Souza AR, Snyder RE, Marlow MM, Pinto TC, Teixeira LM, Riley LW. Population structure of Streptococcus pneumoniae colonizing children before and after universal use of pneumococcal conjugate vaccines in Brazil: emergence and expansion of the MDR serotype 6C-CC386 lineage. J Antimicrob Chemother. 2018;73(5):1206–12.
30. O'Brien KL, Bronsdon MA, Dagan R, Yagupsky P, Janco J, Elliott J, Whitney CG, Yang Y-H, Robinson L-GE, Schwartz B. Evaluation of a medium (STGG) for transport and optimal recovery of Streptococcus pneumoniae from nasopharyngeal secretions collected during field studies. J Clin Microbiol. 2001;39(3):1021–4.
31. Heid CA, Stevens J, Livak KJ, Williams PM. Real time quantitative PCR. Genome Res. 1996;6(10):986–94.
32. Usuf E, Bojang A, Camara B, et al. Maternal pneumococcal nasopharyngeal carriage and risk factors for neonatal carriage after the introduction of pneumococcal conjugate vaccines in The Gambia. Clinical microbiology and infection. 2018;24(4):389-95.
33. Ousmane S, Diallo BA, Ouedraogo R, Sanda AA, Soussou AM, Collard JM. Serotype distribution and antimicrobial sensitivity profile of Streptococcus pneumoniae carried in healthy toddlers before PCV13 introduction in Niamey, Niger. PLoS One. 2017;12(1):e0169547.
34. Usuf E, Bottomley C, Adegbola RA, Hall A. Pneumococcal carriage in sub-Saharan Africa--a systematic review. PLoS One. 2014;9(1):e85001.
35. Rutebemberwa E, Mpeka B, Pariyo G, Peterson S, Mworozi E, Bwanga F, Kallander K. High prevalence of antibiotic resistance in nasopharyngeal bacterial isolates from healthy children in rural Uganda: a cross-sectional study. Ups J Med Sci. 2015;120(4):249–56.
36. Satzke C, Turner P, Virolainen-Julkunen A, Adrian PV, Antonio M, Hare KM, Henao-Restrepo AM, Leach AJ, Klugman KP, Porter BD, et al. Standard method for detecting upper respiratory carriage of Streptococcus pneumoniae: updated recommendations from the World Health Organization pneumococcal carriage working group. Vaccine. 2013;32(1): 165–79.
37. Coles CL, Rahmathullah L, Kanungo R, Katz J, Sandiford D, Devi S, Thulasiraj RD, Tielsch JM. Pneumococcal carriage at age 2 months is associated with growth deficits at age 6 months among infants in South India. J Nutr. 2012; 142(6):1088–94.
38. Usuf E, Badji H, Bojang A, Jarju S, Ikumapayi UN, Antonio M, Mackenzie G, Bottomley C. Pneumococcal carriage in rural Gambia prior to the introduction of pneumococcal conjugate vaccine: a population-based survey. Trop Med Int Health : TM & IH. 2015;20(7):871–9.
39. Mirzaei Ghazikalayeh H, Moniri R, Moosavi SG, Rezaei M, Yasini M, Valipour M. Serotyping, antibiotic susceptibility and related risk factors aspects of nasopharyngeal carriage of Streptococcus pneumoniae in healthy school students. Iran J Public Health. 2014;43(9):1284–90.
40. Hussey S, Purves J, Allcock N, Fernandes VE, Monks PS, Ketley JM, Andrew PW, Morrissey JA. Air pollution alters Staphylococcus aureus and Streptococcus pneumoniae biofilms, antibiotic tolerance and colonisation. Environ Microbiol. 2017;19(5):1868–80.
41. Verhagen LM, Hermsen M, Rivera-Olivero IA, Sisco MC, de Jonge MI, Hermans PWM, de Waard JH. Nasopharyngeal carriage of respiratory pathogens in Warao Amerindians: significant relationship with stunting. Tropical Med Int Health. 2017;22(4):407–14.
42. Rylance J, Kankwatira A, Nelson DE, Toh E, Day RB, Lin H, Gao X, Dong Q, Sodergren E, Weinstock GM. Household air pollution and the lung microbiome of healthy adults in Malawi: a cross-sectional study. BMC Microbiol. 2016;16(1):182.
43. Adetifa IM, Antonio M, Okoromah CA, Ebruke C, Inem V, Nsekpong D, Bojang A, Adegbola RA. Pre-vaccination nasopharyngeal pneumococcal carriage in a Nigerian population: epidemiology and population biology. PLoS One. 2012;7:e30548.
44. Assefa A, Gelaw B, Shiferaw Y, Tigabu Z. Nasopharyngeal carriage and antimicrobial susceptibility pattern of Streptococcus pneumoniae among pediatric outpatients at Gondar University hospital, north West Ethiopia. Pediatr Neonatol. 2013;54(5):315–21.
45. Kamng'ona AW, Hinds J, Bar-Zeev N, Gould KA, Chaguza C, Msefula C, Cornick JE, Kulohoma BW, Gray K, Bentley SD, et al. High multiple carriage and emergence of Streptococcus pneumoniae vaccine serotype variants in Malawian children. BMC Infect Dis. 2015;15:234.
46. Kandasamy RGM, Thapa A, Ndimah S, Adhikari N, Murdoch DR, et al. Multi-Serotype Pneumococcal Nasopharyngeal Carriage Prevalence in Vaccine Naïve Nepalese Children, Assessed Using Molecular Serotyping. PloS one. 2015;10(2):e0114286 doi:10.1371/journal. pone.0114286(PLoS ONE 10(2): e0114286. doi:10.1371/journal. pone.0114286):PLoS ONE 10(12): e0114286. doi:0114210.0111371/journal. pone.0114286.
47. Kellner JD, McGeer A, Cetron MS, Low DE, Butler JC, Matlow A, Talbot J, Ford-Jones EL. The use of Streptococcus pneumoniae nasopharyngeal isolates from healthy children to predict features of invasive disease. Pediatr Infect Dis J. 1998;17(4):279–86.
48. Vallès X, Flannery B, Roca A, Mandomando I, Sigaúque B, Sanz S, Schuchat A, Levine M, Soriano-Gabarró M, Alonso P. Serotype distribution and antibiotic susceptibility of invasive and nasopharyngeal isolates of Streptococcus pneumoniae among children in rural Mozambique. Tropical Med Int Health. 2006;11(3):358–66.
49. Adegbola RA, Hill PC, Secka O, Ikumapayi UN, Lahai G, Greenwood BM, Corrah T. Serotype and antimicrobial susceptibility patterns of isolates of Streptococcus pneumoniae causing invasive disease in the Gambia 1996–2003. Tropical Med Int Health. 2006;11(7):1128–35.
50. Rivera-Olivero IA, Blommaart M, Bogaert D, Hermans PW, de Waard JH. Multiplex PCR reveals a high rate of nasopharyngeal pneumococcal 7-valent conjugate vaccine serotypes co-colonizing indigenous Warao children in Venezuela. J Med Microbiol. 2009;58(Pt 5):584–7.
51. Brugger SD, Frey P, Aebi S, Hinds J, Muhlemann K. Multiple colonization with S. pneumoniae before and after introduction of the seven-valent conjugated pneumococcal polysaccharide vaccine. PLoS One. 2010;5(7):e11638.
52. Abdullahi O, Karani A, Tigoi CC, Mugo D, Kungu S, Wanjiru E, Jomo J, Musyimi R, Lipsitch M, Scott JA. The prevalence and risk factors for pneumococcal colonization of the nasopharynx among children in Kilifi District, Kenya. PLoS One. 2012;7(2):e30787.
53. Kobayashi M, Conklin LM, Bigogo G, et al. Pneumococcal carriage and antibiotic susceptibility patterns from two crosssectional colonization surveys among children aged <5 years prior to the introduction of 10-valent pneumococcal conjugate vaccine — Kenya, 2009–2010. BMC Infect Dis. 2017;17:25 10.1186/s12879-016-2103-0(10.1186/s12879-016-2103-0):10. 1186/s12879-12016-12103-12870.
54. Joloba ML, Bajaksouzian S, Palavecino E, Whalen C, Jacobs MR. High prevalence of carriage of antibiotic-resistant Streptococcus pneumoniae in children in Kampala Uganda. Int J Antimicrob Agents. 2001;17:395–400.

55. Mills RO, Twum-Danso K, Owusu-Agyei S, Donkor ES. Epidemiology of pneumococcal carriage in children under five years of age in Accra, Ghana. Infect Dis (Lond). 2015;47(5):326–31.
56. Cheung Y-B, Zaman SM, Nsekpong ED, Van Beneden CA, Adegbola RA, Greenwood B, Cutts FT. Nasopharyngeal carriage of Streptococcus pneumoniae in Gambian children who participated in a 9-valent pneumococcal conjugate vaccine trial and in their younger siblings. Pediatr Infect Dis J. 2009;28(11):990–5.
57. Tsakala T, Tona G, Mesia K, Mboma J, Vangu J, Voso S, Kanja G, Kodondi K, Mabela M, Walo R. Évaluation des prescriptions dans le traitement du paludisme et de la gastroentérite en milieu hospitalier: Cas des hôpitaux Bondeko et St Joseph à Kinshasa (République démocratique du Congo). Cahiers d'études et de recherches francophones/Santé. 2005;15(2):119–24.
58. Huebner RE, Wasas A, Mushi A, Mazhani L, Klugman K. Nasopharyngeal carriage and antimicrobial resistance in isolates of Streptococcus pneumoniae and Haemophilus influenzae type b in children under 5 years of age in Botswana. Int J Infect Dis. 1998;3(1):18–25.

Timely initiation of complementary feeding to children aged 6–23 months in rural Soro district of Southwest Ethiopia: a cross-sectional study

Bereket Yohannes[1,2,3*], Elias Ejamo[1,4], Thilagavathi Thangavel[1] and Mulugeta Yohannis[1,5]

Abstract

Background: Poor complementary feeding practice to infants is one of risk factors for child undernutrition in Ethiopia. This would vary across the culturally and socioeconomically diverse settings in this country. Thus, this study was aimed to determine the proportion of timely initiated complementary feeding practice of women to their children aged 6–23 months in rural Soro district in Southwest Ethiopia.

Methods: A community based crossectional survey was conducted in Soro district from August to September in 2015. Randomly selected 543 women having children aged 6–23 months were the final sampling units for this study. First, local administrative units (kebeles) of residents were randomly selected from such lists in the district. Secondly, the sample size was proportionally allocated to each selected kebele by population sizes. Individual households were selected by systematic random technique. Data was collected by using a structured questionnaire through face to face interview. Descriptive statistics was done for univariate results, and we applied bivariate logistic regression to look for crude association, and multivariate logistic regression to model predictors with effect measures and 95% confidence intervals (CI). Statistical significance was decaled at $P < 0.05$.

Results: The proportion of timely initiated complementary feeding was 34.3% at 95%CI: (30.31, 38.29) in this study. Secondary and above education levels of respondents (AOR = 2.25 95%CI: 1.17, 4.30) and husbands (AOR = 2.33 at 95% CI: 1.06, 5.14), and maternal Postnatal Care visits (AOR = 1.94 at 95% CI: 1.19, 3.16) were found independent predictors for timely initiated complementary feeding practice in this study.

Conclusions: Timely complementary feeding practice in the study area was low compared to the standard recommends for it. Education in general and equipping child bearing women with specific messages on Infant and Child Feeding Practices may improve infant and child feeding practice in the area. Optimizing utilization of Postnatal Care by post partum women and including specific advices on complementary feeding are recommended.

Keywords: Timely initiation, Complementary feeding, Ethiopia

* Correspondence: bkabalo@gmail.com
[1]School of public Health, Wolaita Sodo University, P.o.box 126 Wolaita Sodo, Ethiopia
[2]Centre for international Health, the University of Bergen, Bergen, Norway
Full list of author information is available at the end of the article

Background

Malnutrition is responsible for about two third of all deaths among children under age 5 years. In Ethiopia, over a third of this is associated with inappropriate infant and young child feeding practice [1, 2] which includes suboptimal complementary feeding practice to infants. Complementary feeding means introducing an infant, other foods and liquids when breast milk alone is no longer sufficient [3–5]. After the first 6 months, breast milk alone is no longer adequate to meet the nutritional needs of the infants, therefore timely initiation of complementary foods to child's diet is recommended [6–9]. This means introducing an infant with solid, semi-solid or soft foods at age 6 months. It is optimal or timely if at least initiated for infants aged 6–8 months [6, 7]. Appropriate complementary feeding should include a variety of foods to ensure nutritional requirements [6–9].

Estimates indicate that proper feeding of breast milk alone in the first six months could avert about 15% of infant deaths, and optimal complementary feeding could further reduce 6% of all deaths among children under 5 [10]. Nonetheless, in low income settings, where almost a fifth of all under age 5 dies due to causes that could be averted by proper complementary feeding [2]; suboptimal child feeding remains a risk factor for child undernutrition [8, 9, 11].

Despite its tremendous trend of improvement on some child nutrition indicators, Ethiopia still remains one of the high burden countries in child undernutrition [8, 12]. Only about half of infants in Ethiopia are timely initiated for complementary foods [2, 10, 12, 13]. It is much lower in Southern Ethiopia [8, 12].

Although several surveys documented on Infant and Young Child Feeding (IYCF) practices in Ethiopia, evidence is still limited on timely initiated complementary feeding practice and its specific predictors in its culturally and socioeconomically diverse settings like the Soro district in Southwest Ethiopia. Thus this study was aimed to determine the proportion of timely initiated complementary feeding practice of women to their infants in rural Soro district. The findings of this study might inform programs targeting infants and young children in the area and other similar settings. They are also expected to add on existing knowledge in the area.

Methods

Study design and setting

This study was aimed to determine the proportion of timely initiated complementary feeding practice of women to their infants in rural Soro district. It was a community based crossectional study among mothers who had children aged 6–23 months. The study was carried out in rural community of Soro district in South Ethiopia from August to September in 2015. The total census projected population in the district was estimated to be 239,058 which compose 15.6% children under age 5 years, 8.3% under age 3, and 3.5% infants and young children (6–23 months). About 55,700(23.3%) women in reproductive age group were expected to live in the district [14].

Population and sampling

A sample size of 543 mothers was computed by using OpenEPi software with the assumptions for the design. The assumptions were 31% anticipated proportion of the outcome [13], 95% confidence level, 5% marginal error, and 6% for none-response [15]. First, out of the 46 rural residential kebeles (administrative units in the area) in the district 14 were selected by simple random sampling. Then sample size of study participant was allocated for each of the 14 units by proportion to population size. Then lists of mothers who had children 6–23 months of age in the each selected kebeles were obtained health posts in each kebele. In rural health posts in the area there family demographic and health profile registration folders (Family Folders). Thus we registered eligible mothers from these folders. Finally the study eligible mothers to child pairs were selected from each kebele by systematic random sampling technique.

Data collection

Data was collected by face-to-face interview to mothers (caregivers) who had children aged 6–23 months through home to home visits. The questionnaire was adapted from WHO standard questions and indicators for assessing IYCF practices to suit the study setting [1, 16].

We used a structured questionnaire which was originally prepared in English and then translated to local Hadiya language and back to English by two people to keep consistency. The data collection tool was pretested to 27 mothers in villages which were not included in the study to validate content and language. Data was collected by fourteen nurses under supervision of 2 degree level trained health officers. The field team was trained for two on modules of the tool and field methods. The modules include; the study objective, relevance of the study, contents of the questionnaire, and ethics.

Study variables

Outcome variable

Timely initiated complementary feeding.

Exposure variables (covariates)

Sociodemographic factors: Age, sex, marital status, respondents' educational status, educational status of husbands, occupation of the mother, family size.

Infant's demographic related factors: age and sex of the child.

Household socioeconomic factors: house hold income.

Maternal health related characteristics: ANC follow up, child birth order, birth preparedness, type of delivery assistance and place of birth.

Operational definitions

Timely initiation of complementary feeding

Introduction solid, semi-solid or soft foods to children between 6 and 8 months of age [6, 7].

Untimely initiation of complementary feeding

Introduction of solid, semi-solid or soft foods to infants before 6 months or beyond 8 months [6, 7].

Statistical analysis

Data were checked for completeness and inconsistencies in the field on spot and corrections made. Then data were, entered in EPI info version 3.5.4 statistical software and exported to SPSS. It was cleaned and analysed by using SPSS version 16. Descriptive statistics was carried out for univariate results. Measures of central tendency and dispersion were used for describing the data. Binary logistic regression used to look for crude association between exposure and outcome variables. Exposure variables with $P < 0.25$ were considered as candidates for multivariate logistic regressions to control for confounding. Thus we reported Adjusted Odds Ratio (AOR) along with 95% CI for the effect measure for association, and statistical significance was declared at P-value < 0.05.

Results

Sociodemographic and socioeconomic characteristics

A total of 543 respondents having children aged 6–23 months were interviewed. Among the respondents 539(99.3%) were biological mothers and only 4 (0.7%) were other caregivers. The median (IQR) age of mothers was 28 years (26, 30). The majority of the respondents were Protestant 502(92.4%), and married 537 (98.9%). The median (IQR) age of the child age was 8(9, 17) in months and more than half of the children were male 283 (52.1%). Mothers' who attended formal education was 243 (44.7%) and 330 (60.7%) husbands also attended school. The majority of mothers, 409 (75.3%), were housewives and husbands of 404 (75%) mothers were farmers by occupation. The median family size of the study households was six in number. Of the total households about 84.6% earn an average family monthly income ≤ 1000 Ethiopian Birr. Among the households 434 (79.9%) obtained food from farming followed by small scale business 73(13.4%) and formal employment 12(2.2%). Only 3 (0.6%) households had television and 152 (28%) had radio. It was found that, 22(4.1%) mothers read newspaper, 59(10.9%) mothers listened radio and 5(0.9%) mothers watched Television at least once a week (Table 1).

Maternal health related characteristics

Among the respondents, 445 (82%), mothers had antenatal care follow up at least once during the last pregnancy. Only 134(30.2%) of mothers had at least 4 visits. Almost all of those who had ANC follow up 423 (95.1%) made the first their visit for the service (ANC 1) after second trimester or later. About 439(80.8%) mothers gave their recent child birth at home. Only106 (19.5%) mothers had received postnatal care (PNC) and 298 (54.9%) had complementary feeding counselling during recent pregnancy (Table 2).

Breast feeding practice

Nearly all children541 (99.6%) in this study had ever been breastfed and more than half 301(55.4%) were been initiated to breastfeed timely that is within one hour of birth. Some 501(92.1%) children were continued with breastfeeding at the period of study. Some 42 mothers (7.9%) stopped breast feeding before the child reaches 23 month of age.

Complementary feeding practice

Majority of mothers 541 (99.6%) ever practiced breastfeeding. About 9 in 10 of all mothers 485(89.3%) who had breastfeeding experience had started complementary feeding at the time of the interview. Out of which 48(9.9%) were initiated before six month, 336(69.3%) at six and 101(20.8%) after six month of age. Among the respondents 410(75.5%) had introduced solid, semi solid or soft foods as complementary feeding at the time of the interview. Some 353 reported (65.0%) initiating complementary feeding after the infant's eight months of age.

The result of this study shows the proportion of timely initiated complementary feeding in the study area was 34.3% 95% CI (30.31, 38.29) (Table 3).

Factors associated with timely initiation of complementary feeding

Candidate variables for multivariate technique were identified by using bivariate analysis. The criteria was set to $P < 0.25$ as a yardstick. Accordingly; sociodemographic characteristics such as respondents' achieved educational status, husbands' educational status, and maternal age and maternal health service related characteristics such as Postnatal Care follow up, counselling during recent pregnancy, place of delivery and attendant were identified candidate variables for multivariate technique. We applied multivariate logistic regression for controlling possible confounders.

Table 1 Socio-demographic and socio economic related variables of mothers who had Children of 6–23 months age in rural community of Soro district, South Ethiopia, August, 2015 to September, 2015

Variable *n* = 543	Categories	Frequency	Percentage
Mothers' age	15–24	76	14.0
	25–34	402	74.0
	35–40	65	12.0
Marital status	Married	537	98.9
	Unmarried	2	0.4
	Separated/Divorced	3	0.6
	Widowed	1	0.2
Religion	Protestant	502	92.4
	Orthodox	9	1.7
	Catholic	30	5.5
	Muslim	2	0.4
Ethnicity	Hadiya	526	96.9
	Kambata	11	2.0
	Amhara	3	0.6
	Gurage	1	0.2
	Others	2	0.4
Mothers' educational status	No education	254	46.8
	Read and write	46	8.5
	Primary	186	34.3
	Secondary	52	9.6
	Tertiary	5	0.9
Mothers' occupation	House wife	409	75.3
	Farmer	48	8.8
	Government employer	5	0.9
	Small business	65	12.0
	Causal work	16	2.9
Husbands' Occupation (*n* = 539)	Not employed	20	3.7
	Farmer	404	75
	Employed	19	3.5
	Small scale trading	81	15
	Casual labour	11	2.0
	Daily labour	4	0.8
Monthly income	<=500	299	55.1
	501–1000	160	29.5
	1001–1500	25	4.6
	1501–2000	10	1.8
	2001 and above	9	1.7
	Don't know	40	7.4
Source of monthly income	Farming	434	79.9
	Formal employment	12	2.2
	Casual labour	24	4.4
	Small scale business	73	13.4

Table 1 Socio-demographic and socio economic related variables of mothers who had Children of 6–23 months age in rural community of Soro district, South Ethiopia, August, 2015 to September, 2015 *(Continued)*

Variable *n* = 543	Categories	Frequency	Percentage
Head of household	Husband	522	96.1
	Wife	16	2.9
	Oldest brother/sister	4	0.7
	Others	1	0.2

The findings of this study show mothers who had secondary school and above education were 2 folds more likely to timely initiate complementary feeding to their infants compared to those who did not attend formal education(AOR = 2.25 at 95% CI: 1.17, 4.30). Mothers living with their husbands trained to the level ability to read and write had also above 2 folds greater odds of timely initiating complementary foods to their infants compared to those who did not have formal education and were not able to read and write(AOR = 2.33 at 95%CI: 1.06, 5.14). On the other hand those mothers who had postnatal care were about 2 times more likely to timely initiate complementing food to their infants(AOR = 1.94 at 95%CI: 1.19, 3.16) compared to those who did not use the service (Table 4).

Discussion

The proportion of timely initiated complementary feeding in study was 34.3%. Parental education and maternal postnatal care follow-up were independent predictors for the outcome. The timely initiated complementary feeding practice in this study was much lower than findings from India(55%), Nepal (70%), Bangladesh (71%), Sirlanka (84%), and Kenya (80.6%) [17–19]. The observed disparity might be due to cultural barriers, and socioeconomic and health care access disparities.

Much lower proportion of infants in Soro were timely initiated to complementary feeding in compared the national figure for Ethiopia in 2011(51%) [12] and in 2016(56%) [8]. Similarly it was also lower than data from Tigray (48.4%) in Northern Ethiopia [13], Sidama (72.2%) [20] in the South. This might be due to sociodemographic differences including the low level of parental education in our settings. It might also be explained by the low coverage and utilization of maternal health services; particularly poor postnatal care utilization in Soro coupled missed opportunities during visits for maternal services. On the other hand, timely initiated complementary feeding practice in this study is in line with 'alive thrive survey' report for Southern Ethiopia in 2011 (31.2%) [13]. This might imply that timely initiation of complementary feeding would be low in Southern Ethiopia's across the different

Table 2 Obstetrics and maternal health service utilization related variables of mothers who had children 6–23 months of age in rural community of Soro district, South Ethiopia, August, 2015 to September, 2015

Variable	Categories	Frequency	Percentage
ANC follow up	Yes	445	82.0
	No	98	18
Number of ANC visit(N = 445)	Only once	53	11.9
	2–3 times	258	57.9
	>or = 4 times	134	30.2
Place of delivery	Home delivery	439	80.8
	Hospital	17	3.1
	Health center	68	12.52
	Health post	17	3.1
	Private clinic	2	0.4
Individual who assisted the delivery	Skilled Provider (Nurse/midwife/HO/Doctor)	94	17.3
	HEWs	17	3.1
	Non professionals (TBA and other persons)	432	79.6
Postnatal care	Yes	106	19.5
	No	437	80.5
Months of pregnancy during Initiation of ANC (n = 445	1–3	22	4.9
	4+	423	95.1
Counselling on complementary feeding	Yes	298	54.9
	No	237	43.6
	Don't know	8	1.5

Table 3 Child feeding practices of mothers who had children 6–23 months of age in rural community of Soro district, South Ethiopia, August to September, 2015

Variable	Categories	Frequency	Percentage
Ever breastfed	Yes	541	99.6
	No	2	0.4
Initiation of breast feeding	Immediately within 1st hour	301	55.4
	After 1st hour	234	43.1
	Don't remember	8	1.5
Prelacteal feeding	Yes	18	3.3
	No	525	96.7
Ever started any CF	Yes	485	89.3
	No	58	10.7
Ever started solid,semi solid or soft foods	Yes	410	75.5
	No	133	24.5
Initiation of liquid foods(cow milk gruel)	Early	48	8.8
	Timely	419	77.2
	Lately	76	14
Initiation of solid, semi solid or soft foods	Early	4	0.7
	Timely	186	34.3
	Lately	353	65

settings and the disparity might also vary with the diversity and socioeconomic variations.

This study indicated that mothers educated to secondary and above levels were above two folds more likely to timely initiate complementary feeding to infants compared to those who did not attend any school level. Similar findings were reported from Mekelle town in North Ethiopia, Nairobi in Kenya [21, 22], and Nepal [17]. The better educated mothers would have good knowledge about the importance of complementary feeding practice; they might also better understand the message. They might have better connection to nutrition information sources.

Paternal education also enhances mothers to timely initiate complementary feeding by more than 2 folds compared to who had husband with no formal education. Similar finding was reported from Axum town in North Ethiopia [23]. This might be argued that education might enable the husbands to better understand their wives and provide help by approving what mothers would like to do to keep their children healthy. The educated husbands might enhance wives awareness on to timely initiation of complementary feeding to their infant.

Postnatal care user mothers were almost 2 times more likely to timely initiate complementary feeding to their infants compared to those who did not follow the service. Similar finding was reported from Kamba district in Southwest Ethiopia [15]. Mothers who had no postnatal care follow up would start complementary feeding earlier (before 6 months) or later (after 8 months) compared to mothers who followed the care. A postnatal period could be an ideal time to counsel mothers on optimal complementary feeding practice [21, 23, 24].

Some level of recall bias was expected while interviewing respondents particularly none-mother ones in this study. The study was also limited in scope for exploring socio-cultural and behavioural factors. Using WHO guidelines and indicators might be strength in this study.

Conclusions

Only about a third of mothers in this study timely initiated complementary feeding to their infants, which was much lower than the national figure for Ethiopia and also far lower than the WHO recommendations. Higher (secondary and above) parental educational status, and better postnatal care utilization were associated with timely initiation of complementary feeding. Maternal education to higher might have enabled them to comprehend packages of routine messages pertaining to

Table 4 Factors associated with Timely initiation of complementary feeding among mothers who had 6–23 months children in Soro district, South Ethiopia, Aug 2015 to Sept, 2015

Variables	Category	Complementary feeding timely Yes	No	COR [95% C.I	AOR [95% C.I]
Mothers' age	15–24	27	49	1.83(0.87, 3.86)	1.87(0.85,4.11)
	25–34	144	258	1.86(1.01,3.43)*	1.85(0.96,3.47)
	35–40	15	50	1	
Mothers' educational status	No education	78	176	1	
	Read and write	19	27	1.58(0.83,3.02)	1.15(0.57,2.32)
	Primary	57	129	0.99(0.66,1.50)	0.81(0.51,1.29)
	Secondary and above	32	25	2.88(1.60,5.19)***	2.25(1.17,4.30)**
Educational status of husband($n = 539$	No education	48	125	1	
	Read and write	17	19	2.33(1.11,4.85)*	2.33(1.06,5.14)*
	Primary	83	146	1.48(0.96,2.27)	1.35(0.84,2.16)
	Secondary and above	38	63	1.57(0.93,264)	1.20(0.67,2.18)
PNC follow up	Yes	53	53	2.28(1.48,3.52)***	1.94(1.19,3.16)**
	No	133	304	1	
Place of delivery	Home delivery	140	299	1	
	Institutional delivery	46	58	1.69(1.10,2.62)*	1.40(0.36,5.38)
Assistant of the delivery	Non professional	138	294	1	
	Health professional	48	63	1.62(1.06,2.48)*	0.79(0.21,2.99)
Counselling on complementary feeding	Yes	118	180	1.62(1.18,2.45)**	1.48(1.00,2.19)
	No	68	170	1	

Foot note * = $p < 0.05$ ** = $p < 0.01$ *** = $p < 0.001$

complementary feeding. Husbands' education was also equally important for timely complementary feeding to their infants. Authors recommend health workers should give special emphasis to mothers with low literacy while giving services. Postnatal care utilization should be strengthened on one hand and it should get due emphasis for counselling mothers on appropriate optimal complementary feeding practices. Further studies are recommended to evaluate the association between maternal prenatal (ANC) and delivery service utilization with appropriate complementary feeding practice. Further evidence is also needed on its socio-cultural and behavioural barriers in the area and beyond.

Abbreviations

ANC: Antenatal care; AOR: Adjusted Odds Ratio; BF: Breast Feeding; CF: Complementary Food; CI: Confidence Interval; EDHS: Ethiopian Demographic Health Survey; FMOE: Federal Ministry of Education; HEW: Health Extension Worker; HO: Health Officer; IYCF: Infant and Young Child Feeding; NORHED: Norwegian Programme for Capacity Development in Higher Education and Research for Development; PNC: Postnatal Care; PPS: Proportional to Population Size; SENUPH: South Ethiopia Network Universities in Public health; SNNPR: Southern Nation Nationality Peoples Region; SPSS: Statistical Package for Social Sciences; TBA: Traditional Birth Attendant; WHO: World Health Organization

Acknowledgments

We thank the 'South Ethiopia Network Universities in Public health' (SENUPH_NORHED) project for financial support. This study would have been impossible without facilitation of the school of public health in Wolaita Sodo University. We appreciate the genuine cooperation of Soro district Health Office for this project. We thank data collectors and supervisors involved in the project. We are grateful to mothers responded to the study.

Funding

This study was financial supported by the 'South Ethiopia Network Universities in Public health' (SENUPH_NORHED) project, and the fund was facilitated Wolaita Sodo University.

Authors' contributions

EE: drafted the study protocol, contributed in data entry and analysis and wrote the draft manuscript. TT was involved in the design of the protocol, and write up of the manuscript. BY was involved in the design and write up of the protocol, did major statistical analysis, revised the manuscript and re-wrote it to scientific correspondence. MY, had valuable contributions in statistical analysis, and interpretation of findings. BY and MY also dealt with language, editorial and reviewer matters in all across this manuscript. All authors read and approved the manuscript.

Authors' information

EE is currently working in a district health office in Southwest Ethiopia. He was a graduate of MSc in Human Nutrition from Wolaita Sodo University in Ethiopia. TT is an associate professor of applied human nutrition in the School of Public Health at Wolaita Sodo University. BY is a PhD Fellow in the Centre for International Health at the University of Bergen in Norway jointly with Hawassa University in Ethiopia. He has been working as an assistant Professor in the School of Public at Wolaita Sodo University, and MY is a graduate of MSc in Human Nutrition from the School of Public in Wolaita Sodo University.

Ethics approval and consent to participate

Ethical clearance was obtained from Research Ethics Committee at College of Health Sciences and Medicine in Wolaita Sodo University. The committee due the virtue of its mandate evaluated the written consent feasibility in relation to respondents' education in rural Soro district and gave as approval for informed verbal consent. Thus, official letter of cooperation in attachment with ethical clearance was submitted to Soro District health office for permission. Through official communications to the lower administrative structures we reached to the study respondents. The nature of the study was explained to the study participants to obtain their verbal informed consent prior to participation. Confidentiality of participants was secured through anonymous codes of questionnaire. Any one sick in the household during the survey was linked to the nearby health facility in the area.

Competing interests

The authors declare that they have no competing interests.

Author details

[1]School of public Health, Wolaita Sodo University, P.o.box 126 Wolaita Sodo, Ethiopia. [2]Centre for international Health, the University of Bergen, Bergen, Norway. [3]School of Public Health, Hawassa University, Hawassa, Ethiopia. [4]Soro district Health office, Hosanna, Ethiopia. [5]Damot Pulasa district, Wolaita Sodo, Ethiopia.

References

1. Organization, W.H. and Unicef, Global strategy for infant and young child feeding. 2003.
2. UNICEF., Infant and young child feeding, nutrition section program. 2011, UNICEF:. New York.
3. Lutter C. Meeting the challenge to improve complementary feeding. SCN news. 2003;27:4–9.
4. Organization, W.H. Strengthening action to improve feeding of infants and young children 6–23 months of age in nutrition and child health programmes. in Report of proceedings. 2008.
5. Organization, P.A.H., Guiding principles for complementary feeding of the breastfed child. 2003, Washington, DC: Pan American Health Organization.
6. Daelmans B, Dewey K, Arimond M. New and updated indicators for assessing infant and young child feeding. Food & Nutrition Bulletin. 2009; 30(2):S256.
7. Organization, W.H., Guiding principles for complementary feeding of the breastfed child. 2001, World Health Organization: Geneva: .
8. [Ethiopia], C.S.A.C. and ICF, Ethiopia Demographic and Health Survey 2016, in Final report. 2017, Central statistical authority: Addis Ababa Ethiopia, Rockville, Maryland, USA.
9. Institute, I.F.P.R. Global Nutrition Report 2016, in From promise to impact 2016, international food policy research institute: Washington. DC.
10. Lutter CK, et al. Undernutrition, poor feeding practices, and low coverage of key nutrition interventions. Pediatrics. 2011;128(6):e1418–27.
11. Kumar D, et al. Influence of infant-feeding practices on nutritional status of under-five children. The Indian Journal of Pediatrics. 2006;73(5):417–21.
12. Macro, C.S.A.E.a.O., Ethiopia Demographic and Health Survey. 2011, central statistical agency and ORC macro: Addis Ababa. Maryland: Ethiopia and Calverton; 2011.
13. Ali, D., et al., Alive and thrive baseline survey report: Ethiopia. 2011.
14. office, S.w.H., Soro woreda Health sector planning,monitoring and evalution core process. 2014.
15. Agedew, E., et al., Early Initiation of Complementary Feeding and Associated Factors among 6 Months to 2 Years Young Children. Kamba Woreda, South West Ethiopia: A Community–Based Cross-Sectional Study. J Nutr Food Sci, 2014. 4(314): p. 2.
16. Organization, W.H., Indicators for assessing infant and young child feeding practices: part 2: Measurement 2010.
17. Joshi N, et al. Determinants of inappropriate complementary feeding practices in young children in Nepal: secondary data analysis of demographic and health survey 2006. Maternal & child nutrition. 2012;8(s1): 45–59.
18. Senarath U, et al. Determinants of inappropriate complementary feeding practices in young children in Sri Lanka: secondary data analysis of demographic and health survey 2006–2007. Maternal & child nutrition. 2012;8(s1):60–77.
19. Ogunlesi T, et al. Determinants of timely initiation of complementary feeding among children aged 6-24 months in Sagamu, Nigeria. Niger J Clin Pract. 2015;17(6):785–90.
20. Tessema M, Belachew T, Ersino G. Feeding patterns and stunting during early childhood in rural communities of Sidama, South Ethiopia. Pan African Medical Journal. 2013:14(1).
21. Shumey A, Demissie M, Berhane Y. Timely initiation of complementary feeding and associated factors among children aged 6 to 12 months in northern Ethiopia: an institution-based cross-sectional study. BMC Public Health. 2013;13(1):1050.
22. Kimani-Murage EW, et al. Patterns and determinants of breastfeeding and complementary feeding practices in urban informal settlements. Nairobi Kenya BMC Public Health. 2011;11(1):396.
23. Yemane S, Awoke T, Gebreslassie M. Timely initiation of complementary feeding practice and associated factors among mothers of children aged from 6 to 24 months in Axum town, north Ethiopia. Sciences. 2014;3(5):438–42.
24. Abera K. Infant and young child feeding practices among mothers living in Harar, Ethiopia. Harar bulletin of Health Sciences. 2012;4

26

Differences upon admission and in hospital course of children hospitalized with community-acquired pneumonia with or without radiologically-confirmed pneumonia

Raquel Simbalista[1], Dafne C. Andrade[2], Igor C. Borges[2], Marcelo Araújo[3] and Cristiana M. Nascimento-Carvalho[1,2,4*]

Abstract

Background: The use of chest radiograph (CXR) for the diagnosis of childhood community-acquired pneumonia (CAP) is controversial. We assessed if children with CAP diagnosed on clinical grounds, with or without radiologically-confirmed pneumonia on admission, evolved differently.

Methods: Children aged ≥ 2 months, hospitalized with CAP diagnosed on clinical grounds, treated with 200,000 IU/Kg/day of aqueous penicillin G for ≥ 48 h and with CXR taken upon admission, without pleural effusion, were included in this retrospective cohort. One researcher, blinded to the radiological diagnosis, collected data on demographics, clinical history and physical examination on admission, daily hospital course during the first 2 days of treatment, and outcome, all from medical charts. Radiological confirmation of pneumonia was based on presence of pulmonary infiltrate detected by a paediatric radiologist who was also blinded to clinical data. Variables were initially compared by bivariate analysis. Multi-variable logistic regression analysis assessed independent association between radiologically-confirmed pneumonia and factors which significantly differed during hospital course in the bivariate analysis. The multi-variable analysis was performed in a model adjusted for age and for the same factor present upon admission.

Results: 109 (38.5 %) children had radiologically-confirmed pneumonia, 143 (50.5 %) had normal CXR and 31 (11.0 %) had atelectasis or peribronchial thickening. Children without radiologically-confirmed pneumonia were younger than those with radiologically-confirmed pneumonia (median [IQR]: 14 [7–28 months *versus* 21 [12–44] months; $P = 0.001$). None died. The subgroup with radiologically-confirmed pneumonia presented fever on D1 (33.7 *vs.* 19.1; $P = 0.015$) and on D2 (31.6 % *vs.* 16.2 %; $P = 0.004$) more frequently. The subgroup without radiologically-confirmed pneumonia had chest indrawing on D1 (22.4 % *vs.* 11.9 %; $P = 0.027$) more often detected. By multi-variable analysis, Fever on D2 (OR [95 % CI]: 2.16 [1.15-4.06]) was directly and independently associated with radiologically-confirmed pneumonia upon admission.

Conclusion: The compared subgroups evolved differently.

* Correspondence: nascimentocarvalho@hotmail.com
[1]Postgraduate Program in Pathology, Federal University of Bahia School of Medicine, Salvador, Brazil
[2]Postgraduate Program in Health Sciences, Federal University of Bahia School of Medicine, Salvador, Brazil
Full list of author information is available at the end of the article

Background

Community acquired pneumonia (CAP) is the leading cause of mortality in children aged less than 5 years, accounting for 1.1 million childhood deaths every year – more than AIDS, measles and malaria all together [1]. Considering CAP control a fundamental step to achieve the Millennium Development Goal 4 of "reducing by two-thirds, between 1990 and 2015, the under-five mortality rate" [2], the World Health Organization (WHO) proposed in 1990 a standardized case-management protocol for CAP, based solely on symptoms and signs [3]. In 2005, a standardized manual for pneumonia recognition on chest radiograph (CXR) was also produced specifically for epidemiological studies [4].

However, the use of CXR in the lack of a simple gold-standard exam for pneumonia has been questioned in the literature as a practice able to improve clinical outcome [5]. So far, the evidence suggests that an admission CXR has no effect on the outcome of paediatric outpatients with CAP [6]. The inability to distinguish between viral and bacterial aetiology in CAP represents another limitation of CXR analyses [7]. The interpretation of CXR may also be difficult in young children, when a poor inter-observer concordance between attending physicians at the emergency room is demonstrated [8]. Considering the aforementioned aspects of CXR, the British Thoracic Society recommended that CXR should not be considered a routine investigation in children thought to have CAP [9].

Of note, the Pediatric Infectious Diseases Society and the Infectious Diseases Society of America's guidelines state that CXR (postero-anterior and lateral views) should be obtained in all children hospitalized for management of CAP [10]. It is important to realize that a significant proportion of paediatric CAP cases diagnosed on clinical grounds actually have a normal CXR. For example, in Pakistan, 82 % of the children aged 2–59 months with CAP diagnosed according to the WHO criteria had a normal CXR [11]. To the best of our knowledge, the differences in progression of symptoms and signs between children with CAP diagnosed on clinical grounds with or without radiological confirmation has been assessed only once. That study included 382 children with non-severe CAP, and demonstrated earlier resolution of the symptoms in children with normal CXR. It was also reported that persistence of symptoms such as fever and tachypnoea was predictive of radiologically-confirmed pneumonia [12].

The use of aqueous penicillin G is the recommended antibiotic therapy for all children with CAP who require hospitalization [10]. The rationale for this approach is to treat the bacterial CAP cases caused by *Streptococcus pneumoniae*, which is the most frequent aetiological agent of CAP [13]. Moreover, aqueous penicillin G has treated successfully a massive majority of children hospitalized with CAP [14].

In this context, the aim of this study was to assess if there were differences in hospital course and in outcome between groups of children hospitalized with CAP, diagnosed on clinical grounds, treated with aqueous penicillin G, with or without radiologically-confirmed pneumonia on admission.

Methods

This retrospective cohort included children aged ≥ 2 months hospitalized with CAP and treated intravenously with 200,000 IU/Kg/day of aqueous penicillin G for at least 48 h, and with CXR taken on admission, in a 37-month period (from October 2002 to October 2005), at the Federal University of Bahia Hospital, in Salvador, North-eastern Brazil. The exclusion criteria comprised underlying debilitating conditions such as heart disease with hemodynamic repercussion, chronic lung disease except asthma, severe malnutrition, immunodeficiency, nosocomial pneumonia from another hospital, transfers to other hospitals during aqueous penicillin G treatment, presence of pleural effusion upon admission and radiological diagnoses other than pneumonia or normal CXR or atelectasis or peribronchial thickening. In accordance with the recommendation from the Brazilian Society of Paediatrics, aqueous penicillin G was the standardized treatment for all children hospitalized with a clinical diagnosis of CAP [15]. Sample size was estimated considering a smaller expected frequency of 15 % and an expected difference between the compared frequencies of 10 %. The sample size was thus estimated as 250 cases in the study group, considering a significance level of 0.05 (95 Confidence Interval [95 %CI]) and power of 80 %.

Based on the hospital admittance log-book, which contained the list of all hospitalized children and the respective cause of hospitalization, one researcher (RS) identified all children hospitalized with CAP during the study period and collected data from the medical charts whilst being blinded to the radiological diagnosis. A paediatric radiologist (MA) blinded to clinical data read the CXR taken on admission and registered the findings in a standardized form for the purpose of this study. He looked for the presence of pulmonary infiltrate, pleural effusion, atelectasis, hyperinflation, abscess, peribronchial thickening, pneumatocele and pneumothorax, taking into account previously published definitions [4]. The final radiological confirmation of pneumonia was based on the presence of pulmonary infiltrate [4].

Data on demographics, clinical history, physical examination on admission, treatment, daily hospital course during the first 2 days of treatment (cough, breathlessness, axillary temperature, respiratory rate, cyanosis, chest indrawing, chest retraction, somnolence, nasal flaring, grunting, seizure), and outcome were collected from the medical charts and recorded on a predefined form. For axillary temperature and respiratory rate (RR), the highest registered grade was collected. Fever was defined as axillary temperature ≥ 37.5 °C [16] and tachypnoea as RR ≥ 50 breaths/min in children aged 2–11 months, RR ≥ 40 breaths/min in children from 12 to 59 months of age [17], and RR ≥ 30 in children aged ≥ 60 months [18]. Nutritional evaluation was performed using the software Anthro, version 1.02

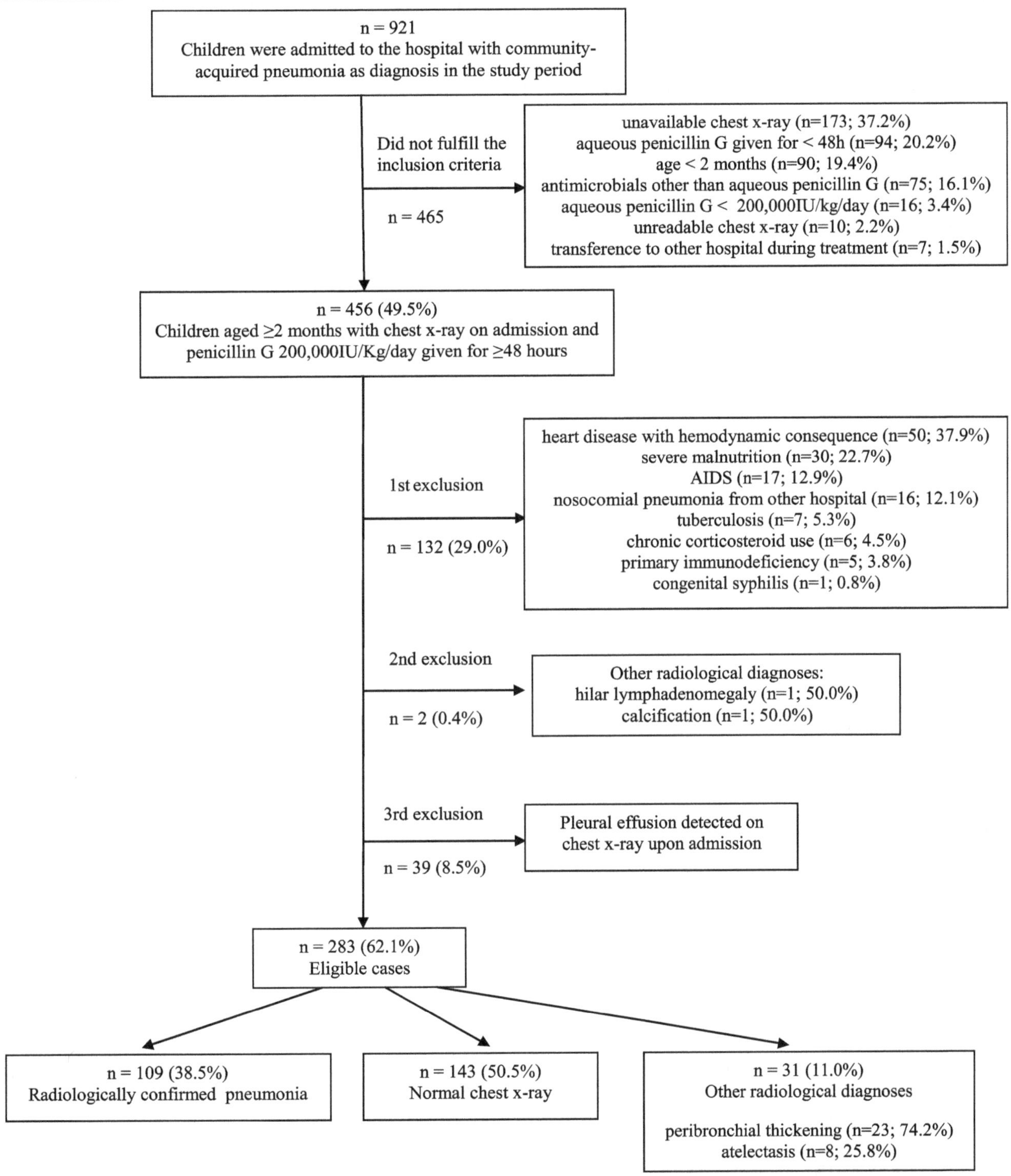

Fig. 1 Flow-chart of the step-by-step selection of children hospitalized with community-acquired pneumonia diagnosed on clinical grounds

(CDC [Center for Disease Control and Prevention] and WHO) and malnutrition and severe malnutrition were defined as Z-score for weight-for-age index under −2.00 or −3.00, respectively, using the National Centre for Health Statistics standard [19].

CAP was classified as non-severe, severe or very severe according to WHO guidelines: patients with chest indrawing were classified as severe CAP and patients with somnolence, seizures, grunting when calm, nasal flaring, cyanosis, or inability to drink were classified as very severe CAP [17]. If a child had chest indrawing along with any item that would classify him/her as very severe CAP, the final classification was very severe CAP.

We compared the frequency of demographic and clinical findings detected upon admission and on each day of hospital course up to the 2nd day between patients with radiologically-confirmed pneumonia and those with normal CXR or without radiologically-confirmed pneumonia.

Table 1 Baseline and clinical characteristics of children hospitalized with community-acquired pneumonia diagnosed on clinical grounds

Characteristics	Radiologically-confirmed pneumonia				
	Yes ($n = 109$)	Normal CXR ($n = 143$)	P	No[e] ($n = 174$)	P
Gender male[a]	70 (64.2)	77 (53.8)	0.098	87 (50.0)	0.019
Age strata[a, b]					
2-11 months	28 (25.7)	63 (44.1)	0.003	73 (42.0)	0.005
1-4 years	67 (61.5)	68 (47.6)	0.028	87 (50.0)	0.059
≥ 5 years	14 (12.8)	12 (8.4)	0.250	14 (8.0)	0.188
History of current illness					
fever[a]	100 (91.7)	112 (78.3)	0.004	140 (80.5)	0.010
duration of fever[c]	$n = 79$	$n = 80$		$n = 105$	
	5 (3–7); 1-30	4(2–6); 1-20	0.093	4(2–7);1-20	0.299
cough[a]	92 (84.4)	123 (86.0)	0.720	152 (87.4)	0.483
duration of cough[c]	$n = 59$	$n = 80$		$n = 93$	
	7 (4–9); 1-45	4.5 (3–7); 1-31	0.022	5(3–7.5);1-31	0.053
breathlessness[a]	67 (61.5)	104 (72.7)	0.058	124 (71.3)	0.087
duration of breathlessness[c]	$n = 46$	$n = 77$	.	$n = 93$	
	2 (1–6); 1-30	3 (1–4.5); 1-30	0.894	3(1–5);1-30	0.504
Physical examination findings					
tachypnoea[a]	68/85[d] (80.0)	79/106[d] (74.5)	0.372	98/131[d] (74.8)	0.377
fever[a]	52/99[d] (52.5)	62/121[d] (51.2)	0.849	79/148[d] (53.4)	0.895
crackles[a]	42 (38.5)	86 (60.1)	0.001	100 (57.5)	0.002
wheezing[a]	32 (29.4)	86 (60.1)	<0.001	99 (56.9)	<0.001
chest retraction[a]	38 (34.9)	53 (37.1)	0.719	69 (39.7)	0.418
Severity according to WHO[b]					
non-severe[a]	76 (69.7)	76 (53.1)	0.008	97 (55.7)	0.019
severe[a]	22 (20.2)	47 (32.9)	0.025	55 (31.6)	0.036
very severe[a]	11 (10.1)	20 (14.0)	0.351	22 (12.6)	0.515
chest indrawing[a]	30 (27.5)	58 (40.6)	0.032	67 (38.5)	0.058
nasal flaring[a]	7 (6.4)	17 (11.9)	0.143	19 (10.9)	0.202
somnolence[a]	1 (0.9)	1 (0.7)	1.000	1 (0.6)	1.000
seizure[a]	1 (0.9)	1 (0.7)	1.000	1 (0.6)	1.000
cyanosis[a]	2 (1.8)	1 (0.7)	0.580	1 (0.6)	0.561

CXR indicates chest radiograph
WHO indicates World Health Organization
[a]Data are shown as n (%)
[b]The frequencies in each age stratum or in the severity groups according to WHO were compared as dichotomic variables
[c]Data are shown as median (IQR); minimum-maximum
[d]Different denominators are due to missing data
[e]Includes normal CXR plus CXR with atelectasis or peribronchial thickening

This last group comprised patients with normal CXR or CXR with atelectasis or peribronchial thickening. A subgroup comparison was performed when wheezers were excluded. We also compared the frequency of length of hospital stay and treatment as well as the final outcome upon discharge between these groups. Categorical variables were compared by using chi-square or Fisher exact test as appropriate, and continuous variables were assessed by using Mann–Whitney U test due to non-parametrical distribution. Multi-variable logistic regression analysis by enter method was used to assess independent association between radiologically-confirmed pneumonia and factors which significantly differed during hospital course in the bivariate analysis. The multi-variable analysis was performed in a model adjusted for age and for the same factor present upon admission. The statistical tests were two tailed, with a significance level of 0.05. The software SPSS (version 9.0, IBM, Armonk, New York) was used for the analysis. The exclusion criteria were chosen for the purpose of addressing potential confounders. Blinding to the radiological diagnosis during medical charts review was performed to address potential bias.

The study was conducted according to the principles expressed in the Declaration of Helsinki and it was approved by the Ethics Committee at Federal University of Bahia. Informed consent was deemed unnecessary due to the retrospective collection of data. Identification of the patients was kept confidential.

Results

During the study period, 921 cases were detected and 456 patients fulfilled the inclusion criteria. After excluding 132 (29.0 %) cases due to underlying debilitating illnesses, a further 39 (8.5 %) with pleural effusion detected on the CXR taken upon admission, and an additional 2 (0.4 %) due to other radiological diagnoses such as calcification and hilar lymphadenomegaly (Fig. 1), the final study group comprised 283 (62.1 %) patients. Overall, 157 (55.5 %) patients were males, the median age was 17 months (IQR [interquartile range]: 9–34 months; minimum 2 months; maximum 9.2 years) and 101 (35.7 %) patients were aged under 1 year. Upon admission, the most common complaints were cough (86.2 %), fever (84.8 %), breathlessness (67.5 %), and the most frequent findings were tachypnoea (76.9 %), fever (53.0 %), crackles (50.2 %), wheezing (46.3 %), chest retraction (37.8 %) and chest indrawing (34.3 %). CAP was severe or very severe among 77 (27.2 %) and 33 (11.7 %) patients, respectively. Malnutrition was detected in 21 (7.4) cases and severe malnutrition in 1 (0.4 %) case.

The compared subgroups included 109 (38.5 %) children with radiologically-confirmed pneumonia, 143 (50.5 %) children with normal CXR and 31 (11.0 %) with other radiological diagnoses (atelectasis or peribronchial thickening). In the radiologically-confirmed pneumonia subgroup, pulmonary infiltrate was classified as alveolar (94.5 %), alveolar-interstitial (3.7 %) or interstitial (1.8 %). Additional radiological findings were

Table 2 Significant differences during hospital course of children hospitalized with community-acquired pneumonia diagnosed on clinical grounds

Characteristics	Radiologically-confirmed pneumonia				
	Yes	Normal CXR	*P*	No[d]	*P*
D1[a]	$n = 109$[b]	$n = 143$[b]		$n = 174$	
Fever	29/86[c] (33.7)	17/107[c] (15.9)	0.004	25/131 (19.1)	0.015
Chest indrawing	13 (11.9)	31 (21.7)	0.043	39 (22.4)	0.027
D2[a]	$n = 109$[b]	$n = 143$[b]			
Fever	31/98[c] (31.6)	16/119[c] (13.4)	0.001	24/148 (16.2)	0.004
Without wheezers					
D1[a]					
Fever	26/62 (41.9)	9/46 (19.6)	0.014	14/59 (23.7)	0.033
Chest indrawing	6/77 (7.8)	9/57 (15.8)	0.147	12/75 (16.0)	0.117
D2[a]					
Fever	28/69 (40.6)	10/50 (20.0)	0.017	15/68 (22.1)	0.020

Data are shown as n (%)

CXR indicates chest radiograph

[a]*D1* is the first day after aqueous penicillin G has been initiated (24 h of treatment), *D2* is the second day after aqueous penicillin G has been initiated (48 h of treatment)

[b]*n* = number of evaluated patients in each subgroup on the respective day of hospital course

[c]Different denominators due to missing data

[d]Includes normal CXR plus CXR with atelectasis or peribronchial thickening

atelectasis (2.8 %) and peribronchial thickening (3.7 %). The baseline characteristics are compared in Table 1. Children without radiologically-confirmed pneumonia were younger than those with radiologically-confirmed pneumonia (median [IQR]: 14 [7–28 months *versus* 21 [12–44] months; $P = 0.001$). No difference was found in the frequency of malnutrition (10 [9.2 %] *versus* 11 [6.3 %]; $P = 0.373$).

Overall, the median duration of hospitalization was 7 days (IQR: 5–10; minimum 2; maximum 31), and the median duration of aqueous penicillin G use was 4 days (IQR: 3–6; minimum 2; maximum 17). Children with radiologically-confirmed pneumonia stayed in hospital for as long as children without radiologically-confirmed pneumonia (median 7 days [IQR: 4–10] *versus* median 7 days [IQR: 5–9]; $P = 0.903$). No difference was found between the two subgroups regarding duration of penicillin use (radiologically-confirmed pneumonia: median 4 days [IQR: 3–6] *versus* no radiologically-confirmed pneumonia: median 4 days [IQR: 3–6]; $P = 0.402$). Overall, aqueous penicillin G was substituted by other antibiotics in 29 (10.2 %) cases. Children with radiologically-confirmed pneumonia had aqueous penicillin G substituted more frequently than those without radiologically-confirmed pneumonia (15.6 % *versus* 6.9 %; $P = 0.019$).

No patient died and everyone was discharged after improvement. Table 2 presents the significant differences found during progression of disease between children with or without radiologically-confirmed pneumonia or normal CXR during aqueous penicillin G treatment. Those with substitution of aqueous penicillin G were excluded. The comparison of the symptoms and signs during hospital course which did not demonstrate significant difference is shown in Table 3. Table 4 depicts the multi-variable analysis of factors whose difference was significant in the bivariate analysis presented in Table 2.

Table 3 Symptoms and signs without significant differences during hospital course of children hospitalized with community-acquired pneumonia diagnosed on clinical grounds

Characteristics	Radiologically-confirmed pneumonia				
	Yes	Normal CXR	*P*	No[d]	*P*
D1[a]	$n = 109^b$	$n = 143^b$		$n = 174^b$	
Tachypnoea	54/90[c] (60.0)	51/107[c] (47.7)	0.084	65/132[c] (49.2)	0.115
Cyanosis	0	0	-	0	-
Chest retraction	21 (19.3)	29 (20.3)	0.842	37 (21.3)	0.685
Somnolence	1 (0.9)	1 (0.7)	1.000	1 (0.6)	1.000
Nasal flaring	4 (3.7)	4 (2.8)	0.730	5 (2.9)	0.737
Grunting	0	1 (0.7)	1.000	1 (0.6)	1.000
Seizure	0	0	-	0	-
Cough	41 (37.6)	44 (30.8)	0.255	55 (31.6)	0.299
Breathlessness	18 (16.5)	33 (23.1)	0.199	42 (24.1)	0.127
D2[a]	$n = 109^b$	$n = 143^b$		$n = 174^b$	
Tachypnoea	45/93[c] (48.4)	52/119[c] (43.7)	0.496	67/145[c] (46.2)	0.742
Cyanosis	1 (0.9)	0	0.433	0	0.385
Chest indrawing	11 (10.1)	14 (9.8)	0.937	19 (10.9)	0.826
Chest retraction	14 (12.8)	16 (11.2)	0.688	20 (11.5)	0.734
Somnolence	2 (1.8)	0	0.186	0	0.148
Nasal flaring	1 (0.9)	1 (0.7)	1.000	1 (0.6)	1.000
Grunting	0	1 (0.7)	1.000	1 (0.6)	1.000
Seizure	0	0	-	0	-
Cough	44 (40.4)	65 (45.5)	0.419	79 (45.4)	0.406
Breathlessness	25 (22.9)	28 (19.6)	0.517	34 (19.5)	0.494

Data are shown as n (%)

CXR indicates chest radiograph

[a]*D1* is the first day after aqueous penicillin G has been initiated (24 h of treatment), *D2* is the second day after aqueous penicillin G has been initiated (48 h of treatment)

[b]*n* = number of evaluated patients in each subgroup on the respective day of hospital course

[c]Different denominators due to missing data

[d]Includes normal CXR plus CXR with atelectasis or peribronchial thickening

Table 4 Multi-variable analysis of factors associated with radiologically-confirmed pneumonia during hospital course in bivariate analysis, adjusted for age and for the same factor upon admission, among children hospitalized with community-acquired pneumonia diagnosed on clinical grounds

	Compared subgroup					
	Normal CXR		CXR without pneumonia		Without wheezers	
Characteristics	OR (95 % CI)	*P*	OR (95 % CI)	*P*	OR (95 % CI)	*P*
Fever on D1[a]	2.18 (1.07-4.43)	0.031	1.75 (0.92-3.34)	0.091	2.00 (0.89-4.48)	0.094
Age	1.00 (1.00-1.00)	0.062	1.00 (1.00-1.00)	0.023	1.00 (0.99-1.00)	0.089
Report of fever upon admission	4.01 (1.54-10.42)	0.004	3.47 (1.35-8.94)	0.010	1.75 (0.58-5.23)	0.317
Chest indrawing on D1[a]	0.65 (0.31-1.37))	0.259	0.60 (0.29-1.22)	0.160	0.60 (0.20-1.77)	0.354
Age	1.00 (1.00-1.00)	0.033	1.00 (1.00-1.00)	0.024	1.00 (1.00-1.00)	0.072
Chest indrawing upon admission	0.67 (0.38-1.19)	0.174	0.74 (0.43-1.28)	0.281	0.67 (0.30-1.46)	0.311
Fever on D2[a]	2.66 (1.32-5.36)	0.006	2.16 (1.15-4.06)	0.016	2.24 (1.04-4.79)	0.039
Age	1.00 (1.00-1.00)	0.086	1.00 (1.00-1.00)	0.044	1.00 (0.99-1.00)	0.116
Report of fever upon admission	4.15 (1.61-10.67)	0.003	3.65 (1.44-9.23)	0.006	2.01 (0.69-5.83)	0.199

Multi-variable analysis by logistic regression
CXR indicates chest radiograph
CXR without pneumonia includes normal CXR plus CXR with atelectasis or peribronchial thickening
[a]*D1* is the first day after aqueous penicillin G has been initiated (24 h of treatment), *D2* is the second day after aqueous penicillin G has been initiated (48 h of treatment)

Discussion

This study provides evidence that children hospitalized with CAP diagnosed on clinical grounds treated with aqueous penicillin G, present differences during hospital course when radiologically-confirmed pneumonia cases are compared to others without radiologically-confirmed pneumonia or with normal CXR. Notably, patients with radiologically-confirmed pneumonia were significantly more feverish on admission and during the first 2 days of aqueous penicillin G use. This finding remained when wheezers were excluded from the analysis. It is important to recall that children included in this study were otherwise healthy and had no significant comorbidity.

Several methodological constraints should be highlighted in this investigation. As data were collected retrospectively, there was no control on variables measurement and, as patients were evaluated by different observers, standardization of evaluations could not be guaranteed. Also, no aetiological agent was determined. However, strict criteria for enrolling and grouping the cases were used, and those with potential confounding variables were excluded. Moreover, the study was performed in a teaching hospital where the same standardized procedures for assistance have been used over the period of the study [15]. Interestingly, all children included in the analysis had pneumonia diagnosed and were admitted to hospital by paediatricians.

The presence of fever has been lately associated with radiologically-confirmed pneumonia. A recent study has estimated that presence of fever increases the chance of children hospitalized with lower respiratory tract disease to have radiologically-confirmed pneumonia by 2.5 times [20]. Additionally, it has been demonstrated that the inclusion of fever in the WHO criteria for the clinical diagnosis of CAP substantially increases its specificity, particularly in children with wheezing [21]. The history of fever has also been recognized as the symptom with the greatest sensitivity for the presence of pulmonary infiltrates [22]. Our data provide evidence that persistence of fever up to the second day of treatment is also more frequent among hospitalized children with radiologically-confirmed pneumonia.

In a previous investigation which compared the progression of symptoms among children with non-severe acute lower respiratory tract infection with and without a radiological diagnosis of pneumonia, tachypnoea persisted longer during treatment among those with radiologically-confirmed pneumonia [12]. Herein, this finding was not found, possibly due to sample size. Children without radiologically-confirmed pneumonia had higher frequency of wheezing, which is a potential confounding factor for the diagnosis of CAP among children with tachypnoea [23, 24]. The high frequency of children with a clinical diagnosis of CAP and without radiologically-confirmed pneumonia is in accordance with previous studies. Up to 82 % of children with tachypnoea and wheezing had normal CXR in Pakistan [11]. The prescription of antibiotics based on only tachypnoea should be restricted to settings where CXR performance is not feasible. The lower frequency of fever [23] and the younger age [25] in the subgroup without radiologically-confirmed pneumonia may also guide the clinical suspicion to lower respiratory tract diseases other than CAP, for example bronchiolitis.

The evidence that there is no effect of an admission CXR in the outcome of paediatric outpatients with CAP was provided in a study in which all those children, irrespective of having CXR taken, received antibiotics. That means, those who needed antibiotics received antibiotics, as well as those who did not need antibiotics but instead had a self-limited disease [6]. It has been recently shown that radiologically-confirmed pneumonia is associated with bacterial infection [26]. Although CXR is undoubtedly limited in determining the aetiology of pneumonia [7], it may help identify children with a lower respiratory tract disease and a probable non-bacterial aetiology, such as bronchiolitis, who can benefit from not receiving unnecessary antibiotics.

Conclusions

This is the first study to demonstrate the differences in hospital course between hospitalized children with CAP diagnosed on clinical grounds with or without radiologically-confirmed pneumonia. We highlight differences on the hospital course between the studied subgroups. The performance of CXR may be a tool to select patients who would not benefit from receiving antibiotics and could be followed-up instead.

Competing interests

The authors declare that they have no competing interests.

Authors' contributions

CMN-C designed the study, RS reviewed the medical charts, collected and entered the data, MA read the chest radiographs, DCA and ICB analyzed the data. All authors contributed to the interpretation of the results. RS drafted the manuscript. DCA, ICB and MA contributed to the writing and CMN-C proofread the manuscript. All authors read and approved the final manuscript.

Acknowledgments

There was no funding for this investigation. The authors thank the medical chart unit of the Federal University of Bahia Hospital, in Salvador, Brazil for their cooperation in getting the medical charts to be reviewed.

Author details

[1]Postgraduate Program in Pathology, Federal University of Bahia School of Medicine, Salvador, Brazil. [2]Postgraduate Program in Health Sciences, Federal University of Bahia School of Medicine, Salvador, Brazil. [3]Image Diagnosis, Image Memorial Unit and Bahia Hospital, Salvador, Brazil. [4]Department of Paediatrics, Federal University of Bahia School of Medicine, Salvador, Brazil.

References

1. Walker CL, Rudan I, Liu L, Nair H, Theodoratou E, Bhutta ZA, et al. Global burden of childhood pneumonia and diarrhea. Lancet. 2013;381:1405–16.
2. World Health Organization. The United Nations Children's Fund. Global Action Plan for Prevention and Control of Pneumonia. 2009. http://www.whqlibdoc.who.int/hq/2009/WHO_FCH_CAH_NCH_09.04_eng.pdf. Accessed 20 May 2012.
3. World Health Organization. Programme for the control of acute respiratory infections. Acute respiratory infections in children: case management in small hospitals in developing countries. 1990. http://www.whqlibdoc.who.int/hq/1990/WHO_ARI_90.5.pdf. Accessed 26 May 2013.
4. Cherian T, Mulholland EK, Carlin JB, Ostensen H, Amin R, Campo M, et al. Standardized interpretation of paediatric chest radiographs for the diagnosis of pneumonia in epidemiological studies. Bull World Health Organ. 2005;83:353–9.
5. Swingler GH, Zwarenstein M. Chest radiograph in acute respiratory infections. Cochrane Database of Syst Rev 2008, Issue 1. Art. No.: CD001268. doi: 10.1002/14651858.CD001268.pub3. http://www.onlinelibrary.wiley.com/doi/10.1002/14651858.CD001268.pub3/abstract. Accessed 14 June 2012.
6. Swingler GH, Hussey GD, Zwarenstein M. Randomised controlled trial of clinical outcome after chest radiograph in ambulatory acute lower-respiratory infection in children. Lancet. 1998;351:404–8.
7. Korppi M, Don M, Valent F, Canciani M. The value of clinical features in differentiating between viral, pneumococcal and atypical bacterial pneumonia in children. Acta Paediatr. 2008;97:943–7.
8. Johnson J, Kline JA. Intraobserver and interobserver agreement of the interpretation of pediatric chest radiographs. Emerg Radiol. 2010;17:285–90.
9. Harris M, Clark J, Coote N, Fletcher P, Harnden A, McKean M, et al. British Thoracic Society guidelines for the management of community acquired pneumonia in children: update 2011. Thorax. 2011;66:1–23.
10. Bradley JS, Byington CL, Shah SS, Alyerson B, Carter ER, Harrison C, et al. The management of community-acquired pneumonia in infants and children older than 3 months of age: clinical practice guidelines by the Pediatric Infectious Diseases Society and the Infectious Diseases Society of America. Clin Infect Dis. 2011;53:25–76.
11. Hazir T, Nisar YB, Qazi SA, Khan SF, Raza M, Zameer S, et al. Chest radiography in children aged 2–59 months diagnosed with non-severe pneumonia as defined by World Health Organization: descriptive multicentre study in Pakistan. BMJ. 2006;333:629.
12. Fontoura MS, Matutino AR, Silva CC, Santana MC, Nobre-Bastos M, Oliveira F, et al. Differences in evolution of children with non-severe acute lower respiratory tract infection with and without radiographically diagnosed pneumonia. Indian Pediatr. 2012;49:363–9.
13. Gentile A, Bardach A, Ciapponi A, García-Marti S, Aruj P, Glujovsky D, et al. Epidemiology of community-acquired pneumonia in children of Latin America and the Caribbean: a systematic review and meta-analysis. Int J Infect Dis. 2012;16:5–15.
14. Simbalista R, Araújo M, Nascimento-Carvalho CM. Outcome of children hospitalized with community-acquired pneumonia treated with aqueous penicillin G. Clinics. 2011;66:95–100.
15. Nascimento-Carvalho CM, Souza-Marques HH. Recommendation of the Brazilian Society of Pediatrics for antibiotic therapy in children and adolescents with community-acquired pneumonia. Rev Panam Salud Publica. 2004;15:380–7.
16. El-Radhi AS, Barry W. Thermometry in paediatric practice. Arch Dis Child. 2006;91:351–6.
17. World Health Organization. Integrated Management of Childhood Illness chart booklet (WC 503.2). 2008. http://www.whqlibdoc.who.int/publications/2008/9789241597289_eng.pdf. Accessed 15 January 2009.
18. Nascimento-Carvalho CM. Physical signs in children with pneumonia. Indian Pediatr. 2001;38:307–8.
19. World Health Organization. Training Course on Child Growth Assessment. 2008. http://www.whqlibdoc.who.int/publications/2008/9789241595070_A_eng.pdf. Accessed 13 July 2009.
20. Key NK, Arajo-Neto CA, Cardoso MR, Nascimento-Carvalho CM. Characteristics of radiographically diagnosed pneumonia in under-5 children in Salvador, Brazil. Indian Pediatr. 2011;48:873–7.
21. Cardoso MR, Nascimento-Carvalho CM, Ferrero F, Alves FM, Cousens SN. Adding fever to WHO criteria for diagnosing pneumonia enhances the ability to identify pneumonia cases among wheezing children. Arch Dis Child. 2011;96:58–61.
22. Lynch T, Platt R, Gouin S, Larson C, Patenaude Y. Can we predict which children with clinically suspected pneumonia will have the presence of focal infiltrates on chest radiographs? Pediatrics. 2004;113:e186–9.
23. Mathews B, Shah S, Cleveland RH, Lee EY, Bachur RG, Neuman MI. Clinical predictors of pneumonia among children with wheezing. Pediatrics. 2009;124:e29–36.
24. Castro AV, Nascimento-Carvalho CM, Ney-Oliveria F, Araújo-Neto CA, Andrade SC, Loureiro LL, et al. Additional markers to refine the World Health Organization algorithm for diagnosis of pneumonia. Indian Pediatr. 2005;42:773–81.

Attitudes of pediatricians toward Children's consumption of ionic beverages

Akihisa Okumura[1,2*], Shinobu Ida[3], Masaaki Mori[4], Toshiaki Shimizu[2] and On behalf of the Committee on Pediatric Nutrition of The Japanese Pediatric Society

Abstract

Background: The aim of our study was to clarify the attitudes of pediatricians toward children's consumption of ionic beverages.

Methods: A questionnaire survey of pediatric practitioners' attitudes toward the consumption of ionic beverages was administered to 537 doctors under 60 years of age who were members of the Japanese Pediatric Society.

Results: We received 215 valid responses from 182 board-certified pediatric specialists and 31 non-specialists. Approximately 60% of respondents recommended ionic beverages either often or sometimes. About half of all respondents cautioned patients about excessive consumption. About 40% had experienced at least one instance of excessive consumption characterized by acute symptoms including vomiting, diarrhea, and pyrexia. Specialists were more likely to recommend ionic beverages for oral rehydration than did non-specialists. Non-specialists more often recommended ionic beverages to patients with pyrexia.

Conclusions: Pediatricians' attitudes toward children's consumption of ionic beverages were generally appropriate. Pediatric specialists' attitudes were more appropriate than were those of non-specialists.

Keywords: Vitamin B1 deficiency, Ionic beverages, Excessive consumption, Attitude

Background

We have reported vitamin B1 deficiency (VB1D) caused by excessive consumption of ionic beverages in Japan [1]. The patients with VB1D were infants and young children who continued to drink a large amount of ionic beverages every day for several months, some of whom were raised in a non-nurturing environment [2–8]. VB1D caused by excessive soft drink consumption is presumed to be unique to Japan, where ionic beverages are popular and are widely used on a daily basis. It cannot be ignored that doctors' recommendations of ionic beverages have triggered excessive consumption by some children with VB1D [1, 2]. Oral fluid replacement is widely accepted as important in patients with dehydration caused by infectious diseases such as acute viral gastroenteritis [9, 10]. Several suitable ionic beverages are commercially available in Japan [11, 12]. Appropriate oral fluid replacement is essential to treat and prevent dehydration in children. On the other hand, the annual sales of ionic beverages are increasing in Japan. Some promotions target children, potentially creating a risk of excessive consumption. Parents and caregivers must learn how to prevent excessive consumption by children. However, the repetitive occurrence of VB1D due to excessive ionic beverage consumption among children suggests that parents and caregivers may lack adequate knowledge.

Few studies have evaluated the attitudes of pediatricians toward children's consumption of ionic beverages. The aim of the present study was to explore the attitudes of pediatricians toward consumption of ionic beverages; appropriate attitudes should help prevent excessive consumption. Thus, we surveyed the attitudes of pediatric practitioners toward consumption of ionic beverages.

Methods

We identified 537 doctors who met the following four criteria: 1) membership in the Japanese Pediatric Society; 2) working in Tokyo, Osaka, or Aichi Prefecture; 3) in

* Correspondence: okumura.akihisa.479@mail.aichi-med-u.ac.jp
[1]Department of Pediatrics, Aichi Medical University, Nagakute, Japan
[2]Department of Pediatrics, Juntendo University Faculty of Medicine, Tokyo, Japan
Full list of author information is available at the end of the article

daily practice; and, 4) under 60 years of age. This study was approved by the Ethics Committee of the Japanese Pediatric Society. Informed consent was obtained from all participants when they returned the completed questionnaires by mail.

The questionnaires were mailed to 532 pediatricians; the other 5 had moved. All subjects were asked to complete the questionnaire and return it by mail. In this study, sports drinks, ionic beverages, and oral rehydration solutions were collectively termed "ionic beverages" to minimize the redundancy of questions and to simplify analysis of the responses. Brand names are not mentioned below; we are sensitive to possible marketing issues. Instead, brief mentions of each brand are provided in the footnote to Table 1.

The contents of the questionnaire were as below.

Q1. Do you recommend ionic beverages to infants?

often, sometimes, infrequently, rarely, never.

Q2. Please write the brand names of ionic beverages which you recommend to infants.

Q3. Have you ever been consulted from the parents for excessive consumption of ionic beverages of their infants?

no, yes.

Q4. Do you know about the health problems of infants due to excessive consumption of ionic beverages?

know in detail, know, know a little, know very little, do not know.

Q5. To those who answered "often" or "sometimes" to Q1.

Which situations do you recommend ionic beverages to infants?

vomiting and/or diarrhea, pyrexia, failure to thrive, after bath, hot weather,

after sweating, others.

Q6. To those who answered "often" or "sometimes" to Q1.

Do you warn caregivers for their children not to take ionic beverages excessively?

always, sometimes, infrequently, rarely, never.

Table 1 The frequency of recommending ionic beverage, recommended brands, consultation of excessive consumption, and knowledge of health problems

	All participants $N = 215$	Pediatric specialists $N = 182$	Non-specialists $N = 31$	
Q1. The frequency of recommending ionic beverages				
Often	34 (15%)	27 (15%)	6 (19%)	NS
Sometimes	91 (42%)	80 (44%)	10 (32%)	
Infrequently	51 (24%)	44 (24%)	7 (23%)	
Rarely	28 (13%)	23 (13%)	5 (16%)	
Never	11 (5%)	8 (4%)	3 (10%)	
Q2. The brand names of ionic beverages which you recommend				
Brand A	130 (48%)	108 (59%)	20 (65%)	NS
Brand B	47 (22%)	43 (24%)	2 (6%)	$P < 0.05$
Brand C	22 (10%)	14 (8%)	7 (23%)	$P < 0.05$
Brand D	16 (7%)	12 (7%)	3 (10%)	NS
Brand E	10 (5%)	7 (4%)	3 (10%)	NS
Other brands	4 (2%)	4 (2%)	0	N/A
Anything	2 (1%)	2 (1%)	0	N/A
Not particular	46 (21%)	40 (22%)	6 (19%)	N/A
Q3. Consultation of excessive consumption of ionic beverages				
Yes	75 (35%)	68 (37%)	7 (23%)	NS
No	139 (65%)	113 (62%)	24 (77%)	
No answer	1 (0.5%)	1 (0.5%)	0	
Q4. Knowledge on the health problems due to excessive consumption of ionic beverages				
know in detail	16 (7%)	14 (8%)	2 (6%)	NS
know	96 (45%)	84 (46%)	12 (39%)	
know a little	56 (26%)	46 (25%)	10 (32%)	
know very little	35 (16%)	29 (16%)	6 (19%)	
do not know	9 (4%)	8 (4%)	1 (3%)	
No answer	1 (0.5%)	1 (0.5%)	0	

NS: not significant, N/A: not assessed

Brand A: An oral rehydration solution mainly sold in hospitals and pharmacies, containing energy 100 kcal/l, sodium ion 50 mEq/l, and potassium ion 20 mEq/l; Brand B: Several types are available. Some are categorized into soft drinks for infants, and others into oral rehydration solution, containing energy 160 kcal/l, sodium ion 35 mEq/l, and potassium ion 20 mEq/l; Brand C: One of the most popular sport drinks in Japan. Several types are available,, containing energy 250 kcal/l, sodium ion 21 mEq/l, and potassium ion 5 mEq/l;. Brand D: Oral rehydration powder prescribed in clinics and hospitals. Its solution can be available commercially, containing energy 130 kcal/l, sodium ion 60 mEq/l, and potassium ion 20 mEq/l;. Brand E: One of the most popular sport drinks in Japan, containing energy 190 kcal/l, sodium ion 17 mEq/l, and potassium ion 2 mEq/l;. Several types are available

We explored whether the responses differed between specialized pediatricians certified by the Japanese Pediatric Society and others. The chi-squared test was used to explore the significance of between-group differences; a p-value < 0.05 was considered to indicate statistical significance. We excluded missing or invalid data, and we did not analyze between-group differences if fewer than 10 responses were received from either group.

Results

We received 215 valid responses (response rate, 40%) from 182 board-certified pediatric specialists and 31 non-specialists. Of all responders, 34 (15%) frequently recommended ionic beverages, and 91 (42%) did so sometimes (Table 1). Brand A was the most commonly recommended (Table 1). Responders who recommended such beverages frequently or sometimes indicated that patients usually presented with acute symptoms including vomiting, diarrhea, and pyrexia. Most respondents reported that they cautioned against excessive consumption (Table 2). Sixteen respondents (7%) reported that they were very familiar with the fact that health could be compromised by excessive consumption, and 96 (45%) replied that they were familiar to some extent with the potential problem (Table 1). Of the recommended beverages, the favorite brand for both specialists and non-specialists was Brand A. Brand B was recommended more frequently by specialists, while brand C was recommended more frequently by non-specialists (Table 1). We found no significant difference in the other variables between specialists and non-specialists (Table 1).

Of all respondents, 75 (35%) had been consulted on excessive consumption of ionic beverages (Table 1). Among them, non-specialists recommended beverages to patients with pyrexia more often than did specialists. We found no difference in terms of the frequency of cautioning against excessive consumption between specialists and non-specialists (Table 2).

Discussion

We explored the attitudes of practicing members of the Japanese Pediatric Society toward consumption of ionic beverages by children. It became clear that most participants of this study have appropriate attitude towards ionic beverages among children. Approximately 60% of respondents stated that they recommended ionic beverages often or sometimes. The beverages most often recommended were those developed for oral rehydration (Brands A and B). Brands C and E, which are less suitable in this respect, were recommended infrequently (about 15% of the time). A 2008 survey of members of the Society of Ambulatory and General Pediatrics of Japan found that approximately 20% of respondents recommended inappropriate beverages such as Brands C and E [13]. In the present survey, the incidence of inappropriate recommendations was less.

Commonly, ionic beverages were recommended to treat acute symptoms including vomiting, diarrhea, and pyrexia. Cautions against excessive consumption were given by about half of the respondents who recommended ionic beverages either often or sometimes. Therefore, a simple recommendation that an ionic beverage should be consumed is unlikely to trigger excessive consumption. However, about 40% of respondents had been consulted by patients about excessive consumption, suggesting that such consumption is not unusual. About 60% of the participants were familiar with the health problems attributable to excessive consumption; the extent of awareness thus seems to be adequate. A large majority of respondents prescribed ionic beverages in a responsible manner.

We found that specialists recommended appropriate ionic beverages more often than did non-specialists. In

Table 2 Situation where the participants recommend ionic beverages and caution for excessive consumption

	Participants who recommend ionic beverages frequently or sometimes			
	All $N = 125$	Pediatric specialists $N = 107$	Non-specialists $N = 16$	
Q5. Situation where the participants recommend ionic beverages				
Vomiting and/or diarrhea	122 (98%)	104 (97%)	16 (100%)	NS
Pyrexia	39 (31%)	30 (28%)	9 (56%)	P < 0.05
After bath	1 (1%)	1 (1%)	0	N/A
Hot weather	5 (4%)	3 (3%)	2 (13%)	N/A
After sweating	6 (5%)	5 (5%)	1 (6%)	N/A
Failure to thrive	0	0	0	N/A
Others	9 (7%)	9 (8%)	0	N/A
Q6. Caution for excessive consumption of ionic beverages				
Always	38 (30%)	31 (29%)	6 (38%)	NS
Sometimes	26 (21%)	25 (23%)	1 (6%)	
Infrequently	25 (20%)	22 (21%)	3 (19%)	
Rarely	22 (18%)	17 (16%)	5 (31%)	
Never	14 (11%)	12 (11%)	1 (6%)	

NS: not significant, N/A: not assessed

contrast, non-specialists recommended ionic beverages to patients with pyrexia more often than did specialists, suggesting that specialists recommended more appropriate beverages than did non-specialists and were more sensitive to the possibility of over-consumption.

It remains unclear whether doctor recommendations influence the consumption of ionic beverages. A survey of sports drinks consumption in nursery school children found that doctors' advice triggered such consumption in 65% of children, suggesting that the influence of doctors' recommendations was strong [14]. In a study on how excessive soft drink consumption could be curbed, parents replied that they would reduce consumption if a doctor so recommended [15]. Although the cited work was performed in an effort to control caloric intake and the purpose thus differed from that of the present study, the cited work showed that doctors' advice may alter the children's consumption behaviors. Kawashita et al. found that most parents of 3-year-old children who consumed sports drinks stated that pediatricians had recommended the drinks; however, the consumption levels of these children were significantly lower than those of children whose parents had not received such recommendations [16]. Annual ionic beverage sales are increasing in Japan, and children are targeted in some promotions. The effects of ionic beverages on children, especially infants and young children, needs to be better understood. Appropriate advice by pediatricians is important in this context.

There are several limitations to our study. First, both the number of subjects approached and the questionnaire response rate were inadequate. It would be unwise to seek to apply our results to all populations of pediatricians. It is important to survey more pediatricians and increase the response rate. In particular, the proportion of non-specialist respondents in the present study was low. Thus, the power of our statistical analyses may be inadequate. We targeted members of the Japanese Pediatrics Society. However, presently, many doctors who treat children are not members of the Society. Those doctors must also be surveyed to more accurately evaluate children's consumption of ionic beverages.

Conclusions

The attitudes of pediatricians toward children's consumption of ionic beverages were generally appropriate. The attitudes of pediatric specialists were more appropriate than those of non-specialists. To prevent excessive consumption, it is important that pediatric specialists impart correct information. Academic societies must encourage pediatricians to understand circumstances under which ionic beverages are required and the potential risks involved.

Abbreviations

VB1D: Vitamin B1 deficiency

Acknowledgements

The members of The Committee on Pediatric Nutrition of The Japanese Pediatric Society were as follows; Shinobu Ida (chairperson), Setsuko Ito, Mikako Inokuchi, Toshihiro Ohura, Akihisa Okumura, Mitsuyoshi Suzuki, Kimitaka Takitani, Kazushige Dobashi, Mitsuhiko Hara, Toru Kikuchi, Shigetaka Sugihara, Nobuo Yoshiike, Tomoo Okadan, Kazunari Kaneko, Chiharu Tsutsumi, Yuriko Ohta, Keiichi Hanaki, Kazue Kawakami, Yoshio Hanawa, Hiroaki Inomata, Tatsuya Oguni, Atsuyuki Yamataka, Yuko Bito, Keiichi Uchida, Hiroko Kodama, Masaaki Mori, and Toshiaki Shimizu. We deeply thank all participants of this study. This study was supported by the Japanese Pediatric Society.

Funding

This research received no specific grant from any funding agency in the public, commercial, or not-for-profit sectors.

Authors' contributions

AO conceptualized and designed the study, drafted the initial manuscript, and approved the final manuscript as submitted. SI and MM collected data and performed the initial analyses, reviewed and revised the manuscript, and approved the final manuscript as submitted. TS coordinated and supervised the data collection process, critically reviewed the manuscript, and approved the final manuscript as submitted. This study was conducted by the Committee on Pediatric Nutrition of The Japanese Pediatric Society.

Competing interests

Masaaki Mori has received lecture fees from MSD K.K and Accvie LLC, and consulting fees from Daiichi Sankyo Co., Ltd. and Taisho Pharmaceutical Co., Ltd. For the remaining authors, none is declared.

Author details

[1]Department of Pediatrics, Aichi Medical University, Nagakute, Japan. [2]Department of Pediatrics, Juntendo University Faculty of Medicine, Tokyo, Japan. [3]Department of Pediatric Gastroenterology and Endocrinology, Osaka Medical Center and Research Institute for Maternal and Child Health, Osaka, Japan. [4]Department of Lifetime Clinical Immunology, Graduate School of Medical and Dental Sciences, Tokyo Medical and Dental University, Tokyo, Japan.

References

1. Okumura A, Ida S, Mori M, Shimizu T. Committee on Pediatric Nutrition of the Child Health Consortium of Japan. Vitamin B1 Deficiency Related to Excessive Soft Drink Consumption in Japan. J Pediatr Gastroenterol Nutr. 2018;66:838–42.
2. Hiraki A, Kikuchi M. Wernicke's encephalopathy due to excessive intake of isotonic drink; report of 2 cases. No To Hattatsu. 2014;46:34–8. [in Japanese]
3. Saeki K, Saito Y, Komaki H, Sakakibra T, Nakagawa E, Sugai K, et al. Thiamine-deficient encephalopathy due to excessive intake of isotonic drink or overstrict diet therapy in Japanese children. Brain and Development. 2010; 32:556–63.
4. Shioda T, Watanabe, Kyogoku T, Kato H, Okumura Y, Aida HA. Case of pediatric Wernicke's encephalopathy due to excesive intake of isotonic drinks. The Journal of the Japan Pediatric Society. 2014;118:930–6. [in Japanese]
5. Kataoka H, Arakaki Y, Waki K, Hayashi T, Ogino K, Hananoka Y, et al. Beriberi presenting reversible severe pulmonary hypertension by excessive intake of isotonic drink. The Journal of the Japan Pediatric Society. 2012;116:1228–32. [in Japanese]
6. Fujii T, Hojo A, Nakamura T, Iwasaki J, Takayanagi T, Uemura S, et al. Rapid improvement of echocardiographic and electrocardiographic findings in a

1-year-old patient with beriberi heart. The Journal of the Japan Pediatric Society. 2012;116:84–91. [in Japanese]
7. Takemoto M, Hanai T, Kamata A, Gondo K. A 20-momth-old infant with beriberi caused by excessive intake of isotonic drink. The Journal of the Japan Pediatric Society. 2008;112:1710–2. [in Japanese]
8. Fujita I, Sata T, Gondo K, Fukazawa M, Kukita J, Zaitsu A, et al. Cardiac beriberi (shoshin beriberi) caused by excessive intake of isotonic drink. Acta Paediatr Jpn. 1992;34:466–8.
9. Spandorfer PR, Alessandrini EA, Joffe MD, Localio R, Shaw KN. Oral versus intravenous rehydration of moderately dehydrated children: a randomized. controlled trial Pediatrics. 2005;115:295–301.
10. Hartling L, Bellemare S, Wiebe N, Russell K, Klassen TP, Craig W. Oral versus intravenous rehydration for treating dehydration due to gastroenteritis in children. Cochrane Database Syst Rev. 2006:CD004390.
11. Ohtsuka Y, Ohtomo Y, Niijima S, Arii N, Obinata K, Kubagawa T, et al. Oral rehydration solution (ORS) therapy for infants with mild dehydration due to viral gastroenteritis. Japanese Journal of Pediatrics. 2007;60:2035–41. [in Japanese]
12. Kiyomasu T, Oh S, Abe J, Fujiwara H, Uenishi T, Hanamoto N, et al. A questionnaire-based survey of OS-1. Japanese Journal of Pediatrics. 2007;60: 2043–6. [in Japanese]
13. Furukawa Y, Igarashi M, Ito J, Kaji H, Shida K, Takaragi S, et al. Survey of pediatrician treatment of acute gastro-enteritis in infants. Gairai Shounika. 2008;11:126–34. in Japanese
14. Nagatani N, Hata Y, Tateno H, Ide M, Sasaki M, Nishimura Y, et al. A survey of sports drink intake among children at a nursery school in Sapporo and the opinions of mothers: comparison of the results from 2001 and 2010. Kanagawa Shigaku. 2011;46:183–92. [in Japanese]
15. Rader RK, Mullen KB, Sterkel R, Strunk RC, Garbutt JM. Opportunities to reduce children's excessive consumption of calories from beverages. Clin Pediatr. 2014;53:1047–54.
16. Kawashita Y, Fukuda H, Kawasaki K, Kitamura M, Hayashida H, Furugen R, et al. Pediatrician-recommended use of sports drinks and dental caries in 3-year-old children. Community Dent Health. 2011;28:29–33.

28

Clinical features and outcomes of invasive pneumococcal disease in a pediatric intensive care unit

Hsiang-Ju Hsiao[1,2], Chang-Teng Wu[2,3], Jing-Long Huang[2,4], Cheng-Hsun Chiu[2,5], Yhu-Chering Huang[2,6], Jainn-Jim Lin[2,7], I-Anne Huang[1,2], Oi-Wa Chan[2,7], I-Jun Chou[2,3] and Shao-Hsuan Hsia[2,7*]

Abstract

Background: Invasive pneumococcal disease (IPD) results in high morbidity and mortality globally each year, although it is a vaccine-preventable disease. This study aimed to characterize the clinical features of IPD in a pediatric intensive care unit (PICU) in Taiwan. The seven-valent pneumococcal conjugate vaccine (PCV7) was introduced in the private sector in October 2005. The estimated coverage rate of PCV7 vaccination in 2010 was 45.5 % among children <5 years of age.

Methods: We conducted a retrospective study at a single center in northern Taiwan for invasive pneumococcal disease in a PICU from 2009 to 2013. Demographic characteristics, clinical courses, serotype, antibiotic susceptibility, and outcomes were analyzed.

Results: Over the 5-year study period, 2167 patients were admitted to the PICU; 48 (2.2 %) had IPD. There were 29 female and 19 male patients. Their mean age was 3.7 years (range 0.7–12.5 years, with the peak age at 2–5 years; $n = 30$, 63 %). Pneumonia was the most frequent type ($n = 38$, 79 %), followed by meningitis ($n = 10$, 21 %). In total, three patients died, all within 72 h after admission; the final diagnoses were all meningitis. Thirty-four children with pneumonia received chest tube insertion for pleural effusion drainage. Of them, 22 (65 %) finally still underwent video-assisted thoracoscopic surgery. Eight (17 %) children had hemolytic uremic syndrome, and seven of them underwent hemodialysis. In total, 37 serotypes were detected; 95 % were covered by PCV13. Serotype 19A was most common (54 %) overall; however, in those with meningitis, serotype 19 F was most common.

Conclusions: Meningitis is the most severe type of invasive pneumococcal disease in our pediatric intensive care unit. It may progress rapidly even when subjects are given antibiotics promptly. The most common serotype in meningitis is 19 F, which is vaccine preventable. Thus, universal mass pneumococcal vaccination is still needed.

Keywords: Hemolytic uremic syndrome (HUS), herd immunity, invasive pneumococcal disease, mortality, pediatric intensive care unit, pneumococcal conjugate vaccine, serotype 19 F, *Streptococcus pneumoniae*

Background

Streptococcus pneumoniae is a Gram-positive encapsulated bacterium. It can cause a wide disease spectrum, from otitis media to sepsis and meningitis [1]. Invasive pneumococcal disease (IPD) is defined as *S. pneumoniae* isolated from sterile sites, such as blood, cerebrospinal fluid, pleural fluid, or ascites. IPD results in high global morbidity and mortality each year [2], but it is a vaccine-preventable disease [3–5]. Its incidence decreased after the introduction of a seven-valent pneumococcal conjugate vaccine (PCV7) in the private sector in Taiwan in October 2005 [6, 7]. The estimated coverage rate of PCV7 vaccination was 5.7 % in 2006 and 45.5 % in 2010 among children <5 years of age. PCV13 was introduced in April 2010, and in 2013, a national catch-up program was launched in Taiwan to provide government-funded PCV13 for all children aged 2–5 years [7].

* Correspondence: shsia@cgmh.org.tw
[2]Chang Gung University College of Medicine, Taoyuan, Taiwan
[7]Division of Pediatric Critical Care Medicine, Department of Pediatrics, Chang Gung Memorial Hospital, Linkou, Taiwan
Full list of author information is available at the end of the article

The symptoms and signs of IPD are related to host immunity, *S. pneumoniae* virulence, and the site of infection [1]. Early recognition and prompt diagnosis remain challenges. There have been few studies analyzing the early clinical presentation in severe IPD in children since the introduction of PCV7 in Taiwan. We designed this study to characterize the clinical features and outcomes of IPD in a pediatric intensive care unit (PICU) under partial PCV immunization.

Methods

Hospital setting

Chang Gung Memorial Hospital is a tertiary care hospital in northern Taiwan. Chang Gung Memorial Hospital is the only referral center in Taoyuan County, which has a population of 2 million people. The PICU is a 29-bed ICU serving children over 2 months of age. We reviewed the Chang Gung Memorial Hospital PICU patient database, which listed the name and diagnosis of every patient admitted to the PICU between January 2009 and December 2013. The study was approved by the institution review board (IRB: 100-2984A3).

Clinical features

All children admitted to the PICU of Chang Gung Memorial Hospital with isolation of *S. pneumoniae* from sterile sites (blood, pleural fluid, and cerebrospinal fluid) were included. We collected data including demographics, underlying conditions or illnesses, previous hospitalizations, laboratory data, empiric and definite antimicrobial agents, requirements for and duration of intensive care, surgical intervention, final diagnosis, and outcome.

Pneumonia was defined as the presence of 1) radiological pneumonia plus positive blood culture, 2) *S. pneumoniae* isolates from pleural fluid culture, or 3) positive blood culture plus placement of chest tube for pleural fluid drainage. We defined meningitis as the presence of *Streptococcus pneumoniae* in cerebrospinal fluid or blood in association with a clinical diagnosis of meningitis [8].

The Glasgow Outcome Scale–Extended Pediatric Revision (GOS-E Peds) [9] was used for the assessment of outcome at 3 months after discharge. The GOS-E Peds uses the following eight-point scale: 1. upper good recovery, 2. lower good recovery, 3. upper moderate disability, 4. lower moderate disability, 5. upper severe disability, 6. lower severe disability, 7. vegetative state, and 8. death.

Serotyping of *S. pneumoniae*

Detection of *S. pneumoniae* was first done in the Chang Gung Memorial or other hospital. Since October 2007, IPD has been listed as a notifiable disease in Taiwan [6]. It is mandatory to report IPD cases and for infection control personnel to deliver the isolated *S. pneumoniae* to the Centers for Disease Control, Taiwan (TCDC). Upon receipt, *S. pneumoniae* isolates were subcultured immediately and confirmed by standard microbiological methods, followed by serotyping using the capsular swelling method (Quellung reaction) [6]. The final report was faxed to Chang Gung Memorial Hospital.

Statistical analysis

For analysis of serotype distribution, serotypes were categorized as PCV7 types (4, 6B, 9 V, 14, 18C, 19 F, and 23 F); PCV13 serotypes not included in PCV7 (1, 3, 5, 6A, 7 F, and 19A); and non-vaccine serotypes. Data analysis was performed using the SPSS software (ver. 21.0; SPSS, Chicago, IL). Categorical variables were compared using Fisher's exact test. Descriptive statistics for continuous variables, such as laboratory parameters, were calculated and are reported as the means ± standard deviation (SD). The Mann–Whitney U-test was used to detect continuous variables differences between two groups. Statistical significance was set at $p < 0.05$.

Results

Epidemiology

Over the 5 years study period, 2167 patients were admitted to the PICU; of them, 48 (2.2 %) had IPD (Table 1). There were 29 female and 19 male patients; their mean age was 3.7 years (range, 0.7–12.5 years, with a peak in age 2–5 years ($n = 30$, 63 %). Pneumonia was the most frequent type ($n = 38$, 79 %), followed by meningitis ($n = 10$, 21 %). The mean PICU stay was 11.2 ± 11.9 days; the mean length of hospital stay was 21.6 ± 14.0 days. In total, three cases died, all died within 72 h after admission; the final diagnosis in all was meningitis. The case-fatality rate was 6.3 %. Most survived and recovered with no sequelae. However, there were four children with less than good recoveries (Table 2).

Clinical characteristics

In total, 38 (79 %) patients initially presented with respiratory distress/failure, and all had radiological pneumonia; three of them presented initially with GCS ≤12. Another 10 (21 %) patients presented initially with altered mental status without radiological pneumonia and were finally diagnosed with meningitis; eight of them presented initially with GCS ≤12. Three children had no apparent preceding upper respiratory tract infection before admission; one of them died. Also, 12 children had seizures during the illness; 10 were diagnosed as having meningitis, and the other two as having septic shock with encephalopathy.

In total, 16 (33 %) patients needed intubation; six were 'elective' intubations to protect the airway because of altered mental status, and 10 were intubated because of respiratory failure. Also, 34 children with complicated pneumonia received chest tube insertion for pleural

Table 1 Clinical features of IPDs in 48 children admitted to our pediatric intensive care unit

	Survival ($n = 45$)	Death ($n = 3$)	Total ($n = 48$)	p
Males	18	1	19	1.00
Age (years)				0.18
< 2	9	2	11	
2–5	29	1	30	
6–17	7	0	7	
Received vaccination	11	0	11	1.00
Symptoms and signs[1]				
Fever	45	3	48	
Cough and rhinorrhea	43	2	45	0.18
Vomiting without abdominal pain	15	3	18	0.05
Altered mental status	10	3	13	0.02
GCS <12	8	3	11	0.01
Seizure	9	3	12	0.01
Initial laboratory values				
WBC count (1000 cells/mm^3)	14.7 ± 12.6	4.6 ± 2.1	14.1 ± 12.4	0.16
CRP (mg/L)	243 ± 107	178 ± 84	240 ± 107	0.32
Positive blood culture result	26	3	29	0.27
Disease category				0.01
Pneumonia	38	0	38	
Meningitis	7	3	10	
Length of hospital stay	22.9 ± 13.4	1.7 ± 1.2	21.6 ± 14.0	<0.01
in PICU	11.8 ± 12.1	1.7 ± 1.2	11.2 ± 11.9	<0.01

WBC white blood cells; *CRP* C-reactive protein
[1]All symptoms were at the time of presentation, except seizure, which was during the illness

Table 2 Details of pediatric IPD cases with less than good recoveries

Case	Age (years)	Gender	Initial presentation[1]	Clinical diagnosis	Serotype	Vaccinated	Outcome
1	1.1	M	Status epilepticus GCS:E2V2M4	Meningitis	6B	No	Lower severe disability
2	6.2	M	Respiratory failure	Complicated pneumonia HUS	19 A	No	Upper moderate disability
3	0.7	M	Opitoshtonous GCS: E2V3M4	Meningitis	19 A	No	Lower severe disability
4	1.9	F	Altered mental status GCS: E1V1M2	Meningitis	19 F	No	Death
5	1.2	F	Altered mental status GCS: E3V2M4	Meningitis	23 F	No	Death
6	9.4	F	Altered mental status GCS: E2V2M4	Meningitis + brain abscess	Not available	No	Vegetative state
7	4.6	M	Altered mental status GCS: E3V2M6	Meningitis	19 F	No	Death

[1]All patients had cough and rhinorrhea, with the exception of patients 1 and 5
M male; *F* female; *GCS* Glasgow Coma Scale; *HUS* hemolytic uremic syndrome

effusion drainage. Of them, 22 (65 %) ultimately underwent video-assisted thoracoscopic surgery (VATS). Eleven (23 %) patients (four meningitis and seven pneumonia) developed unstable hemodynamic status and had to be given inotropic agents, including dopamine, epinephrine, milrinone, or norepinephrine. One child (Patient 2, Table 2) had complicated pneumonia and developed respiratory failure with mechanical ventilation; this patient received extra-corporeal membrane oxygenation (ECMO) support. Unfortunately, he also had a stroke during his PICU stay, and had a moderate disability at follow-up. Also, eight (17 %) children had HUS; seven of them received hemodialysis. All were in the pneumonia group.

Vaccination status, serotype, and antimicrobial resistance

The vaccination status of all children was known; 37 had not been vaccinated against IPD. A conjugated pneumococcal vaccine had been administered to 11 children prior to IPD; seven children received PCV7 and four received PCV13. In those who received PCV7, two children suffered from serotype 19A, a 4-year-old female who received one dose of PCV7 suffered from serotype 6A, and in four children, the serotypes were unknown. Of those who received PCV13, a 2-year-old female who received one dose of PCV13 suffered from serotype 6B, a 2-year-old male who received one dose of PCV13 suffered from serotype 19A, one child suffered from a non-typeable type, and in one child, the serotype was unknown. In the meningitis group, no patient had received a pneumococcal conjugated vaccine. However, at least 60 % of serotypes of the patients with meningitis were covered by PCV13 (Table 3).

In total, 37 serotypes were detected; 95 % were covered by PCV13 (Table 3). Serotype 19A was most common in our study. In 2009, serotype 14 was isolated in four children and serotype 19A in two children. In 2010 to 2013, only one serotype 14 cases was isolated; however, serotype 19A was isolated in 18 children. In 2012, serotype 15 was identified. In 2013, one non-typeable strain was identified. We further divided the patients into meningitis and pneumonia groups (Table 3); serotype 19 F was most common and was detected only in the meningitis group, and serotype 19A was most common type in pneumonia group. In those with HUS, serotype 14 was isolated in two children, 19A was isolated in three children, 6B was isolated in one child, and the serotype was not available in two children.

All patients were initially prescribed vancomycin plus ceftriaxone. Antimicrobial sensitivity testing was performed in 55 isolates. No resistance was detected against vancomycin. Only one *S. pneumoniae* with penicillin MIC <0.06 μg/mL was detected, and *S. pneumoniae* with penicillin MIC >2 μg/mL was detected in 20 % of all isolates. Three cases of *S. pneumoniae* with ceftriaxone MIC ≤0.05 μg/mL were detected, and *S. pneumoniae* with ceftriaxone MIC ≥2 μg/mL was detected in 16 % of all isolates; two were isolated from CSF.

Table 3 Demographic characteristics, serotype distribution, and outcomes in those with meningitis and pneumonia

	Meningitis $n = 10$	Pneumonia $n = 38$	p
Male	2	17	0.28
Age (years)			0.05
<2	4	7	
2–5	3	27	
6–17	3	4	
Serotype distribution			
PCV7 serotypes			
6B	1	2	
14	0	5	
19 F	3	0	
23 F	1	1	
PCV13 serotypes not included in PCV7			
6A	0	1	
19A	1	19	
3	0	1	
Other	1[1]	1[2]	
Unknown	3	8	
Survival	7	38	0.01

[1] 15,[2]non-typeable

Outcomes

Three patients died in this study; all had meningitis. The prognostic factors for mortality were GCS < 12 ($p = 0.01$), seizure ($p = 0.01$), and vomiting without abdominal pain ($p = 0.05$). All of these three patients had the same characteristics; therefore, the data did not permit the use of logistic regression due to the lack of "complete separation." Gender, headache, white cell counts, C-reactive protein, and vaccination status were not significantly associated with mortality. Children without good recovery (Table 2) were more frequent in children <2 years (4/11, 36 %) than those between 2 and 5 years old (1/30, 3 %) or those 6–17 years (2/7, 33 %; $p = 0.01$).

Discussion

We provide the first detailed description of the severe IPD in a PICU under partial PCV immunization in northern Taiwan. In our study, we examined a series of 48 patients diagnosed with IPD at a tertiary hospital in Taiwan. Patients with IPD had two distinct types of presentation: 79 % (38/48) had complicated/uncomplicated pneumonia, presenting as respiratory distress/failure, and the most common serotype in pneumonia was 19A. The other 21 % (10/48) children had meningitis, presenting as altered mental status. Of them, three children died within 72 h, and 19 F was the most common serotype in meningitis. All three children who died had the same characteristics, namely GCS <12, seizure, and vomiting without abdominal pain.

Pneumonia was the most common type of IPD in our series. Our study, like others [3, 6, 10, 11], highlights the prevalence of serotype 19A after PCV7 was introduced. This may have been the result of vaccine selection. PCV7 was introduced to Taiwan in 2005, and the estimated coverage rate of PCV7 vaccination was 45.5 % in 2010 among children <5 years of age. [7]. For those with pneumonia, all patients showed good recovery except one child who had moderate disability after dialysis and ECMO. This may be the result of advances in critical care medicine over the past decade [12]. Hemolytic uremic syndrome is one of the most common complications of necrotizing pneumonia in Taiwan [13–16]. In our study, seven patients received hemodialysis because of HUS. In North America, 50 % of pneumococcus HUS was associated with serotype 19A after the introduction of PCV 7 [12, 17]; our study showed similar results.

Meningitis was the second most frequent type of IPD in our study; however, all three children who died had meningitis. Among those with meningitis, no *S. pneumoniae* penicillin MIC <0.06 μg/mL was isolated, and 20 % were resistant to Ceftriaxone . Thus, in those with suspected meningitis, empiric antibiotics, such as vancomycin plus a third-generation cephalosporin, are suggested [18]. We prescribed vancomycin plus ceftriaxone initially, yet three children still died within 72 h. Kanegaye et al. reported that 4 h after parental antibiotics, cerebrospinal fluid sterilization of pneumococcus might occur [19]. These findings indicate that the damage caused by *S. pneumoniae* infections may not be stopped by eradicating *S. pneumoniae*.

The three children who died had the same characteristics, namely seizures, GCS <12, and vomiting without abdominal pain; all of these signs indicate increased intracranial pressure (IICP). *S. pneumoniae* not only results in disruption of the blood brain barrier but also in neuronal and vascular injury, finally leading to IICP and diffuse brain ischemia [20, 21]. Early antibiotic use is essential; aggressive control of IICP is also important. Adjunctive therapy is an important issue for pneumococcal meningitis [22], patients with meningitis due to *S. pneumoniae* who were treated with corticosteroids had a lower death rate [23].

Serotype 19 F was the most common type in the meningitis group in our study. In adults, serotype 19 F has been associated with an elevated risk of meningitis and death [24]. Hsu et al. reported the effects of a pneumococcal conjugate vaccine on pneumococcal meningitis; it showed that serotypes 9 V, 14, and 23 F had better herd immunity than serotypes 4, 6B, 18C, and 19 F [3]. Wei et al. also reported that for all serotypes included in PCV, except serotype 19 F, demonstrated a sustained decreasing trend between 2008 and 2014 in Taiwan [7]. In our study, at least 60 % of the meningitis serotypes were vaccine-preventable. None of the children had an underlying illness; other studies have also shown that most children with IPD were previously healthy [7]. Thus, universal mass pneumococcal vaccination is still needed.

Being aged less than 2 years was not a predictor of mortality, but it may predict those who will not have a good recovery [10]. In 2013, a national catch-up program was launched in Taiwan to provide government-funded PCV13 for children aged 2-5 years [7]. In 2014, the Taiwanese government expanded the age group of children to 1 year of age. In Taiwan, the prevalence of *S. pneumoniae* colonization in children was 14.1 %. By breaking the chain of disease transmission and reducing the nasopharyngeal carriage rate among children, this policy may help to protect children less than 1 year old.

This study had some limitations. First, this was a retrospective, single-center study, and the sample size was limited. Additionally, the three patients who died had the same characteristics, so our data could not support logistic regression analysis due to the absence of "complete separation". Second, some patients had received antibiotics before admission; these resulted in false-negative culture results, and some true IPD cases were likely not included. Polymerase chain reaction (PCR) would improve diagnostic yield [10]. Third, some *S. pneumoniae* serotypes were not available. Taiwan CDC provides the *S. pneumoniae* serotype only to the first hospital reporting IPD; thus, cooperation between hospitals is needed. Fourth, host immunity is an important factor for IPD; in Taiwan, the rate of asymptomatic carriage of *S. pneumoniae* in children aged 2–5 years was 19 % [25], and the incidence of IPD among children aged 2–4 years was 21.1 per 100,000 populations, strongly suggesting that host immunity plays a key role. Gaschignard et al. suggested that children with IPD, particularly those aged >2 years, should undergo immunological investigation [26]. We have been performing immunological investigations since 2012, and we will report those results in future.

Conclusions

Our study showed a wide spectrum of invasive pneumococcal disease in our pediatric intensive care unit. Meningitis is the most severe type. Meningitis can progress rapidly even when subjects are given antibiotics promptly. The most common serotype in meningitis was 19 F, which is vaccine preventable. Thus, universal mass pneumococcal vaccination is still needed. We observed replacement of pneumococcal serotypes, specifically, the prevalence of serotype 19A. Further study on controlling increased intracranial pressure caused by *S. pneumoniae* meningitis is needed.

Abbreviations

ECMO: extra-corporeal membrane oxygenation; GCS: Glasgow Coma Scale; GOS-E Peds: Glasgow Outcome Scale–Extended Pediatric Revision; HUS: hemolytic uremic syndrome; IICP: increased intracranial pressure; IPD: invasive pneumococcal disease; MIC: minimum inhibitory concentration; PCV: pneumococcal conjugate vaccine; PCV7: seven-valent pneumococcal conjugate vaccine; PCV13: 13-valent pneumococcal conjugate vaccine; PICU: pediatric intensive care unit; VATS: video-assisted thoracoscopic surgery.

Competing interests

The authors declare that they have no competing interests.

Authors' contributions

HJH designed the study, collected the data, and participated in data analysis and in writing the manuscript; CTW participated in data analysis and in writing the manuscript; JLH critically reviewed the study protocol, supervised data collection, and participated in writing the manuscript; CHC designed the study, supervised data collection, and participated in writing the manuscript; YCH reviewed the study protocol, supervised data collection, and participated in writing the manuscript; JJL designed the study, collected the data, and participated in data analysis and in writing the manuscript; IAH collected the data and participated in data analysis; OWC participated in data analysis; IJC participated in data analysis; SHH designed the study, supervised data collection, and participated in writing the manuscript. All authors have read and approved the final manuscript.

Acknowledgements

This work was supported by grants from Chang Gung Memorial Hospital (CMRPG3 B0841, CMRPG3 B0842, CMPRG3 B0843). We thank Dr. Chuen-Sheue Chiang, Taiwan Centers for Disease Control, for helpful comments on the study. The English in this document has been checked by at least two professional editors, both native speakers of English. For a certificate, please see: http://www.textcheck.com/certificate/5W22WI

Author details

[1]Department of Pediatrics, Chang Gung Memorial Hospital, Keelung, Taiwan. [2]Chang Gung University College of Medicine, Taoyuan, Taiwan. [3]Division of General Pediatrics, Department of Pediatrics, Chang Gung Memorial Hospital, Linkou, Taiwan. [4]Division of Asthma, Allergy, and Rheumatology, Department of Pediatrics, Chang Gung Memorial Hospital, Linkou, Taiwan. [5]Molecular Infectious Disease Research Center, Division of Pediatric Infection, Chang Gung Memorial Hospital, Linkou, Taiwan. [6]Division of Pediatric Infectious Diseases, Department of Pediatrics, Chang Gung Memorial Hospital, Linkou, Taiwan. [7]Division of Pediatric Critical Care Medicine, Department of Pediatrics, Chang Gung Memorial Hospital, Linkou, Taiwan.

References

1. Hsieh YC, Lee WS, Shao PL, Chang LY, Huang LM. Transforming *Streptococcus pneumoniae* in the 21st century. Chang Gung Med J. 2008;31(2):117–24.
2. O'Brien KL, Wolfson LJ, Watt JP, Henkle E, Deloria-Knoll M, McCall N, et al. Burden of disease caused by *Streptococcus pneumoniae* in children younger than 5 years: global estimates. Lancet. 2009;374(9693):893–902.
3. Hsu HE, Shutt KA, Moore MR, Beall BW, Bennett NM, Craig AS, et al. Effect of pneumococcal conjugate vaccine on pneumococcal meningitis. N Engl J Med. 2009;360(3):244–56.
4. Hampton LM, Zell ER, Schrag S, Cohen AL. Sentinel versus population-based surveillance of pneumococcal conjugate vaccine effectiveness. Bull World Health Organ. 2012;90(8):568–77.
5. Leal J, Vanderkooi OG, Church DL, Macdonald J, Tyrrell GJ, Kellner JD. Eradication of invasive pneumococcal disease due to the seven-valent pneumococcal conjugate vaccine serotypes in Calgary. Alberta Pediatr Infect Dis J. 2012;31(9):e169–175.
6. Chiang CS, Chen YY, Jiang SF, Liu DP, Kao PH, Teng HJ, et al. National surveillance of invasive pneumococcal diseases in Taiwan, 2008–2012: differential temporal emergence of serotype 19A. Vaccine. 2014;32(27):3345–9.
7. Wei SH, Chiang CS, Chiu CH, Chou P, Lin TY. Pediatric invasive pneumococcal disease in Taiwan following a national catch-up program with the 13-valent pneumococcal conjugate vaccine. Pediatr Infect Dis J. 2015;34(3):e71–77.
8. Thigpen MC, Whitney CG, Messonnier NE, Zell ER, Lynfield R, Hadler JL, et al. Bacterial meningitis in the United States, 1998–2007. N Engl J Med. 2011;364(21):2016–25.
9. Beers SR, Wisniewski SR, Garcia-Filion P, Tian Y, Hahner T, Berger RP, et al. Validity of a pediatric version of the Glasgow outcome scale-extended. J Neurotrauma. 2012;29(6):1126–39.
10. Paulke-Korinek M, Kollaritsch H, Kundi M, Schmidle-Loss B, Zwazl I, Laaber B, et al. Characteristics of invasive pneumococcal disease in hospitalized children in Austria. Eur J Pediatr. 2014;173(4):469–76.
11. Shen CF, Wang SM, Lee KH, Ho TS, Liu CC. Childhood invasive pneumococcal disease caused by non-7-valent pneumococcal vaccine (PCV7) serotypes under partial immunization in Taiwan. J Formos Med Assoc. 2013;112(9):561–8.
12. Copelovitch L, Kaplan BS. *Streptococcus pneumoniae*-associated hemolytic uremic syndrome: classification and the emergence of serotype 19A. Pediatrics. 2010;125(1):e174–182.
13. Huang YH, Lin TY, Wong KS, Huang YC, Chiu CH, Lai SH, et al. Hemolytic uremic syndrome associated with pneumococcal pneumonia in Taiwan. Eur J Pediatr. 2006;165(5):332–5.
14. Chen SY, Wu CY, Tsai IJ, Tsau YK, Su YT. Nonenteropathic hemolytic uremic syndrome: the experience of a medical center. Pediatr Neonatol. 2011;52(2):73–7.
15. Lee CS, Chen MJ, Chiou YH, Shen CF, Wu CY, Chiou YY. Invasive pneumococcal pneumonia is the major cause of paediatric haemolytic-uraemic syndrome in Taiwan. Nephrology (Carlton). 2012;17(1):48–52.
16. Janapatla RP, Hsu MH, Hsieh YC, Lee HY, Lin TY, Chiu CH. Necrotizing pneumonia caused by nanC-carrying serotypes is associated with pneumococcal haemolytic uraemic syndrome in children. Clin Microbiol Infect. 2013;19(5):480–6.
17. Banerjee R, Hersh AL, Newland J, Beekmann SE, Polgreen PM, Bender J, et al. *Streptococcus pneumoniae*-associated hemolytic uremic syndrome among children in North America. Pediatr Infect Dis J. 2011;30(9):736–9.
18. van de Beek D, Brouwer MC, Thwaites GE, Tunkel AR. Advances in treatment of bacterial meningitis. Lancet. 2012;380(9854):1693–702.
19. Kanegaye JT, Soliemanzadeh P, Bradley JS. Lumbar puncture in pediatric bacterial meningitis: defining the time interval for recovery of cerebrospinal fluid pathogens after parenteral antibiotic pretreatment. Pediatrics. 2001;108(5):1169–74.
20. Radetsky M. Fulminant bacterial meningitis. Pediatr Infect Dis J. 2014;33(2):204–7.
21. Kastenbauer S, Pfister HW. Pneumococcal meningitis in adults: spectrum of complications and prognostic factors in a series of 87 cases. Brain. 2003;126(5):1015–25.
22. Mook-Kanamori BB, Geldhoff M, van der Poll T, van de Beek D. Pathogenesis and pathophysiology of pneumococcal meningitis. Clin Microbiol Rev. 2011;24(3):557–91.
23. Brouwer MC, McIntyre P, Prasad K, van de Beek D. Corticosteroids for acute bacterial meningitis. Cochrane Database Syst Rev. 2013;6:CD004405.
24. Grabenstein JD, Musey LK. Differences in serious clinical outcomes of infection caused by specific pneumococcal serotypes among adults. Vaccine. 2014;32(21):2399–405.
25. Kuo CY, Hwang KP, Hsieh YC, Cheng CH, Huang FL, Shen YH, et al. Nasopharyngeal carriage of *Streptococcus pneumoniae* in Taiwan before and after the introduction of a conjugate vaccine. Vaccine. 2011;29(32):5171–7.
26. Gaschignard J, Levy C, Chrabieh M, Boisson B, Bost-Bru C, Dauger S, et al. Invasive pneumococcal disease in children can reveal a primary immunodeficiency. Clin Infect Dis. 2014;59(2):244–51.

Permissions

All chapters in this book were first published in PEDIATRICS, by BioMed Central; hereby published with permission under the Creative Commons Attribution License or equivalent. Every chapter published in this book has been scrutinized by our experts. Their significance has been extensively debated. The topics covered herein carry significant findings which will fuel the growth of the discipline. They may even be implemented as practical applications or may be referred to as a beginning point for another development.

The contributors of this book come from diverse backgrounds, making this book a truly international effort. This book will bring forth new frontiers with its revolutionizing research information and detailed analysis of the nascent developments around the world.

We would like to thank all the contributing authors for lending their expertise to make the book truly unique. They have played a crucial role in the development of this book. Without their invaluable contributions this book wouldn't have been possible. They have made vital efforts to compile up to date information on the varied aspects of this subject to make this book a valuable addition to the collection of many professionals and students.

This book was conceptualized with the vision of imparting up-to-date information and advanced data in this field. To ensure the same, a matchless editorial board was set up. Every individual on the board went through rigorous rounds of assessment to prove their worth. After which they invested a large part of their time researching and compiling the most relevant data for our readers.

The editorial board has been involved in producing this book since its inception. They have spent rigorous hours researching and exploring the diverse topics which have resulted in the successful publishing of this book. They have passed on their knowledge of decades through this book. To expedite this challenging task, the publisher supported the team at every step. A small team of assistant editors was also appointed to further simplify the editing procedure and attain best results for the readers.

Apart from the editorial board, the designing team has also invested a significant amount of their time in understanding the subject and creating the most relevant covers. They scrutinized every image to scout for the most suitable representation of the subject and create an appropriate cover for the book.

The publishing team has been an ardent support to the editorial, designing and production team. Their endless efforts to recruit the best for this project, has resulted in the accomplishment of this book. They are a veteran in the field of academics and their pool of knowledge is as vast as their experience in printing. Their expertise and guidance has proved useful at every step. Their uncompromising quality standards have made this book an exceptional effort. Their encouragement from time to time has been an inspiration for everyone.

The publisher and the editorial board hope that this book will prove to be a valuable piece of knowledge for researchers, students, practitioners and scholars across the globe.

List of Contributors

Elizabeth Fitzgerald
Assistant Professor of Pediatrics, University of North Carolina at Chapel Hill, Chapel Hill, USA

Rachel Mlotha-Mitole
University of Malawi College of Medicine, Blantyre, Malawi

Emily J. Ciccone and Alyssa E. Tilly
University of North Carolina at Chapel Hill, Chapel Hill, USA

Jennie M. Montijo
Hawaii Permanente Medical Group, Maui, Hawaii, USA

Hans-Joerg Lang
Médecins sans Frontières - Belgium, Paediatric Referent, Brussels, Belgium

Michelle Eckerle
Assistant Professor of Pediatrics, Cincinnati Children's Hospital Medical Center, Cincinnati, Ohio, USA

Cécile Delecroix and Raja Brauner
Fondation Ophtalmologique Adolphe de Rothschild and Université Paris Descartes, Paris, France

Jean-Claude Souberbielle
Assistance Publique-Hôpitaux de Paris, Hôpital Necker-Enfants Malades, Service d'Explorations Fonctionnelles, Paris, France

Scheilla Bayitondere, Eric Ngabireyimana, Fulgence Nkikabahizi and Evelyne Shema
Ministry of Health, Rwinkwavu District Hospital, Rwinkwavu, Rwanda

Francois Biziyaremye, Catherine M. Kirk, Christine Mutaganzwa and David B. Tugizimana
Partners In Health/Inshuti Mu Buzima, Rwinkwavu, Rwanda

Hema Magge
Boston Children's Hospital, Boston, MA, USA

Kim Wilson
Brigham and Women's Hospital, Boston, MA, USA

Katrina Hann
Partners In Health Sierra Leone, Freetown, Sierra Leone

Ann C. Miller
Harvard Medical School, Boston, MA, USA

Rabha Elmesmari
School of Medicine, College of Medical, Veterinary, and Life Sciences, University of Glasgow, Glasgow G12 8 QQ, UK

Anne Martin
MRC/CSO Social and Public Health Sciences Unit University of Glasgow, Glasgow G12 8 QQ, UK

John J. Reilly
Physical Activity for Health Group, University of Strathclyde, George Street, Glasgow G1 1XQ, UK

Rabha Elmesmari
Al-Fatah Hospital, Medical School, Benghazi University, Benghazi, Libya

James Y. Paton
Office Block, Ground Floor, Zone 1 (Paediatrics) Royal Hospital for Children, 1345 Govan Road, Glasgow G51 4TF, UK

Nadine Kacenelenbogen, M. Schetgen and M. Roland
Université Libre de Bruxelles, General Medicine Department, Campus Facultaire Erasme, Route de Lennik 808/612, 1070 Brussels, Belgium

Michèle Dramaix-Wilmet
Université Libre de Bruxelles, Centre for Research in Epidemiology, Biostatistics and Clinical Research, School of Public Health, Campus Erasme CP598, Route de Lennik 808, 1070 Brussels, Belgium

Isabelle Godin
Université Libre de Bruxelles, Department of Health Information Promotion Education (SIPES), School of Public Health, Campus Erasme CP598, Route de Lennik 808, 1070 Brussels, Belgium

Katherine J. Deans, Peter C. Minneci, Karen Leonhart, Jennifer N. Cooper and Kelly J. Kelleher
The Research Institute at Nationwide Children's Hospital, 700 Children's Drive, FB3145, Columbus, OH 43205, USA

Kristine M. Nacion
National Quality Forum, 1030 15th Street NW, Suite 800, Washington, DC 20005, USA

Sarah Hudson Scholle
National Committee for Quality Assurance, 1100 13th St, NW, Suite 1000, Washington, DC 20005, USA

Taina Mustila
Seinäjoki Central Hospital, Hanneksenrinne 7, 60220 Seinäjoki, Finland

Jani Raitanen
UKK Institute for Health Promotion, Tampere, Finland

Riitta Luoto
Faculty of Social Sciences, University of Tampere, Tampere, Finland

Päivi Keskinen
Pediatric Research Centre, 33014 University of Tampere, Tampere, Finland
Tampere University Hospital, 33521 Tampere, Finland

Dong Keon Yon
Department of Pediatrics, CHA Bundang Medical Center, CHA University School of Medicine, Seongnam, Republic of Korea

Tae Keun Ahn and Dong Eun Shin
Department of Orthopedic Surgery, CHA Bundang Medical Center, CHA University School of Medicine, Seongnam, Republic of Korea

Gwang Il Kim
Department of Pathology, CHA Bundang Medical Center, CHA University School of Medicine, Seongnam, Republic of Korea

Moon Kyu Kim
Department of Pediatrics, Severance Hospital, Yonsei University College of Medicine, Seoul, Republic of Korea

Ana Paula Vanz, Bruna Pinheiro, Marina Zambrano, Evelise Brizola and Têmis Maria Félix
Child and Adolescent Health, Universidade Federal do Rio Grande do Sul, Porto Alegre, Brazil

Juliana van de Sande Lee and Maria Marlene de Souza Pires
Division of Pediatric Endocrinology, Hospital Infantil Joana de Gusmão, Florianópolis, Brazil
Medical Sciences, Universidade Federal de Santa Catarina, Florianópolis, Brazil

Neusa Sicca da Rocha
Medical Sciences: Psychiatry, Universidade Federal do Rio Grande do Sul, Porto Alegre, Brazil

Ida Vanessa D. Schwartz
Medical Sciences, Universidade Federal do Rio Grande do Sul, Porto Alegre, Brazil
Department of Genetics, Universidade Federal do Rio Grande do Sul, Porto Alegre, Brazil
Health Technology Assessment in Clinical Genetics Research Group, Hospital de Clínicas de Porto Alegre, Porto Alegre, Brazil Medical Genetics Service, Hospital de Clinicas de Porto Alegre, Porto Alegre, Brazil

Silvia Seibt
Paediatrics, Taranaki Base Hospital, New Plymouth, New Zealand

Catherine A. Gilchrist, Emma J. Best and Cameron
Department of Paediatrics: Child and Youth Health, Faculty of Medical and Health Sciences, University of Auckland, Private Bag 92019, Wellesley Street, Auckland 1142, New Zealand

Peter W. Reed
Children's Research Centre, Starship Children's Hospital, Auckland, New Zealand

Emma J. Best
Infectious Diseases, Starship Children's Hospital, Auckland District Health Board, Auckland, New Zealand

Anthony Harnden
Nuffield Department of Primary Care Health Sciences, University of Oxford, Oxford, England

Carlos A. Camargo Jr
Emergency Medicine, Massachusetts General Hospital, Harvard Medical School, Boston, USA

Cameron C. Grant
General Paediatrics, Starship Children's Hospital, Auckland District Health Board, Auckland, New Zealand

Weifeng Liang and Hong Yan
Department of Epidemiology and Health Statistics, School of Public Health, Xi'an Jiaotong University College of Medicine, No.76 West Yanta Road, Xi'an, Shaanxi 710061, People's Republic of China

Yuan Xing
Xi'an Center for Disease Control and Prevention, Xi'an, Shaanxi 710054, People's Republic of China

Miaomiao Pang
Shaanxi Provincial Corps Hospital of Chinese People's Armed Police Force, Xi'an, Shaanxi 710054, People's Republic of China

Duolao Wang
Department of Clinical Sciences, Liverpool School of Tropical Medicine, Liverpool L3 5QA, UK

J. F. de Groot, N. Damen, L. van de Steeg, L. Koopmans and C. Wagner
NIVEL Netherlands Institute for Health Services Research, Otterstraat 118-124, 3513 CR Utrecht, the Netherlands

E. de Loos
Netherlands Federation of University Medical Centres-Consortium Quality of Care, NIAZ & CBOimpact Dutch Institute for Healthcare Improvement, Utrecht, the Netherlands

P. Rosias
Zuyderland Medical Centre Sittard, Sittard, the Netherlands

M. Bruijn
Noord West Ziekenhuisgroep, Alkmaar, the Netherlands

J. Goorhuis
Medisch Spectrum Twente, 7500 KA Enschede, the Netherlands

C. Wagner
APH Amsterdam Public Health Institute, VU University Medical Centre, Amsterdam, the Netherlands

L. van de Steeg
Ecorys, 3006 AD Rotterdam, the Netherlands

L. Koopmans
TNO Healthy Living, Schipholweg 77-89, 2316 ZL Leiden, the Netherlands

M. Bruijn
Department of Pediatrics, Northwest Clinics, 1800 AM Alkmaar, The Netherlands

Maria G. Koliou
Department of Paediatrics, Archbishop Makarios III Hospital, Nicosia, Cyprus
School of Medicine, University of Cyprus, Nicosia, Cyprus
Cyprus Institute of Biomedical Sciences (CIBS), Nicosia, Cyprus

Elpidoforos S. Soteriades
Cyprus Institute of Biomedical Sciences (CIBS), Nicosia, Cyprus

Kyriaki Andreou
The Hull IVF Unit, Hull, UK

Demetris Lamnisos and Giagkos Lavranos
Department of Health Sciences, School of Sciences, European University Cyprus, Nicosia, Cyprus

Paris Iakovides and Christos Economou
Private practice, Nicosia, Cyprus

Elpidoforos S. Soteriades
Harvard School of Public Health, Department of Environmental Health, Environmental and Occupational Medicine and Epidemiology (EOME), Boston, USA

Yabwile Mulambia and Neil Kennedy
The College of Medicine, University of Malawi, Chichiri, Blantyre 3, Malawi

Aaron J. Miller
Building Regional Alliances to Nurture Child Health, 2 Gold St, New York, NY 10038, USA

Geraldine MacDonald
Institute of Child Care Research, Queen's University, University Rd, Belfast BT7 1NN, UK

Neil Kennedy
Centre for Medical Education, Queens's University Belfast, University Rd, Belfast BT7 1NN, UK

M. Nordvall-Lassen
The Research Unit of Women's and Children's Health, section 7821, The Juliane Marie Centre, Copenhagen University Hospital, Rigshospitalet, Blegdamsvej 9, DK-2100 Copenhagen, Denmark

H. K. Hegaard
Faculty of Health and Medical Sciences, University of Copenhagen, Copenhagen, Denmark
Child, Family and Reproductive Health, Department of Health Science, Faculty of Medicine, Lund University, Lund, Sweden
Obstetric Clinic, The Juliane Marie Centre, Rigshospitalet, Copenhagen University Hospital, Copenhagen, Denmark

M. Hedegaard
Obstetric Clinic, The Juliane Marie Centre, Rigshospitalet, Copenhagen University Hospital, Copenhagen, Denmark

C. Obel
Institute of General Medical Practice, Department of Public Health, Aarhus University, Aarhus, Denmark

M. S. Lindhard and T. B. Henriksen
Perinatal Epidemiology Research Unit, Department of Paediatrics, Aarhus University Hospital, Skejby, Aarhus, Denmark

Qin Zhang, Qi Guo, Ming Gui, Bo Hu, Ling Lu and Fang Deng
Department of Pediatrics, First Affiliated Hospital of Anhui Medical University, 19th Floor of Medicine and Medical Tech Building, 218 Jixi Road, Hefei 230022, Anhui, China

Zhenhua Ren
Department of Anatomy, School of Basic Medicine, Anhui Medical University, Hefei 230032, Anhui, China

Coral Hanevold, Susan Halbach and Karyn Yonekawa
Department of Pediatrics, Division of Nephrology, University of Washington, Seattle, WA, USA

Jin Mou
MultiCare Institute for Research & Innovation, MultiCare Health System, Tacoma, WA, USA

Xiao-Lan Ying and Chong-Huai Yan
MOE-Shanghai Key Laboratory of Children's Environmental Health, Xinhua Hospital affiliated to Shanghai Jiaotong University School of Medicine, Shanghai 200092, China

Morri Markowitz
Division of Environmental Sciences, Children's Hospital at Montefiore, Albert Einstein College of Medicine, Bronx NY10467, USA

Lisa B. E. Shields
Norton Neuroscience Institute, Norton Healthcare, Louisville, KY 40202, USA

Dennis S. Peppas and Eran Rosenberg
Norton Children's Urology, Norton Healthcare, Louisville, KY 40207, USA

Iole Brunod, Sophie Hassid and Laurent Thomachot
Pediatric and Neonatal Intensive Care Unit, Hôpital Nord, Assistance Publique-Hôpitaux de Marseille, Chemin des Bourrely, 13015 Marseille, France

Barthélémy Tosello and Catherine Gire
Department of Neonatology, Hôpital Nord, Assistance Publique des Hôpitaux de Marseille (APHM), Chemin des Bourrely, 13015 Marseille, France

Barthélémy Tosello
Aix Marseille Univ, CNRS, EFS, ADES, Marseille, France

Michel Panuel
Department of Medical Imaging, Assistance Publique-Hôpitaux de Marseille, Hôpital Nord, Chemin des Bourrely, 13015 Marseille, France

Bo Hyun Park and Hyesook Park
Department of Preventive Medicine, College of Medicine, Ewha Womans University, 1071, Anyangcheon-ro, Yangcheon-ku, Seoul 158-710, Korea

Hye Ah Lee
Clinical Trial Center, Mokdong Hospital, Ewha Womans University, Seoul, Korea

Eun Ae Park, Su Jin Cho and Hae Soon Kim
Department of Pediatrics, College of Medicine, Ewha Womans University, Seoul, Korea

Deniz Baklaci, Ismail Guler, Ihsan Kuzucu, Rauf Oguzhan Kum and Muge Ozcan
Numune Training and Research Hospital, Department of Otolaryngology, 931st Avenue 945st Street No:5/3 Çankaya, Ankara, Turkey

Woosun Choi
Department of Radiology, Chung-Ang University Hospital, Seoul, Republic of Korea

Young Bae Choi
Department of Pediatrics, Chungbuk National University Hospital, Cheongju, Republic of Korea

Matilda Emgård, Rickard Nordén, Ebba Samuelsson, Shadi Geravandi, Lucia Gonzales-Siles, Magnus Lindh, Rune Andersson and Susann Skovbjerg
Department of Infectious Diseases, Institute of Biomedicine, University of Gothenburg, Gothenburg, Sweden

Balthazar Muhigirwa, Eric Munguakonkwa, Jeanière T. Manegabe, Didace Cibicabene, Lambert Morisho, Benjamin Mwambanyi, Jacques Mirindi and Nadine Kabeza
Panzi Hospital, Bukavu, Democratic Republic of the Congo

Théophile Kashosi
Université Evangélique en Afrique, Bukavu, Democratic Republic of the Congo

Rune Andersson
CARe - Center for Antibiotic Resistance Research, Gothenburg University, Gothenburg, Sweden

Archippe M. Birindwa
Hôpital Général de Référence de Panzi, BP: 266 Bukavu, DR, Congo
Université Evangélique en Afrique, Bukavu, Democratic Republic of the Congo
Panzi Hospital, Bukavu, Democratic Republic of the Congo
Department of Infectious Diseases, Institute of Biomedicine, University of Gothenburg, Gothenburg, Sweden

Elias Ejamo, Thilagavathi Thangavel and Mulugeta Yohannis
School of public Health, Wolaita Sodo University, Wolaita Sodo, Ethiopia

Bereket Yohannes
Centre for international Health, the University of Bergen, Bergen, Norway
School of Public Health, Hawassa University, Hawassa, Ethiopia

Elias Ejamo
Soro district Health office, Hosanna, Ethiopia

Mulugeta Yohannis
Damot Pulasa district, Wolaita Sodo, Ethiopia

Dafne C. Andrade, Igor C. Borges and Raquel Simbalista
Postgraduate Program in Health Sciences, Federal University of Bahia School of Medicine, Salvador, Brazil

Marcelo Araújo
Image Diagnosis, Image Memorial Unit and Bahia Hospital, Salvador, Brazil

Cristiana M. Nascimento-Carvalho
Department of Paediatrics, Federal University of Bahia School of Medicine, Salvador, Brazil
Postgraduate Program in Pathology, Federal University of Bahia School of Medicine, Salvador, Brazil

Toshiaki Shimizu
Department of Pediatrics, Aichi Medical University, Nagakute, Japan

Akihisa Okumura
Department of Pediatrics, Juntendo University Faculty of Medicine, Tokyo, Japan
Department of Pediatrics, Aichi Medical University, Nagakute, Japan

Shinobu Ida
Department of Pediatric Gastroenterology and Endocrinology, Osaka
Medical Center and Research Institute for Maternal and Child Health, Osaka, Japan

Masaaki Mori
Department of Lifetime Clinical Immunology, Graduate School of Medical and Dental Sciences, Tokyo Medical and Dental University, Tokyo, Japan

Hsiang-Ju Hsiao
Department of Pediatrics, Chang Gung Memorial Hospital, Keelung, Taiwan
Chang Gung University College of Medicine, Taoyuan, Taiwan

I-Anne Huang and I-Jun Chou
Chang Gung University College of Medicine, Taoyuan, Taiwan

Chang-Teng Wu
Division of General Pediatrics, Department of Pediatrics, Chang Gung Memorial Hospital, Linkou, Taiwan
Chang Gung University College of Medicine, Taoyuan, Taiwan

Jing-Long Huang
Division of Asthma, Allergy, and Rheumatology, Department of Pediatrics, Chang Gung Memorial Hospital, Linkou, Taiwan
Chang Gung University College of Medicine, Taoyuan, Taiwan

Cheng-Hsun Chiu
Molecular Infectious Disease Research Center, Division of Pediatric Infection, Chang Gung Memorial Hospital, Linkou, Taiwan
Chang Gung University College of Medicine, Taoyuan, Taiwan

Yhu-Chering Huang
Division of Pediatric Infectious Diseases, Department of Pediatrics, Chang Gung Memorial Hospital, Linkou, Taiwan
Chang Gung University College of Medicine, Taoyuan, Taiwan

Jainn-Jim Lin, Oi-Wa Chan and Shao-Hsuan Hsia
Division of Pediatric Critical Care Medicine, Department of Pediatrics, Chang Gung Memorial Hospital, Linkou, Taiwan
Chang Gung University College of Medicine, Taoyuan, Taiwan

Index

www.ingramcontent.com/pod-product-compliance
Lightning Source LLC
LaVergne TN
LVHW080715210926
848485LV00003B/467